Cognitive Disorders

NEUROLOGICAL DISEASE AND THERAPY

Series Editor

WILLIAM C. KOLLER
Department of Neurology
University of Kansas Medical Center
Kansas City, Missouri

1. Handbook of Parkinson's Disease, *edited by William C. Koller*
2. Medical Therapy of Acute Stroke, *edited by Mark Fisher*
3. Familial Alzheimer's Disease: Molecular Genetics and Clinical Perspectives, *edited by Gary D. Miner, Ralph W. Richter, John P. Blass, Jimmie L. Valentine, and Linda A. Winters-Miner*
4. Alzheimer's Disease: Treatment and Long-Term Management, *edited by Jeffrey L. Cummings and Bruce L. Miller*
5. Therapy of Parkinson's Disease, *edited by William C. Koller and George Paulson*
6. Handbook of Sleep Disorders, *edited by Michael J. Thorpy*
7. Epilepsy and Sudden Death, *edited by Claire M. Lathers and Paul L. Schraeder*
8. Handbook of Multiple Sclerosis, *edited by Stuart D. Cook*
9. Memory Disorders: Research and Clinical Practice, *edited by Takehiko Yanagihara and Ronald C. Petersen*
10. The Medical Treatment of Epilepsy, *edited by Stanley R. Resor, Jr., and Henn Kutt*
11. Cognitive Disorders: Pathophysiology and Treatment, *edited by Leon J. Thal, Walter H. Moos, and Elkan R. Gamzu*
12. Handbook of Amyotrophic Lateral Sclerosis, *edited by Richard Alan Smith*

Additional Volumes in Preparation

Handbook of Parkinson's Disease: Second Edition, Revised and Expanded, *edited by William C. Koller*

Handbook of Pediatric Epilepsy, *edited by Fereydoun Dehkharghani and Jerome Murphy*

Cognitive Disorders
Pathophysiology and Treatment

edited by

Leon J. Thal

University of California at San Diego
and San Diego Veterans Affairs Medical Center
San Diego, California

Walter H. Moos

Chiron Corporation
Emeryville, California

Elkan R. Gamzu

Cambridge NeuroScience, Inc.
Cambridge, Massachusetts

Marcel Dekker, Inc. New York • Basel • Hong Kong

Library of Congress Cataloging-in-Publication Data

Cognitive disorders : pathophysiology and treatment /
edited by Leon J. Thal, Walter H. Moos, Elkan R. Gamzu.
p. cm. -- (Neurological disease and therapy ; v. 11)
Includes bibliographical references and index.
ISBN 0-8247-8601-7 (alk. paper)
1. Cognition disorders. I. Thal, Leon J. II. Moos, W. H.
(Walter Hamilton). III. Gamzu, Elkan. IV. Series.
[DNLM: 1. Cognition Disorders--physiopathology. 2. Cognition
Disorders--therapy. W1 NE33LD v. 11]
RC994.C4C64 1991
616.8'3-dc20
DNLM/DLC
for Library of Congress 91-46988
CIP

This book is printed on acid-free paper.

MARCEL DEKKER, INC.
270 Madison Avenue, New York, New York 10016

Current printing (last digit):
10 9 8 7 6 5 4 3 2 1

PRINTED IN THE UNITED STATES OF AMERICA

Preface

Cognitive dysfunction is a common manifestation of many different disease states ranging from autism and dyslexia in children to Alzheimer's and Parkinson's diseases in the elderly.

A number of scientists and clinicians are interested in the cognitive manifestations of these diseases, but usually focus on the disease state itself. Thus there are many chapters and books on cognitive disorders in Alzheimer's disease or cognitive disorders as a consequence of head injury, for example.

Similarly, those scientists interested in cognitive dysfunction as a process are often interested in specific disease states (primary or secondary lesions for example) as a means to study the process. Thus there are many books on memory that focus on animal studies and use human disease states as exemplars.

The intent of this book is to make available to the clinician a comprehensive series of scientific reviews of the major disease states that involve cognitive dysfunction. That is to say, the primary focus is a clinical one. Secondarily, we hope that the compilation of such a book will broaden the horizons of both clinical and basic researchers whose interest in cognitive dysfunction is secondary to their other goals.

To the best of our knowledge, this is the first book of its kind. Most books on memory and cognition are targeted almost exclusively to the academic, basic research market. While this book would also appeal to many of those researchers, we seek a broader public among the many health care professionals who have to deal with the manifestations of cognitive disorders on a daily basis, and we hope to provide them with a scientifically derived compendium of facts that will help in diagnosis and treatment.

Leon J. Thal, M.D.
Walter H. Moos, Ph.D.
Elkan R. Gamzu, Ph.D.

Contents

Contributors

M. Flint Beal, M.D. Neurochemistry Research Unit and Huntington's Disease Clinic, Massachusetts General Hospital, Boston, Massachusetts

Thomas H. Crook III, Ph.D. President, Memory Assessment Clinics, Inc., Bethesda, Maryland

Jeffrey L. Cummings, M.D. Neurobehavior Unit, Department of Neurology, West Los Angeles Veterans Affairs Medical Center, and Department of Neurology, UCLA School of Medicine, Los Angeles, California

Frank Dahlke, M.D. Department of Clinical Psychiatry, Schering AG, Berlin, Germany

Robert E. Davis, Ph.D. Department of Neuroscience Pharmacology, Parke-Davis Pharmaceutical Research Division, Warner-Lambert Co., Ann Arbor, Michigan

Theodora Duka, M.D., Ph.D. Department of Human Pharmacology, Schering AG, Berlin, Germany

Douglas Galasko, M.D. Department of Neuroscience and Neurology, University of California at San Diego, and San Diego Veterans Affairs Medical Center, San Diego, California

Elkan R. Gamzu, Ph.D. President and Chief Operating Officer, Cambridge NeuroScience, Inc., Cambridge, Massachusetts

Felicia C. Goldstein, Ph.D. Department of Neurology, Neurobehavioral Program, Emory University School of Medicine, Atlanta, Georgia

Franz F. Hefti, Ph.D. Division of Neurogerontology, Andrus Gerontology Center, University of Southern California, Los Angeles, California

John S. Kennedy, M.D., F.R.C.P.(c) Department of Psychiatry, University Hospitals of Cleveland, Case Western Reserve University, Cleveland, Ohio

John T. Kenny, Ph.D. Department of Psychiatry, University Hospitals of Cleveland, Case Western Reserve University, Cleveland, Ohio

Susan K. Klein, M.D. Departments of Pediatrics and Neurology, Case Western Reserve University, Cleveland, Ohio

Glenn J. Larrabee, Ph.D. Department of Neuropsychological Research, Memory Assessment Clinics, Inc., Sarasota, Florida, and private practice, Hill View Park Medical complex, Sarasota, Florida

Paul D. Leber, M.D. Potomac, Maryland

Harvey S. Levin, Ph.D. Division of Neurosurgery, University of Texas Medical Branch, Galveston, Texas

William J. McEntee, M.D. Vice President for Medical Research, Memory Assessment Clinics, Inc., Sarasota, Florida

Walter H. Moos, Ph.D. Vice President, Research and Development, and Director of Chemical Therapeutics, Chiron Corporation, Emeryville, California

Mary Anne Muriello, M.D. Pediatric Resident, Rainbow Babies and Children's Hospital, Cleveland, Ohio

Christopher F. O'Brien, M.D. Department of Neurology, University of Rochester Medical Center, Rochester, New York

Isabelle Rapin, M.D. Saul R. Korey Department of Neurology, Department of Pediatrics, and Rose F. Kennedy Center for Research in Mental Retardation and Human Development, Albert Einstein College of Medicine, Bronx, New York

G. Webster Ross, M.D. Neurobehavior Unit, West Los Angeles Veterans Affairs Medical Center, and Department of Neurology, UCLA School of Medicine, Los Angeles, California

Harold A. Sackeim, Ph.D. Department of Biological Psychiatry, College of Physicians and Surgeons, Columbia University, and New York State Psychiatric Institute, New York, New York

Lon S. Schneider, Ph.D. Division of Neurogerontology, Andrus Gerontology Center, University of Southern California, Los Angeles, California

Ira Shoulson, M.D. Department of Neurology and Pharmacology, University of Rochester Medical Center, Rochester, New York

David N. Stephens, Ph.D. Department of Neuropsychopharmacology, Schering AG, Berlin, Germany

Elsdon Storey, D.Phil., F.R.A.C.P. Neurochemistry Research Unit and Huntington's Disease Clinic, Massachusetts General Hospital, Boston, Massachusetts, and Department of Neurology, The University of Melbourne, Victoria, Australia

Leon J. Thal, M.D. Departments of Neuroscience and Neurology, University of California at San Diego, and Chief, Neurology Division, San Diego Veterans Affairs Medical Center, San Diego, California

I

COGNITIVE DISORDERS OF CHILDHOOD

1

Developmental Disabilities: Mental Deficiency, Autism, and Dysphasia

Isabelle Rapin *Albert Einstein College of Medicine, Bronx, New York*

I. INTRODUCTION

Developmentally disabled is a term applied to otherwise seemingly normal children who do not acquire complex abilities, such as finely coordinated sensorimotor skills, focused attention, language, scholastic achievements, sociability, and other cognitive skills, at the expected age. Although overt lesions and other brain insults typically associated with obvious sensorimotor deficits, seizures, and other neurologic signs also impair these complex abilities, the term *developmental disability,* by common accord, is restricted to children without such signs.

The label, developmental disability, carries with it the implication that it is not the result of an acquired brain abnormality. As a result, the developmental disabilities are often assumed to represent no more than a lag in brain development, the consequences of which will disappear with time. It is indeed true that many developmentally disabled children eventually acquire skills they did not develop at the same age as their peers, but detailed neuropsychological testing often reveals persistent, although subtle, cognitive deficits. Compensation has occurred through the use of less efficient strategies that become available because of plasticity in the development and organization of the immature brain (1). In such cases, "catching up" does not denote a delay in otherwise normal maturation, but deviance in brain organization.

A. Brain Development and Plasticity

Fetal life and childhood are the periods of life during which the brain grows in size and organizational complexity. Childhood ends when the body and brain have reached their full development, at ages that differ for different brain systems and that occur latest for regions of the association cortex subserving the most complex cognitive skills. The more immature the brain, the greater its plasticity, that is, the greater its potential for major reorganization in the face of an insult or in response to environmental influences. Plasticity persists longer in later-developing systems, such as those sustaining higher cognitive functions, than in earlier-maturing ones such as sensorimotor systems. Plasticity at the subcellular level persists throughout life and is thought to be responsible for learning (2).

The potential of the brain for major reorganization is relative. It is quite limited in the visual system in which there is a high degree of topologic concordance between the retina and the visual cortex. There is some plasticity in the sensorimotor system, in the sense that lesions, which would produce permanent motor deficits in adults, produce less severe ones if sustained during fetal life or early childhood, although large lesions produce predictable and permanent deficits similar to those of adults. Plasticity is greatest for complex functions, such as language, which is genetically linked to left hemispheric function in most persons, but can be sustained by the right hemisphere in cases of large early lesions of the perisylvian cortex on the left (3).

The earlier the developing brain sustains damage, the less the pathological consequences of an insult will resemble those that would follow the same insult to the mature brain. Insults to the fetal brain may leave no discernible scar, but will result in maldevelopment. Maldevelopment may range from subtle subcellular neuronal changes (e.g., spine dysgenesis; 4), to alterations of the cellular architecture of the cortex or subcortical areas (e.g., migration cell defects and altered connectivity), and to major malformations such as agenesis of the corpus callosum, neural tube defects, or septo-optic dysplasia. The type of defect depends on the severity, extent, type, and timing of the injury.

Lesions acquired in childhood produce deficits similar to those of adults, but tend to have a better prognosis than in adulthood, when the brain has lost most of its plasticity. Acquired lesions of childhood will not be considered in this chapter. Instead the focus is the so-called developmental disorders of brain function, most of which are believed to have a prenatal origin and to reflect subtle alterations in brain structure (5) and function. Usually, their etiologies are unknown. A significant proportion are probably genetic (6,7).

The behavioral symptoms of damage to, or maldevelopment of, the immature brain are a function of the severity and brain systems affected, as well as of the timing of the damage. Symptoms are not a function of the etiology of the damage, beyond some that are very selective for particular brain systems, such as the selective affinity of unconjugated bilirubin for the vestibular, auditory, and cerebellar nuclei and basal ganglia. Thus, none of the developmental disorders of brain function represents a "disease," although there are particular congenital syndromes, such as Williams syndrome (8), Turner's syndrome (9), and fragile-X (10), that are associated with fairly specific developmental deficits of higher cerebral function. The selectivity of the effects of such disorders on brain development is not yet understood. There are behavioral, if not somatic, phenocopies of these and other behavioral disorders, so that identifying a particular behavioral syndrome is not the equivalent of identifying its etiology.

Because of plasticity in the organization of the immature brain, investigators have been reluctant to assign particular behavioral syndromes of early life to the brain systems that would be likely to be damaged in adults with similar symptoms. Nevertheless, drawing parallels and recognizing differences between behavioral syndromes in children and adults has heuristic value for gaining an understanding of brain–mind relationships and the localization of affected systems.

B. Major Developmental Disabilities

The conditions usually included among the developmental disabilities are listed in Table 1.

This chapter focuses on mental deficiency, developmental language disorders, and autism. Sensorimotor disorders and attention disorders are not discussed as such, but are frequent in children with other developmental disorders, since strict specificity of brain dysfunction is the exception, rather than the rule among the developmental disabilities. The learning disabilities are regularly the consequence of earlier disorders of language and perception.

C. Prevalence and Importance

There are no reliable figures on the prevalence of each of the developmental disorders of brain function. As just stated, children often have more than one type of deficit, for example, mental deficiency and pervasive developmental disorder, or attention deficit disorder, and a learning disabil-

TABLE 1 Major Developmental Disabilities

Motor disorders
- Dyspraxia
- Clumsiness
- Hypotonia
- Minor spasticity
- Minor movement disorders (including postural instability, synkineses, and, perhaps, tics)
- Oromotor dysfunction, dysarthria

Sensory–perceptual disorders
- Impaired somatosensory perception (e.g., haptic perception, tactile localization, perception of the body in space)
- Impaired visual–spatial perception
- Impaired auditory perception (e.g., duration, order, speech–sound discrimination)

Language disorders (dysphasias)
- Developmental language disorders
- Stuttering

Attention disorders
- Attention deficit disorder, with or without hyperactivity

Learning disabilities
- Reading disorders (dyslexias)
- Spelling disorders
- Dysgraphias
- Dyscalculias

Pervasive developmental disorders
- Autistic spectrum disorders

Mental deficiency

ity. Symptoms change with age; what was labeled dysphasia in the preschool years is called dyslexia at school age. The severity of the developmental disabilities varies greatly, from severe handicap to a mild deficit in an otherwise competent child. Prevalence figures vary depending on who is counting—an advocate for handicapped children, or an administrator of scarce educational resources. Owing to the lack of biological markers for the disorders, the need to develop unambiguous diagnostic criteria is clear.

It is reasonable to guess that 5–10% or more of children have some degree of developmental disability. Only a fraction of these children come to medical attention. They may not be referred to physicians unless their disability is severe or progressive or is associated with an attention deficit or other behavioral abnormality that might respond to medication. Unless severe, many are not recognized until school age, which, for many persons, is the most intellectually demanding period of life. There are, no doubt, other developmental disabilities, for example, for music or color discrimination, that simply do not come to attention in our culture because these are not skills required for success in school, which everyone must attend, or in adult life, which offers many niches. Thus, the borderland between pathology and variation in genetic endowment remains fuzzy.

II. MENTAL DEFICIENCY

A. Definition and Severity

The term *mental deficiency,* rather than the more common term *mental retardation,* is preferred because the word "retardation" implies the potential for catching up, an unwarranted assumption that does not apply except in the mildest cases and in those caused by environmental deprivation, which do not concern us here.

The best definition of *mental deficiency* is the inability to live independently as an adult because of inadequate cognitive skills. The definitions used in *DSM III-R* (11) and in ICD-10 (12) stress that not only must the individual have a statistically significant deficit on an IQ test, but she or he must also be impaired in functional adaptation to society.

The most frequent definition of mental deficiency used in childhood is a score on a standardized intelligence test battery that is 2 or more standard deviations (SD) below the mean for the general population (IQ of 100 ± 15; i.e., the child must have an IQ of 70 or below). This definition rests on the assumption that intelligence tests measure skills relevant to independent functioning in society, not only those needed for success in school. This quantitative definition lends itself to partitioning mental deficiency into mild (2 SD or more below the mean or IQs of 55–70), moderate (>3 SD below the mean or IQs of 40–55), severe (>4 SD or IQs 25–40), and profound (>5 SD or more or IQs below 25). Persons with IQ scores within 1–2 SD of the mean (IQ 70–85) are considered borderline, rather than mentally deficient. They are educable, with special help in school, and one can anticipate that most will function independently as adults.

In general, persons with mild mental deficiency are educable to the degree that they can acquire some functional reading and calculating skills and learn to travel and shop, although they are unlikely to be able to make change, and they may be employable in a sheltered environment. They can be expected to be self-sufficient in caring for their own physical needs. Persons with moderate deficiency may learn to read a few words and to count, but will need some supervision in everyday life. Severely deficient persons may be able to dress, have some functional language skills, but will require a sheltered environment. Profoundly mentally deficient persons are generally nonverbal and will usually be unemployable and totally dependent. It is important to keep in mind, however, that aggressive habilitative efforts may enable some severely mentally impaired persons to perform some useful tasks, accordingly, the day of simply warehousing the handicapped has passed (13).

Rather than using test batteries, such as the Wechsler Scales and Stanford Binet, that are highly correlated with success in school, but somewhat less so with success in everyday life, the Revised Vineland Developmental Scale (14) is a questionnaire administered to a parent or caretaker by a trained interviewer who inquires about the person's level of functioning in everyday life. The Vineland covers all ages, from infancy to adult life, and provides information on motor skills, language, adaptive skills, sociability, and maladaptive behaviors. It is particularly useful for assessing uncooperative and handicapped persons, it is extremely well standardized, and it provides relevant data when planning for the future of a developmentally impaired person.

The differential diagnosis between developmental dysphasia or learning disability and mild mental deficiency is not straightforward. By definition, *learning disability* implies normal intelligence, with a circumscribed deficit for a school-related ability, such as reading, spelling, writing, or mathematics, with or without an associated deficit in attention, whereas *mental deficiency* implies overall intellectual incompetence (15). However, circumscribed deficits in language, visual–spatial skills, or attention are likely to lower scores on one or more of the subtests of the intelligence test battery and, thereby, its mean summary score. There is often an overlap in the IQ scores of borderline or mildly mentally deficient and learning-disabled persons. A profile with wide variability among subtest scores suggests learning disability, whereas a flatter profile suggests mental deficiency.

B. Causes of Mental Deficiency

Mental deficiency may be the consequence of overall damage or maldevelopment of the brain, or of multifocal abnormalities. It is rarely the consequence of a single focal brain lesion. Unfortunately, the correlation between localization and size of lesions visible on neuroimaging tests and level of intellectual competence is low. Some reasons for this low correlation is that microscopic lesions and biochemical lesions do not produce discernible neuroimaging pathology and that the relationship between subcortical abnormality and cognitive development remains ill-defined. It is possible, for example, that pathology in limbic circuits critical for learning might result in profound mental deficiency without producing a motor deficit or a lesion visible by neuroimaging (16). In general, however, the more severe the mental deficiency, the more likely a neuroimaging test will be abnormal and an etiologic diagnosis made. This stems from the greater likelihood that the deficiency is due to some gross maldevelopment or damage to the brain or to a recognizable systemic disease affecting brain development and function diffusely.

Mental deficiency is a static condition. Progressive loss of intellectual milestones implies *dementia,* even when it occurs in infancy or early childhood. It may be difficult to decide in a very young child, especially on initial evaluation, whether she or he is retarded or demented, because progressive disease starting in utero may preclude any meaningful development and, therefore, give the impression of a static condition. Under those circumstances, progressive appearance of spasticity, loss of reflexes, seizures, a movement disorder, or optic atrophy, and signs of progressive brain deterioration on serial neuroimaging tests suggest a progressive disease, that is, a dementia, rather than a static condition such as mental deficiency.

It is not possible to list all the conditions that may result in mental deficiency. In general, diffuse maldevelopment or pathology of the cortex, for example, lissencephaly, micrencephaly, or severe anoxia, is associated with severe or profound mental deficiency. Diffuse involvement of the white matter has more variable consequences. There are children with severe hydrocephalus and markedly thinned white matter whose intelligence is normal or near normal, whereas others are significantly mentally deficient.

Perinatal pathology, notably prematurity, anoxia, and trauma are frequently blamed for the occurrence of mental deficiency. Data from the Collaborative Project, which tracked prospectively more than 50,000 pregnancies and infants until aged 7 years, indicate that this is an overestimated cause of mental deficiency (and cerebral palsy) (17). A recent estimate is that perinatal pathological events, including prematurity, probably account for no more than 10% of developmental disorders, inborn errors of metabolism for 5% or fewer, and early brain maldevelopment for 10% (18). The more severe the mental deficiency, the more likely that the child will have motor signs, seizures, communication deficits, autistic behaviors, or combination thereof, since severe mental deficiency denotes widespread and often nonselective damage to the developing brain.

C. Workup

The first step is to make an exact diagnosis, if possible, and to assess the severity of the mental deficiency. The more severely affected the child, the greater the likelihood of making a diagnosis by history, physical examination, neuroimaging, biochemical tests, or high-resolution chromosomal analysis. How much testing to do in mildly affected children is controversial. Although the causes of mental deficiency are legion, many are extraordinarily rare, and it is impossible to screen for all of them. One must rely on the clinical findings for guidance. A number of conditions, for example, tuberous sclerosis, Down syndrome, Williams syndrome, fragile-X, de Lange's syndrome, and many others can be diagnosed with high probability by the physical examination alone. Useful reference books exist, the best known of which is *Smith's Recognizable Patterns of Human Malformation* (19), with excellent pictures of various syndromes and an index that lists abnormalities, both of which are of great help in arriving at a specific diagnosis. Chromosomal studies are most likely to be fruitful in children with frank malformations or three or more minor ones (20). McKusick's *Mendelian Inheritance in Man* (21) is equally helpful if a mendelian trait is suspected.

Blind screening for aminoacidurias; organic acidurias; lactate, pyruvate, long-chain fatty acids; and lysosomal enzymes is as unlikely to yield a diagnosis as chromosomal studies in a child in whom neither the history nor the examination provides clues. Neuroimaging is also unlikely to be helpful in unstigmatized children with normal classic neurological examinations. The electroencephalogram (EEG) provides no data to help in the diagnosis of mental deficiency, although it is invaluable in children suspected of having seizures.

Psychological or, better, neuropsychological testing is required for a quantitative assessment of the child's cognitive skills and to highlight skills that may be used to circumvent deficits in planning educational intervention (22). Psychological testing in infancy, which has yielded crucial data on the development of infantile competence, has limited predictive validity. The same is true of tests in toddlers and preschoolers, although test results have immediate usefulness in planning remediation. The predictive validity of the IQ increases with age, but there are many pitfalls in testing handicapped children with sensorimotor deficits, attention deficits, pervasive developmental disorders, and other problematic behaviors.

D. Management of Mental Deficiency

Mental deficiency is not amenable to pharmacologic treatment. It is preventable by dietary manipulation or the administration of certain vitamins or other supplements in a few conditions such as some of the aminoacidurias and organic acidurias that can be diagnosed in utero or soon after birth, before they have had a chance to damage the brain (23). Mental deficiency can be prevented by selective abortion of fetuses detected prenatally to have severe structural anomalies of the brain by ultrasonography. Amniocentesis or chorionic villus sampling enables prenatal diagnosis of chromosomal abnormalities, such as trisomies or fragile-X, or of genetic–metabolic diseases of the brain, such as lysosomal, peroxisomal, mitochondrial, and a variety of other metabolic diseases, including spongy degeneration of the brain (Canavan's disease). Unfortunately, in most of these rare conditions, the diagnosis is not suspected unless there are risk factors, a positive family history, or there already is an affected sibling. From a public health standpoint, immunization against rubella, adequate prenatal care and nutrition, and cessation of smoking, alcohol consumption, and use of street drugs would have the greatest impact on the prevention of mental deficiency.

Management of the mentally deficient child is educational and is mandated by Public Law 94-142. Early stimulation enhances cognitive development and increases the probability that the child will reach his or her potential. There are now infant, toddler, and preschool programs for children with a diagnosis of mental deficiency or who are suspected of being mentally deficient. Early referral is highly desirable to relieve the parents' burden and enrich the child's environment. There is great need for parental counseling, both in terms of planning for the child, managing behavioral problems adequately, and prevention. Genetic counseling is essential in appropriate cases. Parent groups are often very helpful, not only for emotional support, but because parents have much to learn about management of behavior problems and gaining access to resources from other parents who have faced problems similar to theirs.

III. AUTISM AND PERVASIVE DEVELOPMENTAL DISORDERS

A. Definition

According to *DSM III-R* (11) and ICD-10 (12), the hallmark of these disorders is a *qualitative* impairment in sociability and communication skills, with preoccupations and a narrow range of interests. This definition is broader than the image of the autistic child many professionals carry in their mind, that of a nonverbal child who rocks in a corner, oblivious to those around, and who is severely mentally deficient, with the possible exception of a narrow island of superior, but meaningless, competence (splinter skill) such as doing jig-saw puzzles. The *DSM III-R* lists a series of behaviors in each of the behavioral categories mentioned earlier and specifies how many in each category must be present to diagnose classic autism (Table 2). Children with

TABLE 2 *DSM III-R* Criteria for Autistic Disorder

At least 8 of the following 16 items are present, these to include at least 2 items from A, 1 from B, 1 from C.

Note: Consider a criterion to be met *only* if the behavior is abnormal for the person's developmental level.

A. Qualitative impairment in reciprocal social interaction as manifested by the following:
(The examples within parentheses are arranged so that those first mentioned are more likely to apply to younger or more handicapped, and the later ones to older or less handicapped persons with this disorder.)
   1. Marked lack of awareness of the existence or feelings of others (e.g., treats a person as if he or she were a piece of furniture; does not notice another person's distress; apparently has no concept of the need of others for privacy)
   2. No or abnormal seeking of comfort at times of distress (e.g., does not come for comfort even when ill, hurt, or tired; seeks comfort in a stereotyped way, e.g., says "cheese, cheese, cheese" whenever hurt)
   3. No or impaired imitation (e.g., does not wave bye-bye; does not copy mother's domestic activities; mechanical imitation of others' actions out of context)
   4. No or abnormal social play (e.g., does not actively participate in simple games; prefers solitary play activities; involves other children in play only as "mechanical aids")
   5. Gross impairment in ability to make peer friendships (e.g., no interest in making peer friendships; despite interest in making friends, demonstrates lack of understanding of conventions of social interaction, e.g., reads phone book to uninterested peer)

B. Qualitative impairment in verbal and nonverbal communication and in imaginative activity, as manifested by the following:
(The numbered items are arranged so that those first listed are more likely to apply to younger or more handicapped, and the later ones, to older or less handicapped, persons with this disorder.)
   1. No mode of communication, such as communicative babbling, facial expression, gesture, mime, or spoken language
   2. Markedly abnormal nonverbal communication, as in the use of eye-to-eye gaze, facial expression, body posture, or gestures to initiate or modulate social interaction (e.g., does not anticipate being held, stiffens when held, does not look at the person or smile when making a social approach, does not greet parents or visitors, has a fixed stare in social situations)
   3. Absence of imaginative activity, such as play-acting of adult roles, fantasy characters, or animals; lack of interest in stories about imaginary events
   4. Marked abnormalities in the production of speech, including volume, pitch, stress, rate, rhythm, and intonation (e.g., monotonous tone, questionlike melody, or high pitch)

TABLE 2 Continued

5. Marked abnormalities in the form or content of speech, including stereotyped and repetitive use of speech: for example, immediate echolalia or mechanical repetition of television commercial; use of "you" when "I" is meant (e.g., using "You want cookie?" to mean "I want a cookie"); idiosyncratic use of words or phrases (e.g., "Go on green riding" to mean "I want to go on the swing"); or frequent irrelevant remarks (e.g., starts talking about train schedules during a conversation about sports)
6. Marked impairment in the ability to initiate or sustain a conversation with others, despite adequate speech (e.g., indulging in lengthy monologues on one subject regardless of interjections from others)

C. Markedly restricted repertoire of activities and interests, as manifested by the following:
1. Stereotyped body movements (e.g., hand-flicking or hand-twisting, spinning, head-banging, complex whole-body movements)
2. Persistent preoccupation with parts of objects (e.g., sniffing or smelling objects, repetitive feeling of texture of materials, e.g., insists on carrying around a piece of string)
3. Marked distress over changes in trivial aspects of environment (e.g., when a vase is moved from usual position)
4. Unreasonable insistence on following routines in precise detail (e.g., insisting that exactly the same route always be followed when shopping)
5. Markedly restricted range of interests and a preoccupation with one narrow interest (e.g., interested only in lining up objects, in amassing facts about meteorology, or in pretending to be a fantasy character)

D. Onset during infancy or childhood.

Specify if childhood onset (after 36 months of age).

Pervasive Developmental Disorder—Not Otherwise Specified

This category should be used when there is a qualitative impairment in the development of reciprocal interaction and of verbal and nonverbal communication skills, but the criteria are not met for autistic disorder, schizophrenia, or schizotypal or schizoid personality disorder. Some people with this diagnosis will exhibit a markedly restricted repertoire of activities and interests, but others will not.

Source: Ref. 11.

fewer deficits are called pervasive developmental disorder—not otherwise specified (PDD-NOS). Both autism and PDD–NOS fall under the umbrella term *pervasive developmental disorder* (PDD). The term *autistic spectrum disorder* is another way to stress both the commonality of symptoms and the marked variability in their severity among children on the spectrum. In this chapter, the term *autism* is used in this broad sense.

Like other developmental disorders, autism is not a disease, but a behaviorally defined syndrome, the manifestations of which reflect the extent and severity of the underlying brain dysfunction. The more severe the brain damage, the more likely it is to produce autistic symptoms, because it is more likely to affect those systems responsible for autistic symptomatology. Autism is appropriately considered pervasive because, in addition to the many symptoms it shares with other developmental disorders, it affects aspects of behavior that these other disorders typically spare, notably sociability, drive, and affect. Furthermore, it does so in quite characteristic ways. What distinguishes an autistic child from a mentally deficient one, or an intelligent autistic child from a learning-disabled or dysphasic one, is the abnormal quality of the child's interpersonal interaction, impairment of his or her ability to play, the almost universal presence of stereotypies, which, in low-functioning children, may take on a self-abusive character.

A great deal of variability exists among autistic children. As one would expect, the most severely cognitively deficient children are those whose sociability is also most deficient and who are most likely to be nonverbal and to have no play skills. These children are also the ones with the most prominent stereotypies and self-abuse, although these behavioral domains are not necessarily proportionately affected in the autistic population. Wing and Gould (24) divided autistic children into three subgroups on the basis of their social skills. Allen (25) proposed that there may be five subgroups on the basis of autistic children's sociability, type of language deficit, and the characteristics of their play.

In addition to the symptoms listed in *DSM III-R,* autistic children often have a variety of other symptoms. There is considerable debate among investigators, some of whom postulate that autism reflects a single basic dysfunction affecting many aspects of behavior, whereas others see it as a widespread disorder causing malfunction of distinct brain systems. Autistic children may be highly distractible or have overfocused attention for what interests them. Many have disordered sleep patterns. As a group they tend to be anxious and to have unusual fears. Their affective responses may be labile or blunted, and they may not perceive pleasure and pain as vividly as others. Motor stereotypies (often referred to as self-stimulation) are almost universal. Hypotonia and toe-walking are frequent.

It is estimated that 70% of autistic children have IQs below 70. However, mental deficiency is not a defining feature of the syndrome, since some autistic children have superior intelligence. Even these gifted autistic children can be shown to have uneven cognitive skills. Most autistic children have lower verbal than performance skills, since all of them have a language disorder, at least in the preschool years. There are, however, a smaller number of children whose nonverbal skills are considerably lower than their verbal skills, and who are also likely to be clumsy and apraxic. The term Asperger's syndrome is often used for such children (26). Whether such children have selective impairment of the right hemisphere or of the white matter (27), and whether they constitute a specific genetic syndrome (28), remains to be seen.

Allen and Rapin (25,29,30) hypothesize that the clinically defined subtypes of language disorders in preschool autistic children are the same as those of nonautistic dysphasic children (see next section), with the proviso that all autistic children have impaired comprehension and that the prevalence of two of the subtypes, verbal auditory agnosia (VAA) and the semantic pragmatic syndrome, is higher in the autistic than the nonautistic population.

All autistic children have deficient language use (pragmatics). Nonverbal children do not use communicative gestures acquired by normal children early in the second year, such as pointing and vocalizing to indicate wants, shaking the head to indicate no, and nodding to indicate yes. Instead they may simply cry, or look at what they want, or get it for themselves, or bring their mother's hand to the desired object. They often do not look up when called and may not know that people, including themselves, and things have names. Even highly verbal autistic children have deficient pragmatics; they may speak with averted gaze, have difficulty with turn-taking in conversation, and with maintaining topic. Their prosody (i.e., the intonation, rhythm, and melody of speech), the role of which is to indicate the intent of an utterance and the affect of the speaker, is regularly affected. They make speak monotonously, in a high-pitched poorly modulated voice, or in a singsong with statements having the rising intonation appropriate for questions. Autistic children's comprehension of the pragmatics and prosody of those who speak to them is equally deficient so that they may genuinely not know whether a person addressing them is exasperated or happy.

Autistic children who remain mute with very impaired comprehension and production of speech in the face of much better nonverbal skills are likely to have VAA. Their prognosis is worse than that of nonautistic children with VAA because of their pragmatic deficits. They seem unaware that language and gestures provide one with the power to influence the behavior of others to one's advantage. Therefore, they remain essentially without a communication system, unless vigorous efforts are made to engage them in communication through the visual channel.

The other subtype of language disorder that is particularly prevalent in the autistic population is the semantic–pragmatic syndrome. These children speak too much, often with minimal need for a conversational partner so that they speak aloud to themselves. They are echolalic and use overlearned scripts; they perseverate and come back again and again to favorite topics. They have great difficulty formulating language on demand, which limits one's ability to engage them in meaningful conversation. Their excellent expressive skills in spontaneous language are deceptive, since their comprehension is regularly inferior to their expression.

B. Workup

Physicians must be sensitive to the deficits in social interaction and play that will enable differentiation of an autistic child from a language-disordered or mentally deficient one. Observing the child at play with representational toys while taking the history is the most efficient way to obtain a sufficiently representative sample of the child's behavior for making this distinction. The history must include questions about behaviors characteristic of autistic children. It is essential to determine that a child has autistic features in addition to whatever other developmental problems may be present, since this diagnosis clarifies for the parents so many otherwise inexplicable problems with the child's behavior. It is very important to stress that intelligence varies greatly among autistic children, and that reliable assessment of the child's potential may have to await the emergence of language and of the child's ability to accede to an adult's demands. Referral for speech and language evaluation and for detailed neuropsychological testing is essential, but may have to be deferred. In fact, in autistic preschoolers, response to appropriate remediation is the most reliable gauge of the child's potential.

The workup of an autistic child is similar to that of any handicapped child. All autistic children with delayed language acquisition must undergo a definitive test of hearing because autism and hearing loss may coexist (31) and hearing loss mandates specific intervention. As many of these children are difficult or impossible to test behaviorally, most of them should be promptly referred for audiometric testing with brain stem auditory-evoked responses. Autistic children have a significantly higher risk of having seizures than normal children (32,33), accordingly, a referral for a sleep EEG is recommended, especially in autistic children with no language and severely impaired comprehension who may have epileptic aphasia and unrecognized minor absence seizures that warrant antiepileptic treatment. Currently, evoked potential testing, with the exception of its audiometric application, has no clinical usefulness, despite its promise for research purposes.

The yield of neuroimaging is very low, despite recent reports of hypoplasia of the cerebellar vermis in some high-functioning autistic men (34). Neuroimaging abnormalities may ultimately shed some light on the pathophysiology of autistic symptoms, but their clinical usefulness is now very limited. Some cases of autism clearly have a genetic cause (35), but even in families with more than one affected person, genetic markers have yet to be found. Chromosomal studies, including looking for fragile-X, should be performed when there are other developmentally impaired family members or the child, usually, but not invariably, is a boy, and has a long facies and ears (enlarged testes are rarely found before adulthood) (10,36). The yield of shotgun biochemical tests is extremely low.

C. Management

The difficult behaviors of autistic children sooner or later bring up the question of behavior-modifying medication (37). One often needs to resist strong pressure to start autistic children on a psychotropic drug regimen, the efficacy of which is often marginal. Autistic children are not acutely psychotic and have a lifelong deficit; hence, there is no endpoint in the use of such drugs. Also, drugs are, at best, an adjuvant and never a replacement for educational and behavioral intervention.

Lack of understanding of the physiological and biochemical basis of autistic behaviors greatly hinders progress in pharmacologic treatment. A number of neurotransmitter abnormalities, notably of serotonin and dopamine, have been implicated in the pathogenesis of autism (38). Therapy with the serotonin antagonist fenfluramine may modestly improve the sociability, overactivity, distractibility, and stereotypies of some autistic children, but it is not as effective as initially hoped (39). Campbell and associates (40) report that haloperidol is the most effective drug to reduce stereotypies, aggressivity, and agitation and to enhance the child's ability to profit from behavioral intervention. Because of the possible development of long-term, potentially irreversible side effects, such as tardive dyskinesia, in as many as a quarter of children, one must prescribe the smallest effective dose and taper the drug after a few months to assess whether it is still required (41). Campbell and colleagues (40) do not recommend the use of chlorpromazine and thioridazine because of their sedative side effects.

Symptoms of attention disorder may improve with the use of stimulants, such as methylphenidate and pemoline. Caution is in order because of the possible emergence of tics and the worsening of stereotypies, especially with the use of dextroamphetamine. Behaviors such as self-mutilation and unprovoked aggression do not respond well to antipsychotic drugs unless they are used in sedative doses. Propranolol is quite helpful in some autistic children with explosive behavior (42). Desipramine, possibly combined with propranolol, may also help control emotional outbursts (43).

Whether clomipramine, a serotoninergic drug, said to reduce obsessive–compulsive behavior (44), will have a place in the management of autistic children with these traits remains to be seen. Some of the newer benzodiazepines may be helpful, especially in extremely anxious children. The opiate antagonist naltrexone is being used experimentally to mitigate self-mutilation, on the assumption that this behavior may be due to excessively high levels of endogeneous endorphins (45,46). Whether it will improve other autistic behaviors significantly remains to be seen (47).

Dietary manipulation, including the Feingold Diet, is ineffective in autistic children. So is the use of high-dose pyridoxine (vitamin B_6) and magnesium, and of other vitamins, despite the testimonies of parents desperate for an effective treatment for their children.

When all is said and done, one ends up empirically trying various drugs, starting with those least likely to be harmful, and focusing on a particular behavior that one attempts to modify. One must never lose track of the fact that the best one can hope is for drugs to enhance the child's ability to interact and profit from his educational experience.

Special education, in a program that addresses both the communication and behavioral problems of autistic children, is the mainstay of management. Very low functioning autistic children may be appropriately placed in programs for the multiply handicapped. Intelligent autistic children may be able to function in a preschool for children with language disorders, but such programs do not necessarily meet their behavioral needs. In this case, placement in a therapeutic nursery, often affiliated with a department of child psychiatry, may be a superior option (48). Autistic children benefit from highly structured environments, and behavior modification approaches are often helpful for extinguishing unwanted behaviors and fostering more appropriate ones (49–51). Whatever the program, it is essential that educators work closely with the parents who need to learn how to manage their child's tantrums and oppositional behaviors, which are often worse at home than in school. Children with mild autistic traits who have acquired adequate social skills may be able to attend regular classes, although they regularly require explicit teaching of the social skills appropriate for a person of their age. The often superior verbal memory of high-functioning autistic children can be put to good use for teaching them appropriate social scripts.

It is important to refer parents of autistic children to a parent group (52). The Autistic Society of America has chapters in many cities. It is an important advocate for autistic persons, has been instrumental in raising the public's awareness of the syndrome and of the fact that it is not an "emotional" problem reflecting parental mismanagement, but rather a developmental disorder of brain function. Classes for autistic children and group homes for autistic adults, both of which have filled a great need, can now be found in many cities. Unfortunately, autism is still widely considered a stigmatizing diagnosis, and programs for mildly affected children are sadly lacking, so that it may be expedient not to label a mildly affected child autistic for educational purposes. Even in these mild cases, it is essential that parents be told that their child falls on the autistic spectrum, since this knowledge is essential for planning the child's habilitation and long-term future.

IV. DEVELOPMENTAL LANGUAGE DISORDERS (DYSPHASIAS)

A. Definition

Developmental language disorder (DLD) or dysphasia refers to inadequate acquisition of verbal skills in the absence of hearing loss or mental deficiency. As stated in the previous section, DLD is an invariable feature of autism, at least in the preschool years. Developmental language disorder differs from acquired aphasia, which refers to loss of previously acquired language skills following a focal lesion of the dominant hemisphere. Although most dysphasic children eventually acquire normal, or at least serviceable, verbal skills, they continue to experience deficits that impair their acquisition of written language (reading and spelling) and may lower their scores on verbal subtests of intelligence test batteries.

Deciding whether a child is dysphasic or language-delayed may be difficult unless one is aware of the normal milestones of language development. Language learning starts at birth with refining of the infant's ability to make phonemic discriminations relevant to the language he or she is hearing and orientation toward a person speaking to him or her. Responsive turn-taking in cooing is clearly evident before 6 months. Babbling of vowel–consonant sounds develops in the second half of the first year. The average child learns to point, understands a few words, and says his first words by 1 year. By 18 months, most children have a vocabulary of at least a dozen words, and by 2 years they are combining words into meaningful phrases. By 3 years, they are speaking in short grammatical sentences. Comprehension of language usually precedes production. Some children speak in a fluent inflected jargon, whereas others concentrate on developing a large vocabulary of single words before attempting long utterances (53). The use of questionnaires, such as the Early Language Milestone (ELM) screening test (54), and asking mothers to keep a record of their child's utterances are helpful for deciding when a child is probably deviant, rather than simply delayed.

Very little is known about the neurological basis of dysphasia. Asymmetry in hemispheric development, which is already demonstrable in fetal life (55), strongly suggests that specialization of the left hemisphere for language is inborn and genetically determined. The fact that language will develop in the face of even large lesions of the left hemisphere, provided they are sustained in early life, is a strong argument for plasticity in brain organization, since language can be shown to reside in the right hemisphere of such patients (3). Children who become aphasic following a lesion to the left hemisphere usually recover better than adults with similar lesions (56), although subtle deficits are often persistent. These deficits tend to be less pervasive than those of dysphasic children, which has led to the hypothesis that dysphasia denotes the dysfunction of both hemispheres.

It is probably true that, as in adults, expressive disorders with impaired phonology (production of speech sounds) denote dysfunction of more anterior brain systems, since oromotor deficits and deficits in gross and fine motor coordination are more prevalent in these children than in those with receptive and formulation deficits. The syndrome of verbal auditory agnosia, a language deficit specific for language presented to the auditory channel, probably involves temporal auditory association areas (see following section).

As is true of other developmental disorders, dysphasia does not have a single etiology, although it is likely that some types may be genetic. It may or may not be associated with other signs of brain dysfunction, such as minor motor deficits and attention disorder. It is occasionally associated with an unsuspected major brain malformation or acquired lesion (57).

B. Subtypes of Developmental Language Disorders

Language is a complex, multiple-coded system that is vulnerable at several operational levels. The once-held hypothesis that there is but one type of dysphasia has been replaced with several proposed typologies. The one proposed by Allen, Rapin, and colleagues (29,30,58) is based on an aphasiology model that considers input–processing–output disorders at the levels of phonology (sound codes), syntax (rules for producing well-formed sentences), semantics (word meanings or lexicon), and pragmatics (rules for communicative use of language). This is a clinical system that enables the diagnosis of a particular subtype of dysphasia by attending to intelligibility (phonology), comprehension of connected speech, the amount and fluency of the child's speech, and, as an additional feature, but not a decision point, the correctness of syntax (Table 3). The heuristic value of this typology is in attempting to define where in the language system things may have gone wrong and in making hypotheses about the malfunction of specific brain systems by making comparisons with adult aphasia syndromes (59). Such a purely clinical diagnosis requires validation and amplification by formal tests of language.

Verbal auditory agnosia or word deafness is the most severe of the developmental language disorders because it precludes comprehension of lan-

TABLE 3 Developmental Language Deficit Clinical Syndromes

Characteristic	Verbal auditory agnosia	Mixed receptive–expressive	Lexical–syntactic	Semantic–pragmatic	Speech programming	Verbal dyspraxia
Amount of speech	↓↓↓	↓↓	N or ↓	↑↑	N	↓↓↓
Fluency	↓↓↓	↓↓	N or ↓	N	N	↓↓↓
Intelligibility (phonology)	↓↓↓	↓↓	N	N	↓↓	↓↓↓
Comprehension of discourse	↓↓↓	↓↓	↓	↓↓	N	N
Comprehension of words	↓↓	↓	N	N	N	N
Syntax		↓↓	N or ↓	N	N or ↓	
Formulation of discourse		↓ or ↓↓	↓ or ↓↓	N or ↓	N	
Anomia in discourse		+	++	+		

N = normal ↓ = decreased
\+ = present ↑ = increased

guage presented to the acoustic channel and, therefore, the acquisition of language unless it is presented to the visual channel. It is often, but by no means always, associated with autistic features. Verbal auditory agnosia is the exact analogue of word-deafness in adults with bilateral temporal infarcts, except that adults with this syndrome, whose language is highly automatized, continue to speak despite their inability to monitor what they say and to understand what others say to them. Children with VAA are mute or speak only a few misarticulated words and understand little or nothing. As is true of the adults who can read and write, intelligent children with VAA understand gestures and can be taught formal signs and reading, provided they are not severely autistic. This syndrome may be developmental or occur in the context of acquired epileptic aphasia (Landau–Kleffner syndrome) (60). The congenital variant has a guarded prognosis for the acquisition of adequate communication skills. Older children with the acquired variant of VAA have a better prognosis than younger ones, contrary to other forms of acquired aphasia (61). It is the form of DLD that is most likely to be associated with seizures and with a paroxysmal EEG, especially during sleep (33). Control of the clinical seizures, which are by no means always present in either the congenital or the acquired variant, occasionally results in marked improvement of the language disorder.

The *mixed receptive–expressive (phonologic–syntactic) syndrome* is the most common of the dysphasias and may also be associated with autism. Comprehension is equal to or better than production, which is effortful and agrammatic, with a tendency to omit small words (articles, prepositions, pronouns, conjunctions). The children may have oromotor dysfunction with drooling, but dysarthria is not severe enough to account for their impaired production of speech sounds, which varies in different contexts and makes them difficult to understand. Their vocabulary is small, and they tend to speak in short utterances. Children with this syndrome tend to improve considerably before they reach school-age, but are at high risk for later dyslexia.

There are two syndromes in which comprehension is unimpaired or at least dramatically better than expression. One, labeled *verbal* (not oromotor!) *dyspraxia,* comprises extremely dysfluent children who express themselves in single effortful words or short phrases and with very imperfect phonology. These children may or may not have oromotor dysfunction, but again, it is not the cause of their expressive difficulty. Prognosis for fluent speech is guarded (62), but excellent for language acquisition in terms of vocabulary and ability to comprehend sophisticated language. The other is termed the *speech-programming deficit syndrome* because children produce very distorted speech, despite relatively good fluency, vocabulary, and syntax. Prognosis is generally good. Neither of these two syndromes is encountered in autistic children, all of whom have defective comprehension.

There are two higher-order reception–formulation syndromes. The first, which is quite common among both DLD and autistic children, is called the *lexical–syntactic syndrome.* It is characterized by severe word retrieval difficulty, to the point that the child may be mistaken for a stutterer because of multiple hesitations and false starts. The children have difficulty formulating complex discourse, especially when constrained by the need to respond to questions. Their syntax is immature for their age, but better in spontaneous discourse than in reponse to questions. Speech articulation is adequate or mildly immature. Comprehension of complex language is defective. Prognosis is guarded for such skills as reading comprehension and the use of language for complex verbal tasks.

The second higher-order reception–formulation syndrome is the *semantic–pragmatic syndrome* because of prominent deficits in the conversational use of language and in word retrieval The syndrome is most frequent in high-functioning autistic children, but it also occurs in some nonautistic children. Its hallmark is verbosity, which often, but not always, occurs after delayed onset of speech. The children speak clearly, fluently, and incessantly, usually on topics of their choice, without the need for a conversational partner. Syntax and phonology are normal and the vocabulary may be extensive. Prosody is abnormal, speech may be singsong, overprecise, or wooden. Much of what the children say consists of bits and pieces of overlearned phrases and television commercials (delayed echolalia). Echolalia, perseveration, and impaired conversational skills, such as turn-taking, maintenance of topic, and awareness of the interests of others, are prominent. Comprehension of discourse is impaired, and rather than responding to questions, these children frequently repeat the last words of the question (immediate echolalia). Some of them are hyperlexic; that is, they learn to decode written language without special instruction after evincing a precocious interest in letters and numbers. Reading comprehension often remains defective. It is important to be aware of the children's impaired language skills, which are regularly overlooked. Disobedience, an avoidable source of conflict, frequently occurs because of lack of comprehension.

C. Workup

As with autism and mental deficiency, observing the child at play with representational toys and engaging him or her in conversation while at play is the part of the examination most likely to be informative. The ability to imitate movements of the lips, tongue, and jaw and to repeat single and multiple syllables is the part of the sensorimotor examination most likely to be abnormal. Once again, the importance of a definitive test of hearing in all children with inadequate language is stressed. Obtaining a sleep EEG in children suspected of VAA is recommended to make sure not to miss epileptic aphasia. Referral to a speech and language pathologist and to a neuropsychologist is required for school placement and to plan intervention. As in other developmental disorders, neuroimaging and biochemical tests have very little to offer in the absence of other findings.

D. Management

Intervention is entirely educational. For mildly affected children, individual language (not speech) work with a speech and language pathologist may be adequate. More severely affected children will profit from admission to a specialized preschool for language-impaired children (48). Extremely dysfluent children who are unintelligible to all but close family members are often frustrated. The provision of an alternative means for making themselves understood, such as a communication board, formal sign language, or a computer, may help alleviate behavior problems. This tactic does not preclude the development of speech. Quite the contrary, it may facilitate the emergence of more intelligible speech. The provision of language through the visual–manual channel is essential for children with VAA for whom it may be the only means for acquiring language.

E. Stuttering

Stuttering is frequent in preschool children with previously normal speech. It often has a sudden onset and is characterized by dysfluency with blocking in the production of a word, usually associated with multiple repetitions of the first syllable of that word. If children are not corrected, this transient stuttering tends to disappear after several weeks or months. It persists or even appears later, at school age, in a small minority.

Stuttering is not a language disorder, but one affecting the programming of speech acts. Its pathophysiology is not understood. One hypothesis is that there is competition between the two hemispheres for the control of the muscles of phonation and articulation (63). Another is distorted use of auditory feedback for self-monitoring of speech. Rarely, stuttering may appear in the context of a brain disease, notably in adolescents with the juvenile variant of ceroid lipofuscinosis.

There is a voluminous literature on stuttering and its management. There is no indication for a medical workup or for intervention in preschool stutterers. Intervention by a speech and language pathologist is usually deferred until school age or adolescence.

V. SUMMARY

In preschoolers, developmental disabilities that are not associated with obvious motor deficits are most likely to present with a chief complaint of delayed language acquisition. Once hearing loss has been ruled out with a definitive test of hearing, there are three main conditions to consider in the differential diagnosis: mental deficiency, autistic spectrum disorder, and developmental language disability. Children with DLD have adequate social and nonverbal cognitive skills; mentally deficient children have adequate social skills, but have nonverbal as well as verbal cognitive impairments; whereas the hallmarks of children on the autistic spectrum, whatever their intellectual level, are deviant sociability, unusual preoccupations, and stereotypies. Although language comprehension is regularly superior to production in children with DLD and may be intact or almost intact in a sizeable number of them, comprehension is invariably impaired in autistic preschoolers, even in those who are fluent and have a large vocabulary. Autistic preschoolers are thus both dysphasic and autistic. There are at least six clinically recognizable variants of DLD, and the four associated with impaired comprehension are easily recognizable in autistic as well as DLD children. Whether dysphasic syndromes are discernible in mentally deficient preschoolers is not known.

The pathophysiology of the developmental syndromes of brain dysfunction is unknown. They do not have a single etiology, and they are rarely the consequence of gross brain lesions or specific diseases. Genetics may be a frequent etiologic factor. Neuroimaging and investigations for metabolic causes are rarely productive. Sleep EEGs are indicated in children with severe comprehension deficits, especially those with VAA.

Management, which is often very effective, is educational. Since these disorders probably denote subtle static cerebral maldevelopment, functional improvement may be due to the development of alternative strategies. Most dysphasic children speak adequately by school age, but persistent language deficits are likely to reappear in the guise of learning disabilities, notably difficulty learning to read and spell.

In the preschool years, there is a limited need for drug therapy, except in severely affected children on the autistic spectrum. The main indications are severe attention disorder and uncontrollably impulsive behavior. One needs to avoid the long-term use of psychotropic drugs with potentially irreversible side effects in autistic children with uncontrollable behaviors, since the underlying condition is static. There is a great need for alternative behavior-modifying drugs for these children. However, drugs alone cannot be expected to suffice, but must be combined with sophisticated and effective behavior management approaches.

ACKNOWLEDGMENT

Supported in part by Program Project grant NS 20489 from the National Institute of Neurologic Diseases and Stroke, USPHS

REFERENCES

1. Finger S, Stein DG. Brain damage and recovery: research and clinical perspectives. New York: Academic Press, 1982.
2. Kandel ER. Genes, nerve cells, and the remembrance of things past. J Neuropsychiatry 1989; 1:103–125.
3. Milner B. Hemispheric specialization: scope and limits. In: Schmitt FO, Worden FG, eds. The neurosciences: third study program. Cambridge: MIT Press, 1974:75–89.
4. Purpura DP. Pathobiology of cortical neurons in metabolic and unclassified amentias. In: Katzman R, ed. Congenital and acquired cognitive disorders. New York: Raven Press, 1979:43–68.
5. Galaburda AM. The pathogenesis of childhood dyslexia. In: Plum F, ed. Language, communication, and the brain. New York: Raven Press, 1988:127–137.
6. Hallgren B. Specific dyslexia ("congenital word blindness"). A clinical and genetic study. Acta Psychiatr Neurol Scand [Suppl] 1950; 65:1–287.
7. Smith SD, Kimberling WJ, Pennington BF, et al. Specific reading disability: identification of an inherited form through genetic linkage analysis. Science 1983; 291:1345–1347.
8. Bellugi U, Marks S, Bihrle A, Sabo H. Dissociation between language and cognitive functions in Williams syndrome. In: Bishop D, Mogford K, eds. Language development in exceptional circumstances. Edinburgh: Churchill-Livingstone, 1988:177–189.
9. Garron DC. Intelligence among persons with Turner's syndrome. Behav Genet 1977; 7:105–127.
10. Lubs HA, Watson M, Breg R, et al. Restudy of the original marker X family. Am J Med Genet 1984; 17:231–244.
11. American Pyschiatric Association. Diagnostic and Statistical Manual of Mental Disorders, ed. 3, revised. Washington, DC: American Psychiatric Association, 1987.
12. World Health Organization. Mental disorders: glossary and guide to their classification in accordance with the tenth revision (draft) of the international classification of disease. Geneva: WHO, 1989.
13. Rubin IL, Crocker AC. Developmental disabilities: delivery of medical care for children and adults. Philadelphia: Lea & Febiger, 1989.

14. Sparrow S, Balla DA, Cichetti DV. Vineland adaptive behavior scales—revised. Circle Pines, Minn: American Guidance Service, 1984.
15. Rapin I. Children with brain dysfunction: cognition, language, and behavior. New York: Raven Press, 1982:157–173.
16. Geschwind N. Disorders of higher cortical function in children. Clin Proc Child Natl Med Center 1969; 28:262–272.
17. Broman S, Nichols PL, Shaughnessy P, Kennedy W. Retardation in young children: a developmental study of cognitive deficit. Hillsdale, NJ: Laurence Erlbaum, 1987.
18. Freeman JM, ed. Prenatal and perinatal factors associated with brain disorders. Bethesda, Md: National Institutes of Health, 1985.
19. Jones KL. Smith's recognizable patterns of human malformation, 4th ed. Philadelphia: WB Saunders, 1988.
20. de Grouchy J, Turleau C. Clinical atlas of human chromosomes. New York: John Wiley & Sons, 1984.
21. McKusick VA. Mendelian inheritance in man, 9th ed. Baltimore: Johns Hopkins University Press, 1990.
22. Wilson BC. Neuropsychological assessment of the preschool child with developmental deficits. In: Fillskov S, Boll T, eds. Handbook of clinical neuropsychology. New York: John Wiley & Sons, 1986.
23. Nyhan WL, Sakati NO. Diagnostic recognition of genetic disease. Philadelphia: Lea & Febiger, 1987.
24. Wing L, Gould J. Severe impairments of social interaction and associated abnormalities in children: epidemiology and classification. J Autism Dev Disord 1979; 9:11–30.
25. Allen DA. Autistic spectrum disorders: clinical presentation in preschool children. J Child Neurol 1988; 3(suppl):S48–S56.
26. Frith U, ed. Autism and Asperger syndrome. Cambridge: Cambridge University Press, 1991.
27. Rourke BP. Nonverbal learning disabilities: the syndrome and the model. New York: Guilford Press, 1989.
28. DeLong GR, Dwyer J. Correlation of family history with specific autistic subgroups: Asperger's syndrome and bipolar affective disorder. J Autism Dev Disord 1988; 18:593–600.
29. Allen DA, Rapin I, Wiznitzer M. Communication disorders of preschool children: the physician's responsibility. Dev Behav Pediatr 1988; 9:164–170.
30. Rapin I, Allen DA. Developmental dysphasia and autism in preschool children: characteristics and subtypes. In: Proceedings of the first international symposium on specific speech and language disorders in children. England: AFASIC Association for All Speech Impaired Children, 1987:20–35.
31. Jure R, Rapin I, Tuchman RF. Hearing impaired autistic children. Dev Med Child Neurol (in press).
32. Volkmar FR, Nelson DS. Seizure disorders in autism. J Am Acad Child Adolesc Psychiatry 1990; 29:127–129.
33. Tuchman RF, Rapin I, Shinnar S. Autistic and dysphasic children. II. Epilepsy. Pediatrics (in press).

34. Courchesne E, Yeung-Courchesne R, Press AG, et al. Hypoplasia of cerebellar lobules VI and VIII in infantile autism. N Engl J Med 1988; 318:1349–1354.
35. Ritvo ER, Jorde LB, Mason-Brothers A, et al. The UCLA–University of Utah epidemiologic survey of autism: recurrence risk estimates and genetic counseling. Am J Psychiatry 1989; 146:1032–1036.
36. Brown WT, Friedman E, Jenkins EC, et al. Association of fragile-X syndrome with autism. Lancet 1982; 1:100.
37. Holm VA, Varley CK. Pharmacologic treatment of autistic children. In: Dawson G, ed. Autism: nature, diagnosis and treatment. New York: Guilford Press, 1989:386–404.
38. Young JG, Kavanagh ME, Anderson GM, et al. Clinical neurochemistry of autism and associated disorders. J Autism Dev Disord 1982; 12:147–165.
39. Aman MG, Kern RA. Review of fenfluramine in the treatment of developmental disabilities. J Am Acad Child Adolesc Psychiatry 1989; 28:549–565.
40. Campbell M, Anderson LT, Green WH, et al. Psychopharmacology. In: Cohen DJ, Donnellan AM, Paul R, eds. Handbook of autism and pervasive developmental disorders. New York: John Wiley & Sons, 1987:545–565.
41. Perry R, Campbell M, Adams P, et al. Long-term efficacy of haloperidol in autistic children: continuous versus discontinuous drug administration. J Am Acad Child Adolesc Psychiatry 1989; 28:87–92.
42. Jenkins SC, Maruta T. Therapeutic use of propranolol for intermittent explosive behavior. Mayo Clin Proc 1987; 62:204–214.
43. Minshew NJ, Payton JB. New perspectives in autism. Curr Probl Pediatr 1988; 18:561–610, 613–694.
44. Swedo SE, Leonard HL, Rapoport JL, et al. A double-blind comparison of clomipramine and desipramine in the treatment of trichotillomania (hair pulling). N Engl J Med 1989; 321:497–501.
45. Sandman CA, Patta PC, Banon J, et al. Naloxone attenuates self-abusive behavior in developmentally disabled clients. Appl Res Mental Retard 1983; 4:5–11.
46. Herman BH, Hammock MK, Arthur-Smith A, et al. Naltrexone decreases self-injurious behavior. Ann Neurol 1987; 22:550–552.
47. Campbell M, Overall JE, Small AM, et al. Naltrexone in autistic children: an acute open dose range tolerance trial. J Am Acad Child Adolesc Psychiatry 1989; 28:200–206.
48. Allen DA, Mendelson L, Rapin I. Syndrome-specific remediation in preschool developmental dysphasia. In: French JH, Harel S, Casaer P, et al., eds. Child neurology and developmental disabilities. Baltimore: Paul H Brookes, 1989:233–243.
49. Schopler E, Mesibov G, eds. Social behavior in autism. New York: Plenum Press, 19XX.
50. Cohen DJ, Donnellan AM, Paul R, eds. Handbook of autism and pervasive developmental disorders. New York: John Wiley & Sons, 1987.
51. Rogers SJ, Lewis H. An effective day treatment model for young children with pervasive developmental disorders. J Am Acad Child Adolesc Psychiatry 1989; 28:207–214.

52. Hart C. Without reason: a family copes with two generations of autism. New York: Harper & Row, 1989.
53. Bates E, Marchman VA. What is and is not universal in language acquisition. In: Plum F, ed. Language, communication, and the brain. New York: Raven Press, 1988:19–38.
54. Coplan J. The early language milestone scale—revised. Austin, Tx: Pro-Ed, 1989.
55. Chi JG, Dooling EC, Gilles FH. Gyral development of the human brain. Ann Neurol 1977; 1:86–93.
56. Aram DM. Language sequelae of unilateral brain lesions in children. In: Plum F, ed. Language, communication, and the brain. New York: Raven Press, 1988:171–197.
57. Landau WM, Goldstein R, Kleffner FR. Congenital aphasia: a clinicopathologic study. Neurology 1960; 10:915–921.
58. Resnick TJ, Rapin I. Normal and disordered acquisition of language. In: Asbury AK, McKhann GM, McDonald WI, eds. Diseases of the nervous system: clinical neurobiology. Philadelphia: WB Saunders, 1986:759–768.
59. Rapin I, Allen DA. Syndromes in developmental dysphasia and adult aphasia. In: Plum F, ed. Language, communication, and the brain. New York: Raven Press, 1988:57–75.
60. Landau WM, Kleffner FR. Syndrome of acquired aphasia with convulsive disorder in children. Neurology 1957; 7:523–530.
61. Bishop DVM. Age at onset and outcome in acquired aphasia with convulsive disorder (Landau–Kleffner syndrome). Dev Med Child Neurol 1985; 27: 705–712.
62. Ferry PC, Hall SM, Hicks JL. "Dilapidated" speech: developmental verbal dyspraxia. Dev Med Child Neurol 1975; 17 749–756.
63. Jones RK. Observations on stammering after localized cerebral injury. J Neurol Neurosurg Psychiatry 1966; 29:192–195.

2

Developmental Disabilities in School-Aged Children

Susan K. Klein *Case Western Reserve University, Cleveland, Ohio*

Mary Anne Muriello *Rainbow Babies and Children's Hospital, Cleveland, Ohio*

I. INTRODUCTION

Dyslexia (specific reading disability), attention deficit disorder (ADD), and tic disorders associated with learning disabilities are the three most common cognitive disorders that occur in school-aged children, although the effects of developmental disabilities that occur earlier in childhood (Rapin, this volume) are often first encountered when children enter school. This chapter reviews the biology and treatment of these cognitive disorders. ADD and tic disorder have been the subject of many recent reviews linking pathophysiology and treatment (see below), but reviews on dyslexia have been less comprehensive.

As for developmental disabilities in preschool years, developmental disorders in school-aged children have not been classified uniformly with clinical or test score profiles. It is not surprising that clinical trials of drug or behavior therapy have not provided widely applicable results. Identification of clinical subgroups of dyslexia, ADD, or tic disorders based on specific pathophysiological features will aid in testing of new therapies. This chapter reviews current knowledge of the taxonomy, pathophysiology, and treatment of these three conditions.

II. DYSLEXIA

Nearly every modern treatise on dyslexia recognizes that meaningful investigation within any theoretical framework relies on accurate definition. Most investigators have been able to agree on a relatively broad concept of dyslexia, summarized in DSM-III-R as an "impairment in the development of word recognition skills and reading comprehension that is not explainable by Mental Retardation or inadequate schooling and that is not due to a visual or hearing deficit or neurologic disorder" (1, p. 43). Early research sought to expand and refine a universal description of dyslexia. It has become clear over the past several decades, however, that this attempt has failed because dyslexia is not a homogeneous disorder; the idea that subtypes of dyslexia exist is now well established and accepted (2–6). The encouraging implication for treatment is that more effective remediation can be tailored to behaviorally distinct phenotypes. Moreover, well-classified subtypes will enable the research community to design studies that are more likely to engender valid theories of pathogenesis.

Present theories of pathogenesis, particularly neuroanatomical and neurophysiological observations, have not been based on studies that define dyslexic subjects by validated neuropsychological testing. If neurobiological correlates are to be useful in diagnosing and treating reading disorders and other disorders of higher cerebral function, they should reflect variables in behavior and performance because these are the features that bring children to professional attention and best determine the need for intervention (7). Better classification may thus help to resolve the schism between those who believe that neurobiology is relevant to reading disorders and those who do not.

A. History of Dyslexia

Nineteenth-century theories of localization of brain functions greatly influenced the thinking of early neuroscientists who reported cases of isolated cognitive deficits. Kussmaul (8) introduced the expression "word blindness" in a discussion of speech disturbances and alexia, and Morgan (9) was the first to use the term "congenital word blindness" to refer to a case of developmental dyslexia. Hinshelwood (10), an ophthalmologist, applied the same phrase to otherwise bright patients whom he thought were suffering from a "congenital defect in the visual memory center" that prevented them from learning to read. Orton (11,12) agreed that dyslexics were unable to correctly interpret a memory image of written symbols and attributed this to a delay in the normal development of cerebral dominance.

Orton's work was important because it offered the first integrated theory for the pathogenesis of dyslexia. He introduced the intriguing notion that dyslexics perceived letters and words as mirror images, coining the term "strephosymbolia" (twisted symbols) (11), a concept that has permeated the realm of general knowledge to the extent that lay persons mistakenly equate this variable symptom with dyslexia. In Orton's view of dyslexia, word images are normally encoded in the left hemisphere as an exact representation of the stimulus, but a delay in the establishment of normal left-sided cerebral dominance is responsible for an impairment in their retrieval, thereby permitting the abnormal retrieval of a stored mirror image from the right hemisphere.

Orton's proposal was a springboard for many educational interventions and recognized that dyslexics were intelligent, despite their reading difficulties. In the years since Orton's publications, diverse theories (discussed below) have been proposed, but their impact on educational strategies has remained rather limited. This is because the focus on better classification and definition has not been a priority among researchers until fairly recently. Such a trend will help investigators from heterogeneous disciplines formulate common goals and institute directed therapies.

B. Adult Alexia Model

Many have compared the performance of otherwise normal children who fail to learn to read to previously normal brain-damaged adults with acquired reading deficits (i.e., alexia) (6,9,10). Localized brain pathology identified during craniotomy of alexic adults has been used to infer faulty development of corresponding brain regions in dyslexic children (13). Mattis' description (6) of four dyslexia subtypes, corresponding to syndromes of acquired alexia in adults, typifies this approach.

Others (14) suggest that the underlying impairment in dyslexia cannot be strictly equated with a topographic lesion. Adult alexia models do not take into account the effects of age and environmental differences on neuronal plasticity. Physiological changes occur in the fetal and neonatal brain that do not and cannot occur at later points in life (15) and may differentiate developmental disorders from those which are acquired. Witelson (16) reviews the literature on brain-damaged children and adults, who showed different, age-dependent patterns of language recovery. She supports the notion that neuronal plasticity plays a major part in clinical outcomes in both developmental and acquired language disorders.

C. Functional Model

Marshall (17) holds that dyslexics and alexics both make the same types of reading errors, indicating a perturbation of a global reading method. He believes that it is this functional similarity which makes the two groups comparable. His methodological or functional model recognizes that variable neuroanatomy occurs in individuals with dyslexia expressed in a limited number of reading disabilities.

Marshall proposes a universal reading model composed of basic routes that govern how individuals read aloud (18). This idea has emerged from his understanding of the processes underlying normal beginning reading (19). "Developmental lag in the operation of one route will thus have behavioral consequences that are analogous to selective acquired damage to that route" (17, p. 77). In this view, the development of mature reading is seen as an additive process in which new skills are layered into the preexisting substrate without effecting any qualitative changes in the current system. Consequently, the effect of damaging a complete system is equivalent to developmental arrest in the immature system if the composite of functional modules available to the reader is the same (17).

From these considerations, we see that dyslexic subtypes exist for a heterogeneous group of disorders that are also probably not static (3,5,20). Morris and his colleagues (5, p. 374) stress the "developmental nature of the reading-learning process" and anticipate that subtypes of dyslexic children will merge and diverge at different stages. All these authors view the descriptions of current subtypes as probably only a small part of the spectrum which will enlarge with future research.

D. Neuronal Migration Theory and Neuroanatomical Studies

Caviness et al. (15) reviewed the features of neuronal migration that may be altered in developmental disorders such as dyslexia. Cortical neurons proliferate and differentiate themselves from the glial glue before climbing along specialized glial cells to their destined place in the cortex (15). A jungle of disorganized cell processes becomes an intricate communications network through the establishment of synaptic circuits and receptor anatomy. Abnormalities of cortical architecture may occur as early as the beginning of the third trimester, when the critical period of neurogenesis begins, and as late as the first years of life, when myelination is completed (15).

Galaburda and his colleagues (21–23) have related alterations in these processes to the pathogenesis of dyslexia. His group has accumulated evidence to support the notion that critical variations in corticogenesis may result in dysplastic neuronal architectures underlying subtle developmental disorders. Many microdysplastic foci have been found in eight dyslexic brains described in two series from this laboratory (21,23). The first series was comprised of four male brains notable for aberrations of lamination, clusters of ectopic neurons (ectopias), and distortions of gyral patterns (micropolygyria) in excess of those observed occasionally in normal brains. The defects were concentrated in the inferior frontal and superior temporal (i.e., perisylvian) regions and were far more prominent on the left side. A second series has confirmed the presence of similar microdysgenic anomalies and myelinated cortical scars in three female dyslexic brains.

Both studies also revealed consistent dimensional symmetry of the planum temporale, an area located on the right and left superior temporal surface posterior to the transverse auditory gyrus of Heschl. This finding has been corroborated in magnetic resonance imaging evaluation of 19 dyslexic adolescents who were found to have a significantly greater percentage of symmetrical plana than did matched controls according to area measurements reconstructed from successive coronal images of the brain (24).

The planum temporale is a high-order auditory association area within the classical area of Wernicke, thought to be significant in language comprehension. Geschwind and Levitsky (25) found that the planum temporale was typically larger in the left hemisphere in 100 presumably normal adult brains they studied at autopsy. Witelson and Pallie (26) demonstrated that asymmetry was present in this region at birth, suggesting that this structuralization occurs prenatally.

Galaburda proposed that the symmetrical plana found in his collection of dyslexic brains may have occurred by expansion of the smaller side, suggesting that there may be increased numbers of neurons and/or extraneuronal elements in this area (27). Studies of fetal monkeys offer evidence that distant cortical lesions may reduce normal cell death in thus enlarged cortical projection areas (28). Galaburda et al. (21) postulated that this phenomenon may be related to altered synaptic connections between the lesioned cells and the nonadjacent areas of symmetry. These observations offer a possible link between the occurrence of microdysplasias and the symmetry of the planum temporale in dyslexic brains.

Intrauterine factors might incur cortical lesions that alter the development of the brain during neurogenesis and neuronal migration, which may not be unique to dyslexia. We know that normal adult brains exhibit aberrations of neuronal migration without any evidence of associated clinical pathology. Autopsy studies have revealed that between 3 and 30% of brain specimens show isolated foci of misplaced neurons (29–31). Such localized anomalies have also been associated with severe and obvious environmental insults to the human fetus (toxins, radiation, infections, vascular compromise) occurring during neurogenesis and migration (32–35). Animal studies have reproduced these findings experimentally using similarly timed environmental stressors (36–38).

Some studies (39,40) have suggested an increased frequency of learning disabilities and dyslexia in individuals with immune disorders. Conversely, immune disorders may be more prevalent among dyslexics (40). For example, dyslexia and other learning disabilities seem to occur more frequently in the male children of women with systemic lupus erythematosus (41). Animal studies support these clinical observations. Strains of immunologically deficient laboratory mice with focal neuronal ectopias are more likely to have learning difficulties (42,43). Humphreys and colleagues (23) cite this work and their own findings as proof of specific neuropathological change in dyslexia. They found microdysplastic foci encountered in their autopsies of dyslexic brains clustered around centrally perforating cortical arterioles, implicating a possible microangiopathic phenomenon. Their autopsies of patients with systemic lupus erythematosus, a disease known to have a microangiopathic pathogenesis sometimes manifested within the central nervous system, revealed identical, frequently myelinated cortical anomalies. These authors suggest that some forms of dyslexia emanate from a vasculitic disorder that may be immune-mediated. A conceivable hypothesis is that alterations in typical vascular supply patterns secondary to vasculitis in utero might be related to the altered synaptic connections that Galaburda postulates underlie patterns of neuroanatomical symmetry.

E. Genetic Theories

Observations of a greater prevalence of dyslexia among boys have been the basis for proposing a genetic mechanism (10,44). Complex modes of sex-linked transmission have been hypothesized to explain the gender difference (45). However, in a population of previously unscreened classes of schoolchildren, Shaywitz et al. (46) found that the measured ability of both sexes was comparable even though teachers rated boys as having significantly more behavior, language, and academic problems than girls. They suggest that many studies may have been skewed toward male subjects by acquisition bias. This finding was predicted by Finucci and Childs (47) in a review of gender discrepancy in dyslexia.

Hallgren (48), an early advocate of a "dyslexia gene" with an autosomal dominant mode of inheritance, dismissed a sex linkage and attributed the sex difference to heightened parental concern about the academic performance of boys as opposed to girls. In his study of families with at least one dyslexic child, he found male:female ratios of only 1.3:1 and 1.2:1, respectively, in dyslexic sibling and parent groups, although the index group of dyslexic children had shown a 3:1 male:female ratio. A similar study by Vogler et al. (49) reported nearly identical statistics.

Linkage analysis has been used to demonstrate autosomal dominant inheritance in families with multiple generations of dyslexia (50). A positive linkage operates on the genetic principle of crossing over and requires a very high level of statistical significance. Linkage analysis infers location of a phenotypic trait (here, dyslexia) on a specific chromosome if the trait appears to cross over with an identifiable genetic marker locus. A dyslexia locus has thus been demonstrated within chromosome 15 in about 20% of the families studied in this manner. This supports the belief that there are different subtypes of dyslexia, some of which are heritable (51). Abnormalities of chromosome 15 were found in some of these families with dyslexia (51). Some behavioral geneticists propose that difficulty in phonological coding may be a heritable component of dyslexia, although this trait has not yet been localized to any specific chromosome by linkage analysis (52).

F. Treatment of Dyslexia

1. Behavior Therapy

An overview of theory has lent some perspective for critical appraisal of remedial approaches to dyslexia (reviewed in Refs. 14,53). A critique of the numerous educational programs that have been devised to deal with the problem is beyond the scope of this review. Optometric vision training has focused on remediating defective eye movements purported by some optometrists and ophthalmologists to play a role in reading disability (reviewed in Ref. 54).

2. Pharmacological Therapy

Not much is known about the neurochemistry of dyslexia and whether or not it has any relevance for treatment. Methylphenidate has a well-established record in the treatment of ADD (see below), but has not proven to be a panacea for cognitive disorders in the school-aged child (55,56). Dimond and Brouwers (57) encouraged interest in using piracetam to treat cognitive disorders of both children and adults when they reported that the compound enhanced verbal learning in a group of normal college students. Piracetam (2-oxo 1-pyrrolidine acetamide), is structurally similar to gamma-aminobutyric acid (GABA), one of the inhibitory neurotransmitters in the central nervous system. It has been credited, among other things, as being a facilitator of learning in laboratory animals (58) and an enhancer of alertness and cognitive performance.

A number of studies have attempted to document improvement in reading ability of dyslexic children treated with piracetam (59–69). These studies are summarized in Table 1.

All of these investigations report some kind of improvement in piracetam-treated subjects, but the findings must be interpreted cautiously. Although not strictly standardized, selection criteria were very similar across all the studies; however, it is not clear whether the diverse

TABLE 1 Piracetam Effects in Dyslexia

Investigator	Population	Length of treatment	Selection criteria	Measures	Outcome
Wilsher et al., 1979[a]	16 dyslexic boys vs. 14 normal adolescents	3 weeks	Standard	Number of trials needed to master a serial memory verbal learning task with 10 3-letter nonsense syllables	Piracetam-treated groups improved scores by nearly 2 times that of nondyslexic controls. Learning and then forgetting on the next trial decreased by nearly ½ in the dyslexic piracetam group
Simeon et al., 1980[a]	29 learning-disordered boys 8–13 years old	4 weeks	One grade placement behind in reading, spelling, math on WISC-R Full-Scale WISC-R IQ ≥ 80	History and physical exam EEG Psych evaluation Parent and teacher questionnaires Neuropsychological testing: verbal, nonverbal, sensory, and motor tasks	10 subjects treated with piracetam improved on tests of memory, attention span, concentration, and eye-hand coordination though not statistically significant Clinical global impression more favorable in piracetam-treated subjects who had approximately equal verbal and performance IQs Decreased left-hemisphere delta power on EEGs of piracetam-treated subjects

Rudel and Helfgott, 1983[b]	59 dyslexic boys 8–13 years old	12 weeks	Standard	Neimark Memorization Test: Picture Card Recall	Increased verbal memory and decreased forgotten material on delayed-recall tasks in piracetam-treated subjects
Wilsher and Milewski, 1983[b]	60 dyslexic boys 8–13 years old	12 weeks	Standard	Similarities and Vocabulary subtests within WISC-R	Improvement in Similarities in piracetam-treated subjects
Chase et al., 1984[b]	55 developmentally reading-disabled boys 8–13 years old	12 weeks	Standard	Gilmore Oral Reading Test WISC-R subtests for reading accuracy, rate, and comprehension WRAT Spelling Free-writing sample: number of words, % spelling errors Behavioral assessment by parents and school	Improved reading rate in piracetam-treated group Decreased spelling errors in piracetam-treated group
Connors et al., 1984[b]	13 dyslexic boys 8–13 years old	12 weeks	Standard	VER to verbal and shape stimuli	Longer latencies in left parietal leads in response to verbal stimuli in piracetam-treated group, correlating with decreased reaction times, i.e., left-hemisphere effect of piracetam (not statistically significant)
Helfgott et al., 1984[b]	30 dyslexic boys	12 weeks	Standard	Single word WRAT reading scores Gilmore Oral Reading Test	Improved verbal memory for piracetam-treated group No improvement in prose reading or accuracy

TABLE 1 Continued

Investigator	Population	Length of treatment	Selection criteria	Measures	Outcome
Wilsher et al., 1984[b]	46 dyslexic boys 8–13 years old	8 weeks	Standard	Reading speed, accuracy, and comprehension Free writing sample: number of words % spelling errors	No significant difference between placebo and piracetam group Significant improvement pre- and posttreatment in scores of piracetam-treated individuals
DiIanni et al., 1985[b]	257 dyslexic boys 8–13 years old	12 weeks	Standard	Neuropsychological testing	Improved reading fluency with maintained accuracy in piracetam-treated group
Connors et al., 1987[b]	34 dyslexic children 8–13 years old	36 weeks	Standard	VER to verbal and shape stimuli	
Wilsher et al., 1987[b]	225 dyslexic children	36 weeks	Standard	Gray Oral Reading Test Gilmore Oral Reading Test WRAT-R Reading Subtest	Improved reading accuracy, speed, and comprehension in piracetam-treated group

[a] = Double-Blind Crossover Study
[b] = Double Blind Study
Standard selection criteria = English as a primary language; no neurological, sensory, psychiatric, or emotional impairment; no disadvantaged environment; Full-Scale WISC-R IQ $\geq$ 80 with performance or verbal IQ $\geq$ 90; reading quotient (RQ) $\leq$ 0.85, $RQ = \frac{\text{Gilmore Accuracy Reading Age Score}}{\text{chronological age} \times \text{full-scale IQ}} \times 100$.

measures chosen to detect differences between piracetam and placebo groups reflect real improvement in reading ability. Tests used to measure improvement following drug treatment may not have been sensitive to detect better reading skills. For example, Wilsher (67) used two subtests of the WISC-R (Vocabulary and Similarities) to examine the effects of piracetam on dyslexics' verbal conceptualizing ability. These subtests have strong primary verbal factors and were chosen because Wilsher et al. (59) had previously found increases in verbal learning of dyslexics treated with piracetam. The authors state that these were desirable measures because they have high test-retest stability and high split-half reliability. However, the dyslexic subjects were noted to have performed adequately on these tests prior to treatment, leading one to question the relationship between the observed improvement and justification for treating with piracetam.

Thus far, few data support a basis for pharmacological intervention in dyslexia. No animal models for dyslexia are available for validating drug therapies. Scanty investigation with human subjects is partly reflective of reticence to expose individuals to psychoactive drugs that may have uncharted long-term side effects. The studies thus far have not identified any major side effects of piracetam but they are too limited to address the issue of long-term side effects.

Even if an effective pharmacological intervention is found, it is unlikely to work for every dyslexic. This necessarily resurrects the plea for classification. Spontaneous improvement may occur for some, but not all groups of dyslexic children. For others, dyslexia might be a lifelong developmental disorder, which would theoretically imply a lifelong need for any medication. Clearer indications for pharmacological intervention must be developed, and this will not emerge until the disorder itself is better defined.

III. ATTENTION DEFICIT DISORDER

Definition of ADD is often difficult for the pediatrician and neurologist. Most use the DSM-III-R (1) definition, which is based on recognition of short attention span, impulsiveness, and hyperactivity. This definition labels many children with ADD who may have other behavioral disturbances associated with shortened attention span (specific learning disabilities, autistic spectrum disorder, pervasive developmental disorder, or conduct disorder). No single screening test for identification of ADD has been validated for DSM-III-R criteria (70), although many clinicians use the Conners Teacher (71) and Parent (72) rating scales to identify children with attention deficit hyperactivity disorder.

Some children who are appropriately labeled as having ADD may vary with respect to symptoms and response to interventions. For example,

Urion (73) studied 50 boys with ADD who did not respond to methylphenidate therapy. He subtyped them into three groups defined by (1) poor performance on a test of word fluency, (2) low scores on timed motor and language tasks, and (3) poor construction of a complex figure. Children with motor deficits (type 2) improved in behavior when treated with desipramine. As for dyslexia, a common system of classification is needed to identify children with ADD with and without motor hyperactivity (70), so that the pathophysiology of ADD and its amelioration with drug therapy might be better understood.

A. Pathogenesis

The biology of attention has been extensively studied, but is incompletely understood. Mesulam (74) has defined attention as a composite of state and channel operations. State operations include arousal and readiness to respond to environmental stimuli. Attentional state is probably modulated at the level of the reticular activating system (74). Channel operations encompass selection for further preparation of a response (75). Selective attention is controlled in the cerebral cortex. The frontal lobes may play a large role in selective attention (76), as shown by neuroimaging (77) and evoked potential studies (78–81). However, other brain areas are probably also involved. Lou and co-workers (82,83) found hypoperfusion in the area of the head of the caudate nucleus, which increased when they gave methylphenidate to 19 children with ADD whom they studied with an intra-arterial Xe-133 perfusion technique. They concluded that the modulation of multiple sensory inputs that occurs in the striatum is abnormal in children with ADD.

The role of chemical messengers between and within these anatomical centers is unclear. Central monoamines (the catecholamines dopamine and norepinephrine, and serotonin) may be depleted in children with ADD, since children with ADD respond to drugs that have been shown by animal studies to increase monoamine concentration at the synaptic cleft (84). Limited human studies have suggested the monoamine metabolites are decreased in children with ADD (reviewed in Ref. 70). These hypotheses have been the rationale for drug therapy in ADD. All the commonly used drugs probably block reuptake of catecholamines from the synaptic cleft. Amphetamines and methylphenidate stimulate release of catecholamines from presynaptic terminals. Pemoline and the other amines also slow postsynaptic degradation of transmitter. The variable clinical response to these medications suggests that neurotransmitter interactions may differ among subgroups of children with ADD.

B. Treatment

Both behavioral and pharmacological treatment have a role in the treatment of ADD in children. Educational planning, especially identification of coexistent learning disabilities, is the first step in treatment of children with ADD. Cognitive-behavioral training and psychotherapy have been used alone and in conjunction with pharmacological therapy in ADD. The efficacy of behavior therapy alone is controversial (85–87) but probably has some beneficial effect (88–90). Behavioral therapy may be enhanced by addition of pharmacological therapy (70).

Drug therapy regimens for children with ADD have been reviewed extensively (70,91–92). Table 2 represents a synthesis of these approaches. In general, methylphenidate and pemoline are the most widely used. Of the two, methylphenidate has the shorter half-life. An initial dose of 0.03 mg/kg can be given in the morning and increased every 2 weeks to a target dose of 0.6–0.8 mg/kg/day. If a "wearing off" effect occurs in the afternoon, addition of a second 0.03 mg/kg dose 3 hr after the first dose can be as efficacious as increasing the morning dose. Pemoline should be given as 18.75 mg at the outset and increased by 18.75-mg increments (on a daily or twice-daily dosage schedule) to a target of 0.5–3.0 mg/kg/day. In 22 boys with ADD, Pelham and co-workers (93) found long-acting drugs to be more beneficial in managing aggressive behavior and improving social interactions with peers.

There is a growing role for desipramine in the management of ADD (reviewed in Ref. 70). The initial dose of desipramine is 25 mg, and it can be increased by 25 mg/week to a target dose of 0.5–3.0 mg/kg/day. Clonidine has also been used (94), although few studies have substantiated its efficacy in ADD with or without Tourette syndrome.

Some drugs have fallen out of common usage. Because of its abuse, D-amphetamine is rarely used in the treatment of ADD (95). Methylphenidate, especially the longer-acting formulations, may be sold illegally for ADD, and its distribution is being controlled at the state and local level. Long-acting forms of methylphenidate may not be as effective as the shorter-acting form in some children with ADD (96). There is insufficient evidence to conclude that monoamine oxidase inhibitors, piracetam, bupropion, alprazolam, vasopressin, caffeine, tyrosine, tryptophan, or L-dopa is useful in management of ADD (reviewed in Ref. 70).

The short- and long-term risks and benefits of drug therapy in children with ADD are becoming clearer (70,97). The short-term benefits of drug therapy include a decrease in motor fidgeting (85) and accurate and sustained performance on perceptual searching tasks (97). Side effects, such

TABLE 2 Drugs Commonly Used in Treatment of Attention Deficit Disorder

Drug	Sizes	Kinetics		Initial dosage	Incremental dosage	Therapeutic range
		Peak	t½			
Methylphenidate	5 mg 10 mg 20 mg 20 mg (SR)	2.5 hr	2–4 hr	0.03 mg/kg q A.M.	↑ to 0.6–0.8 mg/kg every 2 weeks Add 2nd dose, 0.3 mg/kg at noon or 0.3 mg/kg in afternoon	0.3–1 mg/kg/day (÷ b.i.d. or t.i.d.) ≤ 80 mg/day max
Pemoline	18.75 mg 37.5 mg 75 mg	3 hr	7–8.5 hr	18.75 mg q A.M.	↑ by 18.75 mg every 2 weeks	0.5–3.0 mg/kg/day (÷ b.i.d. or t.i.d.) ≤ 112.5 mg/day max
Desipramine	10 mg 20 mg 50 mg 75 mg 100 mg	2–8 hr	12–24 hr	25 mg/day	↑ by 25 mg/week	0.5–3.0 mg/kg/day (÷ up to q.i.d.) ≤ 5 mg/kg/day or 100 mg/day max
Clonidine	See Table 3					

as mood swings, irritability, anorexia, insomnia, and headaches, are transient and probably dose-related (98). The long-term beneficial effects of stimulant therapy are ill-defined. It is unclear whether drug therapy improves short- or long-term academic achievement, self-esteem, or peer relationships, or decreases antisocial behavior in adolescence and adulthood (see Ref. 97). Although much has been written about the long-term side effects of growth suppression and precipitation of tic disorders, they may not be as serious as once suspected. Growth suppression (with rebound during summer drug holidays) has been documented in children treated with more than 20 mg/day of methylphenidate (99–101). However, adults who were treated with stimulants for ADD as children do not differ significantly in height from those who were not treated (102). Precipitation of tic syndromes by stimulant medication is also controversial (see below).

Shaywitz and Shaywitz (70) comment that nontraditional therapies, such as diet changes, megavitamin therapy, patterning, and remediation of vestibular dysfunction, often diminish the amount of effort that patients and parents can put into more traditional therapies that might be helpful. Educational programming, combined with behavioral and judicious pharmacological therapy, offers the best treatment for this incompletely understood disorder.

IV. TIC DISORDERS OF CHILDHOOD

A tic is defined as a sudden, involuntary movement that is repetitive, purposeless, and stereotyped (103). Tics can be motor, vocal, or sensory. Motor tics may be simple (eye blinking) or complex (knee bending). Vocal tics similarly are simple (throat clearing, sniffing) or complex (echolalia, palilalia, coprolalia). Sensory tics (104) include unusual sensations confined to specific body regions (tickling, pressure) often relieved by movements that appear to be voluntary, but probably are not. Like other disorders of childhood that include behavioral symptoms, tic disorders are believed to range a clinical spectrum including transient tic disorders, multiple tic disorders, and Tourette syndrome (105).

Transient tic disorder of childhood consists of either motor or vocal tics that occur for more than 2 weeks but less than 1 year. At least 40–50% of simple tic disorders remit spontaneously (106), and less than 10% persist into adult life (107). The diagnosis of chronic multiple tic disorder is made when motor or vocal tics occur for more than 1 year, but do not change and do not co-occur (103).

Most of the literature on tic syndromes in childhood has focussed on Tourette syndrome, defined as the occurrence of multiple motor and vocal tics that occur many times a day, vary in type, frequency, and severity, and persist for at least 1 year (1). The diagnosis of Tourette syndrome presumes the exclusion of tics precipitated by other causes (medication) and of the other idiopathic tic disorders. Twenty to thirty percent of cases of Tourette syndrome in childhood remit by adulthood (107).

Tourette syndrome may be associated with other behavioral abnormalities. ADD occurs in 25–35% of patients with Tourette syndrome (108). Use of monoamines for ADD in children may precipitate tics (109) or increase tics in children with Tourette syndrome (110). Golden (108,111) and others (112,113) have suggested that Tourette syndrome in children with ADD was merely unmasked by monoamine therapy.

Surveys of adults with Tourette syndrome suggest that obsessive compulsive disorder may occur in 51–63% of patients (114, 115). Comings (116) proposed that children with Tourette syndrome are 5–20 times more likely to have other associated behavioral disorders, such as conduct disorder, stuttering, dyslexia, panic attacks, phobias, depression, mania, or test anxiety, but this has not been substantiated by others (108). Learning disabilities may be present in at least 35% of children who have Tourette syndrome (117).

A. Pathogenesis

Several theories have been advanced to explain the symptoms of tic disorders. The most popular theory is dopaminergic overactivity (112). Decreased serotonin and serotonin metabolites (5-hydroxyindoleautic acid) have been found in the cerebrospinal fluid of patients with Tourette syndrome (112). Drug therapy with dopamine receptor agonists has formed the cornerstone of therapy in tic disorders (103). Devinsky (118) has provided anatomical corroboration for these observations. He compared the clinical symptoms of encephalitis lethargica to those of Tourette Syndrome. He noted that dopaminergic suprasensitivity (and the emergence of tics) occurred in patients with dopaminergic hyopactivity who were treated with dopamine agonists. He proposed that midbrain (specifically, periaqueductal gray and tegmentum) dysfunction occurred in disorders such as Tourette syndrome, because the midbrain is the site of most central dopaminergic production.

Other neurotransmitters may modulate dopaminergic pathways in tic disorders. Haber and co-workers (119) suggested that the endorphin pathways may also be altered in Tourette syndrome. They found nearly no dynorphin in the globus pallidus, but normal enkephalins and other endogenous opiates in the brain of a patient with Tourette syndrome studied at postmortem.

B. Etiology

The cause of most tic disorders is unknown, though a familial predisposition has been suggested (120,121). Some subtypes of Tourette syndrome are inherited (autosomal dominant gene with sex-specific and incomplete penetrance) (122,123). The locus of the gene has not been characterized further.

C. Treatment

Simple motor tic and chronic multiple tic disorders usually do not require pharmacological therapy. Children with Tourette syndrome may not need to be treated with medication unless their tics are socially or physically disabling. Guidelines for pharmacological treatment of Tourette syndrome are summarized in Table 3 (92,108). Dopamine antagonists (haloperidol, pimozide, fluphenazine) were the first drugs to be used in Tourette syndrome. The initial dose of haloperidol is 0.5 mg given at night. Increases of 0.5 mg every week should be made, and the total dose divided 2–3 times per day, either until the tics have decreased or a maximum of 5–6 mg/day is reached. Most individuals respond to doses in the 2–2.5 mg/day range (107). Side effects include lethargy, blunting of performance, depression, school phobia, increased appetite, anticholinergic effects (blurred vision, dry mouth, constipation), extrapyramidal reactions, photosensitivity, and side effects relating to prolactin elevation (gynecomastia, galactorrhea, menstrual irregularity). Tardive dyskinesia is rare and may dissipate when haloperidol is discontinued (124). Chest pain or choreiform movements can occur when the drug is withdrawn suddenly (withdrawal emergent syndrome).

Pimozide is currently recommended for use in children older than age 12 years. The initial dose of pimozide is 1 mg at bedtime, with increases of 1 mg every week until tics decrease. The maximal dose is 10 mg for children and 20 mg for adolescents. Side effects are similar to those of haloperidol, with equivalence of 2.5 mg of pimozide to 1 mg of haloperidol (125). Although Q-T intervals have been reported to be prolonged with high-dose pimozide therapy, this has not been the experience in younger children (125).

Some (126,127) claim that fluphenazine, a dopamine antagonist that blocks D-2 receptors selectively, decreases tics without the side effects of other dopamine antagonists. The initial dose of fluphenazine is 1 mg/day, with increments of 1 mg every 1–2 weeks and a target dose of 5 mg/day. Side effects are similar to those reported for other dopamine antagonists (127).

Other drugs have a less clear role in the management of Tourette syndrome. Clonidine, an alpha-adrenergic antagonist, may modulate the

TABLE 3 Drugs Commonly Used in Treatment of Tourette Syndrome

Drug	Sizes	Kinetics: Peak	Kinetics: $t\frac{1}{2}$	Initial dosage	Incremental dosage	Therapeutic range
Haloperidol	1 mg 2 mg 5 mg 10 mg	—	11–24 hr	0.5 mg q HS	↑ 0.5 mg/week (÷ b.i.d.)	2–2.5 mg/day ≤ 5–6 mg/day max
Pimozide	2 mg	4–12 hr	55 hr	1 mg q HS	↑ 1 mg/week (÷ b.i.d.)	0.2 mg/kg/day ≤ 10 mg—child ≤ 20 mg—adolescent max
Fluphenazine	1 mg 2.5 mg 5 mg 10 mg	—	20 hr	1 mg q HS	↑ 1 mg/2 weeks (÷ b.i.d. or t.i.d.)	5 mg/day
Clonidine	0.1 mg 0.2 mg 0.3 mg	3–5 hr	6–10 hr	0.05 mg/day	↑ 0.05 mg/q.o.d. (÷ b.i.d.)	0.15 mg/day < 4–5 mg/kg/day max

serotonin and dopamine pathways in the brainstem (128). The initial dose of clonidine is 0.05 mg/day, which should be increased weekly to a total dose of 0.15 mg/day (107). Side effects include lethargy, sleepiness, and rebound hypertension if the medication is stopped abruptly. Rebound hypertension occurs rarely in children if clonidine is withdrawn over 1 week (129). After a controlled trial, Goetz and co-workers (130) concluded that clonidine may be ineffective in treatment of Tourette syndrome. Calcium channel blockers have also been tried in a few patients (131).

Double-blind studies are needed to answer many questions about drug therapy in tic disorders. It is not known whether one particular dopamine antagonist is superior to another in controlling tics. Leckman and co-workers (132) have developed and validated a questionnaire to rate the number and severity of tics. No controlled study has been carried out to determine whether the extrapyramidal side effects of dopamine antagonists are as severe in children as in adults (124), and whether they are less likely to occur with one drug versus another (127).

Because it is clear that stimulant therapy can precipitate tic disorders (reviewed in Ref. 108), treatment of ADD that occurs with Tourette syndrome remains controversial. Hunt and co-workers (133) suggested that treatment of the underlying Tourette syndrome will ameliorate the associated ADD, because of their findings of improvement in Conners' behavior rating scores in 7/10 children with the syndrome treated with clonidine for 3–5 months. These findings have not been replicated in larger groups. Based on their own experience and review of the literature, Sverd and colleagues (113) suggested that children with ADD and Tourette syndrome can be treated safely with methylphenidate.

The treatment of obsessive compulsive disorder in patients with Tourette syndrome also varies. Fluoxetine (20–60 mg/day) (134), neuroleptics, monoamine oxidase inhibitors, clonidine, and tricyclic antidepressants (103) have all been used to treat patients with obsessive compulsive disorder complicating Tourette syndrome.

Response of tics and associated symptoms to less traditional therapy such as self-hypnosis (135) is even less clear.

V. CONCLUSIONS

The pathophysiology of behavioral disorders in school-aged children is incompletely understood, and current therapies are inadequate. Tic disorders are the best understood of the three behavioral disorders reviewed in this chapter. Classification of these disorders is still imperfect but has been helped by understanding of the pathophysiology of related disorders. Research on tic disorders has been subjected to rigorous observation and validation. In contrast, lack of agreement for identification of subgroups and little characterization of the natural history of dyslexia have limited pharmacological and behavioral trials in this area. Little progress beyond stimulant drug therapy in research on ADD has been made for similar reasons. As for all behavioral disorders of childhood, recognition of the heterogeneous nature of these disorders is the first step in testing of any theory on which drug or behavior therapy may be based.

REFERENCES

1. Diagnostic and statistical manual of mental disorders, 3rd ed rev. Washington, DC: American Psychiatric Association, 1987.
2. Boder E. Developmental dyslexia: a new diagnostic approach based on the identification of three subtypes. J School Health 1970; 40:289–90.
3. Mattis S, French JH, Rapin I. Dyslexia in children and young adults: three independent neuropsychological syndromes. Dev Med Child Neurol 1975; 17:150–63.
4. Satz P, Morris R. Learning disability subtypes: a review. In: Pirozzolo FJ, Wittrock MC, eds. Neuropsychological and cognitive processes in reading. New York: Academic Press, 1981:109–41.
5. Morris R, Blashfield R, Satz P. Developmental classification of reading-disabled children. J Clin Exp Neuropsychol 1986; 8:371–92.
6. Mattis S. Dyslexia syndromes: a working hypothesis that works. In: Benton Al, Pearl D, eds. Dyslexia: an appraisal of current knowledge. New York: Academic Press, 1978:45–58.
7. Klein SK, Rapin I. Clinical assessment of pediatric disorders of higher cerebral function. Curr Prob Pediatr 1990; 20:45–51.
8. Kussmaul A. Disturbance of speech. Cyclopedia Pract Med 1877; 14:581–875.
9. Morgan WP. A case of congenital word blindness. Br Med J 1896; 2:1378.
10. Hinshelwood J. Congenital word blindness. Lancet 1900; 1:1506–8.
11. Orton ST. “Word blindness” in school children. Arch Neurol Psychiatry 1925; 14:581–615.
12. Orton ST. Specific reading disability—strephosymbolia. JAMA 1928; 90: 1095–9.
13. Levine DN, Hier DB, Calvanio R. Acquired learning disability for reading after left temporal lobe damage in childhood. Neurology 1981; 31:257–64.
14. Hynd G, Cohen M. Dyslexia: neuropsychological theory, research, and clinical differentiation. New York: Grune & Stratton, 1983.
15. Caviness VS Jr, Misson J, Gadisseux J. Abnormal neuronal patterns and disorders of neocortical development. In: Galaburda AM, ed. From reading to neurons. Cambridge, MA: MIT Press, 1989:405–39.
16. Witelson SF. Neurobiological aspects of language in children. Child Dev 1987; 58:653–88.
17. Marshall JC. The description and interpretation of acquired and developmen-

tal reading disorders. In: Galaburda AM, ed. From reading to neurons. Cambridge, MA: MIT Press, 1989:69–86.
18. Marshall JC. Routes and representations in the processing of written language. In: Keller E, Gopnik M, eds. Motor and sensory processes in language. Hillsdale, NJ: Erlbaum, 1987.
19. Marshall JC. On some relationships between acquired and developmental dyslexias. In: Duffy FH, Geschwind N, eds. Dyslexia: a neuroscientific approach to clinical evaluation. Boston: Little, Brown, 1985:55–66.
20. Satz P, Fletcher J, Clark W, Morris R. Lag, deficit, rate and delay constructs in specific learning disabilities: a reexamination. In: Ansara A, Geschwind N, Galaburda A, Albert M, Gartrell N, eds. Sex differences in dyslexia. Orton Dyslexia Soc 1981:129–50.
21. Galaburda AM, Sherman GF, Rosen GD, Aboitiz F, Geschwind N. Developmental dyslexia: four consecutive patients with cortical anomalies. Ann Neurol 1985; 18:222–33.
22. Galaburda AM, Rosen GD, Sherman GF. The neural origin of developmental dyslexia: implications for medicine, neurology, and cognition. In: Galaburda AM, ed. From reading to neurons. Cambridge, MA: MIT Press, 1989:377–88.
23. Humphreys P, Kaufman WE, Galaburda AM. Developmental dyslexia in women: neuropathological findings in three patients. Ann Neurol 1990; 28:727–38.
24. Larsen JP, Hoien T, Lundberg I, Odegaard H. MRI evaluation of the size and symmetry of the planum temporale in adolescents with developmental dyslexia. Brain Lang 1990; 39:289–301.
25. Geschwind N, Levitsky W. Human brain: left-right asymmetries in temporal speech region. Science 1968; 161:186–7.
26. Witelson SF, Pallie W. Left hemisphere specialization for language in the newborn: neuroanatomical evidence of asymmetry. Brain 1973; 96:641–6.
27. Galaburda AM. The pathogenesis of childhood dyslexia. In: Plum F, ed. Language, communication, and the brain. New York: Raven Press, 1988:127–37.
28. Goldman-Rakic PS, Galkin TW. Prenatal removal of frontal association cortex in the fetal rhesus monkey: anatomical and functional consequences in postnatal life. Brain Res 1978; 152:451–85.
29. Veith G, Schwindt W. Pathologisch-anatomischer Beitrag zum Problem "Nichtsesshaftigkeit." Fortschr Neurol Psychiatr 1976; 44:1–21.
30. Morel F, Wildi E. Dysgenesie nodulaire disseminee de l'encorce frontal. Rev Neurol 1952; 87:251–70.
31. Kaufmann WE, Galaburda AM. Cerebrocortical microdysgenesis in neurologically normal subjects: a histopathologic study. Neurology 1989; 39:238–44.
32. Martin J, Norman RM. Maple syrup urine disease in an infant with microgyria. Dev Med Child Neurol 1967; 9:152–9.
33. Christensen E, Melchior J. Cerebral palsy—a clinical and neuropathological study. London: William Heinemann, 1967.
34. Hicks SP. Developmental malformations produced by radiation: a timetable of development. Am J Roentgenol 1953; 2:272–93.

35. Slotnik V, Brent RL. The production of congenital malformations using tissue antisera. J Immunol 1966; 96:606–10.
36. Dvorak K, Feit J. Migration of neuroblasts through partial necrosis of the cerebral cortex in newborn rats: contribution to the problem of morphological development and developmental period of cerebral microgyria. Acta Neuropathol (Berl) 1977; 38:203–12.
37. Dvorak K, Feit J, Jurankova Z. Experimentally induced focal microgyria and status verrucosus deformis in rat—pathogenesis and interrelation: histological and autoradiographical study. Acta Neurol (Berl) 1978; 44:121–9.
38. Sato H, Sato N, Tamaki N, Matsumoto S. Experimentally induced cranial meningocele and cerebral microgyria. Brain Dev 1982; 4:73–5.
39. Geschwind N, Behan P. Left-handedness: association with immune disease, migraine, and developmental learning disorder. Proc Natl Acad Sci USA 1982; 79:5097–100.
40. Hugdahl K, Synnevag B, Satz P. Immune and autoimmune diseases in dyslexic children. Neuropsychologia 1990; 28:673–9.
41. Lahita RG. Systemic lupus erythematosis: learning disability in the male offspring of female patients and relationship to laterality. Psychoneuroendocrinology 1988; 13:385–96.
42. Sherman GF, Galaburda AM, Geschwind N. Cortical anomalies in brains of New Zealand mice: a neuropathologic model of dyslexia? Proc Natl Acad Sci USA 1985; 82:8072–4.
43. Spencer DG, Humphries K, Mathis D, Lal H. Behavioral impairments related to cognitive dysfunction in the autoimmune New Zealand Black mouse. Behav Neurosci 1986; 100:353–8.
44. Fisher JH. Case of congenital word blindness (inability to read). Ophthal Rev 1905; 24:315.
45. Sladen BK. Inheritance of dyslexia. Bull Orton Soc 1970; 20:30–40.
46. Shaywitz S, Shaywitz BA, Fletcher JM, Escobar MD. Prevalence of reading disability in boys and girls. JAMA 1990; 264:998–1002.
47. Finucci JM, Childs B. Are there really more dyslexic boys than girls? In: Ansara A, Geschwind A, Galaburda AM, Gartrell N, eds. Sex differences in dyslexia. Towson, MD: Orton Dyslexia Society, 1981:1–9.
48. Hallgren B. Specific dyslexia: a clinical and genetic study. Acta Psychiatr Neurol Scand 1950; 65(Suppl):1–287.
49. Vogler GP, DeFries JC, Decker SN. Family history as an indicator of risk for reading disability. J Learn Dis 1985; 419–21.
50. Smith SD, Pennington BF, Lubs HA. Specific reading disability: identification of an inherited form through linkage analysis. Science 1983; 219:1345–7.
51. Pennington BF. Annotation: the genetics of dyslexia. J Child Psychol Psychiatry 1990; 31:193–201.
52. Olson R, Wise B, Conners F, Rack J. Specific deficits in component reading and language skills: genetic and environmental influences. J Learn Dis 1989; 22:339–48.
53. Lerner JW. Educational interventions in learning disabilities. J Am Acad Child Adol Psychiatry 1989; 28:326–31.

54. Beauchamp G. Visual correlates of dyslexia and related learning disabilities. Pediatr Ann 1990; 19:334–41.
55. Amon MG, Werry JS. Methylphenidate and diazepam in severe reading retardation. J Acad Child Psychiatry 1982; 21:31–7.
56. Gittleman R, Klein DF, Feingold I. Children with reading disorders. II. Effects of methylphenidate in combination with reading instruction. J Child Psychol Psychiatry 1983; 24:193–212.
57. Dimond S, Brouwers EYM. Improvement of human memory through the use of drugs. Psychopharmacology (Berl) 1976; 49:307–9.
58. Gamzu ER, Hoover TM, Gracon SI, Nintenan MV. Recent developments in 2-pyrrolidinone-containing nootropics. Drug Dev Res 1989; 18:177–89.
59. Wilsher CR, Atkins G, Mansfield P. Piracetam as an aid to learning in dyslexia: preliminary report. Psychopharmacology (Berl) 1979; 65:107–9.
60. Simeon J, Waters B, Resnick M. Effects of piracetam in children with learning disorders. Psychopharmacol Bull 1980; 16:65–6.
61. Rudel RG, Helfgott E. Effect of piracetam on verbal memory of dyslexic boys. J Am Acad Child Psychiatry 1985:685–9.
62. Wilsher CR, Milewski J. Effects of piracetam on dyslexic's verbal conceptualizing ability. Psychopharmacol Bull 1983; 19:3–4.
63. Helfgott E, Rudel R, Krieger J. Effect of piracetam on the single word and prose reading of dyslexic children. Psychopharmacol Bull 1984; 20:688–90.
64. Chase CH, Schmitt RL, Russell G, Tallal P. A new chemotherapeutic investigation: piracetam effects on dyslexia. Ann Dyslexia 1984; 34:29–48.
65. Conners CK, Blouin AG, Wingles M, Lougee L, O'Donnel D, Smith A. Piracetam and event-related potentials in dyslexic children. Psychopharmacol Bull 1984; 20:667–73.
66. Di Ianni M, Wilsher CR, Blank MS, Conners CK, Chase CH, Funkenstein HH, Helfgott E, Homes JM, Lougee L, Maletta GJ, Milewski J, Pirozzolo FJ, Rudel RG, Tallal P. The effects of piracetam in children with dyslexia. J Clin Psychopharmacol 1985; 5:272–78.
67. Wilsher CR. Effects of piracetam on developmental dyslexia. Int J Psychophysiol 1986; 4:29–39.
68. Conners CK, Reader M, Caldwell L, Clymer R, Reiss A, Adesman A, Caldwell J, Mayer L, Berg M. The effects of piracetam upon visual event related potentials in dyslexic children. Psychophysiology 1987; 24:513–21.
69. Wilsher CR, Bennett D, Chase CH, Conners K, DiIanni M, Feagans L, Hanvik L, Helfgott E, Koplewicz H, Overby P, Reader M, Rudel R, Tallal P. Piracetam and dyslexia: effects on reading tests. J Clin Psychopharmacol 1987; 7:230–7.
70. Shaywitz SE, Shaywitz BA. Attention deficit disorder: current perspectives, In: Kavanagh JF, Truss TJ Jr, eds. Learning disabilities: proceedings of the national conference. Parkton, MD: York Press, 1988:369–498.
71. Conners CK. A teacher rating scale for use in drug studies with children. Am J Psychiatry 1969; 126:864–88.
72. Conners CK. Symptom-patterns in hyperkinetic, neurotic and normal children. Child Dev 1970; 41:667–82.

73. Urion DK. Response to desipramine in attention deficit hyperactivity disorder is predicted by neurological subtype. Ann Neurol 1988; 26:481.
74. Mesulam MM. Attention, confusional states and neglect. In: Mesulam MM, ed. Principles of behavioral neurology. Philadelphia: FA Davis, 1985: 125–68.
75. Rapin I. Children with brain dysfunction. New York: Raven Press, 1982: 95–104.
76. Roland PE. Cortical regulation of selective attention in man: a regional cerebral blood flow study. J Neurophysiol 1982; 48:1059–78.
77. Zametkin AJ, Nordahl TE, Gross M, King AC, Semple WE, Rumsey J, Hamburger S, Cohen RM. Cerebral glucose metabolism in adults with hyperactivity of childhood onset. N Engl J Med 1990; 323:1361–6.
78. Loiselle DL, Stamm JS, Maitinsky S, White SC. Evoked potential and behavioral signs of attentive dysfunctions in hyperactive boys. Psychophysiology 1980; 17:193–201.
79. Peloquin LJ, Klorman R. Effects of methylphenidate on normal children's mood, event-related potentials and peformance in memory scanning and vigilance. J Abnorm Psychol 1986; 95:88–98.
80. Harter MR, Diering S, Wood FB. I. Separate brain potential characteristics in children with reading disability and attention deficit disorder: relevance-independent effects. Brain Cognition 1988; 7:54–86.
81. Harter MR, Anllo-Vento L, Wood FB, Schroeder MM. II. Separate brain potential characteristics in children with reading disability and attention deficit disorder: color and letter-relevance effects. Brain Cognition 1988; 7: 115–40.
82. Lou HC, Henriksen L, Bruhn P. Focal cerebral perfusion in children with dysphasia and/or attention deficit disorder. Arch Neurol 1984; 41:825–9.
83. Lou HC, Henriksen L, Borner H, Nielsen JB. Striatal dysfunction in attention deficit and hyperkinetic disorder. Arch Neurol 1989; 46:48–52.
84. Kuczenski R. Biochemical actions of amphetamines and other stimulants. In: Creese I, ed. Stimulants: neurochemical, behavior, and clinical. New York: Raven Press, 1983:31–63.
85. Abikoff H, Gittelman R. The normalizing effects of methyphenidate on the classroom behavior of ADD vs ADDH children. J Abnorm Child Psychol 1985; 13:33–44.
86. Brown RT, Borden KA, Wynne ME, Schleser R, Clingermann SR. Methylphenidate and cognitive therapy with ADD children: a methodological reconsideration. J Abnorm Child Psychol 1986; 14:481–97.
87. Cohen NJ, Sullivan J, Minde K, Novak C, Helwiog C. Evaluations of the relative effectiveness of methylphenidate and cognitive behavior modification in the treatment of kindergarten-aged hyperactive children. J Abnorm Child Psychol 1981; 9:43–54.
88. Hindshaw SP, Henker B, Whalen CK. Cognitive-behavioral and pharmacological interventions for hyperactive boys: comparative and combined effects. J Consult Clin Psychol 1984; 52:739–49.

89. Hindshaw SP, Henker B, Whalen CK. Self-control in hyperactive boys in anger-inducing situations: effect of cognitive-behavioral training and methylphenidate. J Abnorm Psychol 1984; 12:55–77.
90. Satterfield J, Hoppe CM, Schell AM. A prospective study of delinquency in 110 adolescent boys with attention deficit disorder and 88 normal adolescent boys. Am J Psychiatry 1982; 139:797–8.
91. Ultmann MH, Rapin I. Hyperactivity in children. In: RT Johnson, ed. Current therapy in neurologic disease—2. Toronto: BC Decker, 1987:250.
92. Gilman AG, Goodman LS, Rall TW, Murad F, eds. Goodman and Gilman's the pharmacological basis of therapeutics, 7th ed. New York: Macmillan, 1985.
93. Pelham WE, Greenslade KE, Vodde-Hamilton M, Murphy DA, Greenstein JJ, Gnagy EM, Guthrie KJ, Hoover MD, Dahl RD. Relative efficacy of long-acting stimulants on children with attention deficit hyperactivity disorder: a comparison of standard methylphenidate, sustained release methylphenidate, sustained-release dextroamphetamine and pemoline. Pediatrics 1990; 86:226–37.
94. Cohen DJ, Young JG, Nathanson JA, Shaywitz BA. Clonidine in Tourette's syndrome. Lancet 1979; 2:551–3.
95. Treffert DA, Joranson D. Restricting amphetamines. JAMA 1981; 245: 1336–8.
96. Pelham WE, Sturges J, Hoza J, et al. Sustained release and standard methylphenidate effects on cognition and social behavior in children with attention deficit disorder. Pediatrics 1987; 80:491–501.
97. Jacobvitz D, Sroufe LA, Stewart M, Leffert N. Treatment of attentional and hyperactivity problems in children with sympathomimetic drugs: a comprehensive review. J Am Acad Child Psychiatry 1990; 29:677–88.
98. Klein DF, Gittleman R, Quitkin A, Rifkin A. Side effects of antipsychotic drugs and their treatment. In: Klein DF, Gittleman R, Quitkin A, Rifkin A, eds. Diagnosis and treatment of psychiatric disorder: adults and children, 2nd ed. Baltimore: Williams & Wilkins, 1980:174–214.
99. Safer DJ, Allen RP, Barr E. Depression of growth in hyperactive children on stimulant drugs. N Engl J Med 1972; 287:217–20.
100. Safer DJ, Allen RP. Factors influencing the suppressant effects of two stimulant drugs on the growth of hyperactive children. Pediatrics 1973; 51:660–7.
101. Greenhill L, Puig-Antich J, Chambers W, Rubinstein B, Hapern F, Sachar EJ. Growth hormone, prolactin and growth responses in hyperkinetic males treated with D-amphetamine. J Am Acad Child Psychiatry 1981; 20:84–103.
102. Gittelman-Klein, Mannuzza S. Hyperactive boys almost grown up. III. Methyphenidate effects on ultimate height Arch Gen Psychiatry 1988; 45:1131–4.
103. Kurlan R. Tourette's syndrome: current concepts. Neurology 1989; 39: 1625–30.
104. Shapiro AK, Shapiro ES, Young JG, Feinberg TW, eds. Gilles de la Tourette syndrome, 2nd ed. New York: Raven Press, 1988:356–60.

105. Golden GS. Tic and Tourette's syndrome: a continuum of symptoms? Ann Neurol 1978; 4:731–4.
106. Corbett JA, Matthews AM, Connell PH, et al. Tics and Gilles de la Tourette syndrome. A follow-up study and critical review. Br J Psychiatry 1969; 115:1229–41.
107. Golden GS. Tics in childhood. Pediatr Ann 1983; 12:821–4.
108. Golden GS. Tourette syndrome: recent advances. Neurol Clin 1990; 8:705–14.
109. Golden GS. The effect of central nervous system stimulants on Tourette syndrome. Ann Neurol 1977; 2:69–70.
110. Golden GS. The relationship between stimulant medication and tics. Pediatr Ann 1988; 17:405–7.
111. Golden GS. The effect of central nervous system stimulants on Tourette syndrome. Ann Neurol 1977; 2:69–70.
112. Singer HS, Butler IJ, Tune LE, Seifert WE, Coyle JT. Dopaminergic dysfunction in Tourette syndrome. Ann Neurol 1982; 12:361–6.
113. Sverd J, Gadow KD, Paolicelli LM. Methylphenidate treatment of attention-deficit hyperactivity disorder in boys with Tourette syndrome. J Am Acad Child Adol Psychiatry 1989; 28:574–9.
114. Frankel M, Cummings JL, Robertson MM, Trimble MR, Hill MA, Benson DF. Obsessions and compulsions in Gilles de la Tourette's syndrome. Neurology 1986; 36:378–82.
115. Pittman RK, Green RC, Jenike MA, Mesulam MM. Clinical comparison of Tourette's disorder and obsessive compulsive disorder. Am J Psychiatry 1987; 144:1166–71.
116. Comings DE. A controlled study of Tourette syndrome. VII. Summary: a common genetic disorder causing disinhibition of the limbic system. Am J Hum Genet 1987; 41:839–66.
117. Erenberg C, Cruse RP, Rothner AD. Tourette syndrome: an analysis of 200 pediatric and adolescent cases. Cleve Clin Q 1986; 53:127–31.
118. Devinsky O. Neuroanatomy of Gilles de la Tourette's syndrome: possible midbrain involvement. Arch Neurol 1983; 40:508–14.
119. Haber SN, Kowell NW, Vonsattel JP, Bird ED, Richardson EP. Gilles de la Tourette's syndrome; a postmortem neuropathological and immunohistochemical study. J Neurol Sci 1986; 75:225–41.
120. Kurlan R. The spectrum of Tourette's syndrome. Curr Opin Neurol Neurosurg 1988; 1:294–8.
121. Pauls DL, Patkostis AJ, Kurlan R, et al. Segregation and linkage analysis of Tourette's syndrome and related disorders. J Am Acad Child Adol Psychiatry 1990; 29:195–203.
122. Pauls DL, Leckman JF. The inheritance of Gilles de la Tourette's syndrome and asociated behaviors: evidence for autosomal dominant transmission. N Engl J Med 1986; 315:993–7.
123. Kurlan R, Behr J, Medved L, Shoulson I, Pauls D, Kidd JR, Kidd KK. Familial Tourette's syndrome: report of a large pedigree and potential for linkage analysis. Neurology 1986; 36:772–6.

124. Polizos P, Englehardt DM. Dyskinetic phenomena in children treated with psychotropic medications. Psychopharmacol Bull 1978; 14:65–8.
125. Erenberg G, Cruse RP, Rothner AD. The use of pimozide in young children with Tourette's syndrome. Ann Neurol 1987; 22:435.
126. Goetz CG, Tanner CM, Klawans HL. Fluphenazine and multifocal tic disorders. Arch Neurol 1984; 31:271–2.
127. Singer HS, Gammon K, Quaskey S. Haloperidol, fluphenazine, and clonidine in Tourette syndrome: controversies in treatment. Pediatr Neurosci 1985–6; 12:71–4.
128. Svensson TH, Bunney BS, Aghajanian GK. Inihibition of both noradrenergic and serotonergic neurons in the brain by the alpha adrenergic agnonist clonidine. Brain Res 1975; 92:291–306.
129. Leckman JF, Detlor J, Harcherik DF, et al. Acute and chronic clonidine treatment in Tourette's syndrome: a preliminary report on clinical response and effect on plama and urinary catecholamine metabolites, growth hormone and blood pressure. J Am Acad Child Psychiatry 1983; 22:433–40.
130. Goetz CG, Tanner CM, Wilson RS, et al. Clonidine and Gilles de la Tourette's syndrome: double-blind study using objective rating methods. Ann Neurol 1987; 21:307–10.
131. Micheli F, Gatto M, Lekhuniec E, Mangone C, Pardal MF, Pikielny R, Parera IC. Treatment of Tourette's syndrome with calcium antagonists. Clin Neuropharmacol 1990; 13:77–83.
132. Leckman JF, Riddle MA, Hardin MT, Ort SI, Swartz KL, Stevenson J, Cohen DJ. The Yale Global Tic Severity Scale: initial testing of a clinician-rated scale of tic severity. J Am Acad Child Adol Psychiatry 1989; 28:566–73.
133. Hunt RD, Minderaa RB, Cohen DJ. Clonidine benefits children with attention deficit disorder and hyperactivity: report of a double-blind placebo-crossover therapeutic trial. J Am Acad Child Psychiatry 1985; 24:617–29.
134. Riddle MA, Hardin MT, King R, Scahill L, Wollston JL. Fluoxetine treatment of children and adolescents with Tourette's and obsessive compulsive disorders: preliminary clinical experience. J Am Acad Child Adol Psychiatry 1990; 29:45–8.
135. Kohen DP, Olness KN, Colwell SO, Heimel A. The use of relaxation/mental imagery (self-hypnosis) in the management of 505 pediatric behavioral encounters. J Dev Behav Pediatr 1984; 5:21–5.

II

COGNITIVE DISORDERS OF MIDDLE YEARS

3

Cognitive Function After Closed Head Injury: Sequelae and Outcome

Felicia C. Goldstein *Emory University School of Medicine, Atlanta, Georgia*

Harvey S. Levin *University of Texas Medical Branch, Galveston, Texas*

The cognitive consequences of closed head injury (CHI) consist of alterations in general intellectual functioning, memory, reasoning/problem solving, language, and attention. Despite advances in delineating these sequelae, precise prediction of recovery has remained elusive. Apart from injury characteristics such as the depth and duration of impaired consciousness, features including demographic background, the family and social support system, and access to rehabilitation play a crucial role in outcome (1,2). Cognitive recovery, as inferred from neuropsychological tests, assumes importance as it impinges on the patient's ability to perform activities of daily living or to resume gainful employment (1,3–6). The challenges facing clinicians who evaluate and treat survivors are thus considerable. Not only is the onus on identifying cognitive deficits, but also in obtaining a sense of their eventual recovery and relation to the level of independent functioning.

The purpose of this chapter is to delineate the cognitive sequelae of adult CHI. First, we will provide an overview of the acute injury and extra injury indices that are related to the initial presentation and prolongation of symptoms. Next, the specific cognitive changes will be discussed. Finally, we will address current approaches to the remediation of cognitive deficits that appear to have potential for improving outcome.

I. OVERVIEW OF VARIABLES RELATED TO COGNITIVE OUTCOME

A number of variables contribute to cognitive performance and recovery. These include the severity and complications of the acute injury as well as demographic and premorbid features of the patient.

A. Neurologic Indices

The Glasgow Coma Scale (GCS) of Teasdale and Jennett (7) is widely used to define the depth and duration of impaired consciousness. As depicted in Table 1, the GCS provides a numerical rating of the patient's best eye, motor, and verbal responses. The total score ranges from 3 (no eye opening, no motor response to stimulation, no verbal response) to 15 (spontaneous eye opening, obeying commands, oriented). The duration of coma, determined through serial assessment, consists of the interval in which there is no eye opening, inability to obey commands, and the absence of comprehensible speech. In general, a GCS score ≤ 8 characterizes a severe head injury, 9–12 a moderate head injury, and 13–15 a mild injury (8–10).

Research has indicated relationships between low GCS scores and poor cognitive outcome (10–14). Alexander et al. conducted a comprehensive follow-up study of patients who were admitted to an acute neurosurgical unit (11). One hundred patients who were eventually testable were administered intellectual and memory measures. These investigators found that the highest GCS score within 24 h of admission was predictive of outcome 2 years postinjury. Of the patients with no or minimal cognitive deficits, 80% had GCS scores ranging from 8 to 15, whereas 70% of those exhibiting severe deficits had scores of 3 or 4. The performance of patients with scores between 5 and 7 was difficult to predict, but an association was noted between the time spent in this range and the likelihood of a poor cognitive response. Other investigators have also found that longer durations of impaired consciousness are related to a bleaker prognosis (12,13). Levin and colleagues (12) observed that patients 5–15 months postinjury with impairments in general intellectual functioning and verbal/visual memory had more extended periods of impaired consciousness (median, 18 days; range, < 1–150 days) than those performing within normal limits (median, 1 day; range, 0–90 days).

The integrity of pupillary responses to light and eye movements in comatose patients predicts prolonged disability and neuropsychological impairment (11,12,15–17). Levin et al. (12) found that acute bilaterally nonreactive pupils were related to subsequent memory and intellectual deficits. Of 13 patients with generalized cognitive impairment, 8 initially exhibited pu-

TABLE 1 The Glasgow Coma Scale

Response	Rating	
Eye opening (E)		
None	1	Not attributable to ocular swelling
To pain	2	Pain stimulus is applied to chest or limbs
To speech	3	Nonspecific response to speech or shout, does not imply the patient obeys command to open eyes
Spontaneous	4	Eyes are open, but this does not imply intact awareness
Motor response (M)		
No response	1	Flaccid
Extension	2	"Decerebrate." Adduction, internal rotation of shoulder, and pronation of the forearm
Abnormal flexion	3	"Decorticate." Abnormal flexion, adduction of shoulder
Withdrawal	4	Normal flexor response, withdraws from pain stimulus with abduction of the shoulder
Localizes pain	5	Pain stimulus applied to supraocular region or fingertip causes limb to move in an attempt to remove it
Obeys commands	6	Follows simple commands
Verbal Response (V)		
No response	1	(Self-explanatory)
Incomprehensible	2	Moaning and groaning, but no recognizable words
Inappropriate	3	Intelligible speech (e.g., shouting or swearing), but no sustained or coherent conversation
Confused	4	Patient responds to questions in a conversational manner, but the responses indicate varying degrees of disorientation and confusion
Oriented	5	Normal orientation to time, place, and person
Summed Glasgow Coma Scale Score=E + M + V (3–15).		

Source: Adapted from Ref. 7.

pillary abnormalities versus only 3 of 18 patients with normal cognitive functioning. Eye movements by oculocephalic responses are tested by rotating the head in a side-to-side or up-and-down motion. Normally, both eyes deviate to the opposite side (e.g., the eyes turn to the left when the head is turned to the right). Eye movements may also be tested by injecting cold water into the ear canal. The normal oculovestibular response is for both eyes to move toward the side of the irrigated ear and then back to midline. Alexandre and colleagues (11) reported that oculovestibular responses within 24 h of injury were as predictive of cognitive outcome as the GCS score. Of 58 comatose patients with abnormal eye movements, all but 5 eventually displayed cognitive deficits. In contrast, 35 patients with intact eye movements exhibited mild or no cognitive impairments.

Focal hemispheric mass lesions similarly contribute to the neuropsychological profile. Studies have demonstrated specific cognitive impairments depending upon side of injury (e.g., verbal deficits following dominant left hemisphere lesions; visuospatial deficits following nondominant right hemisphere lesions) and area (e.g., memory deficits after temporal lobe lesions; impaired problem solving/divergent processing with frontal lobe lesions) (8,11,18,19). The ability to establish neuroanatomic–neuropsychological links is improving with advances in neuroimaging. Magnetic resonance imaging (MRI) is advantageous in detecting intracranial abnormalities that are undisclosed by computed tomography (CT), particularly for parenchymal lesions (8,20–24). Figure 1 indicates the superiority of MRI in detecting lesions after mild or moderate head injuries (8). In this sample of 20 patients, CT disclosed 12 lesions versus 56 lesions by MRI. Also displayed are the locations of the lesions that predominated in the temporal and frontal lobes, the most common sites of damage (25,26). Imaging of structural lesions by CT or MRI may not capture the extent of injury that can be appreciated by metabolic measurements such as positron emission tomography (PET) or cerebral blood flow (22,27,28). For

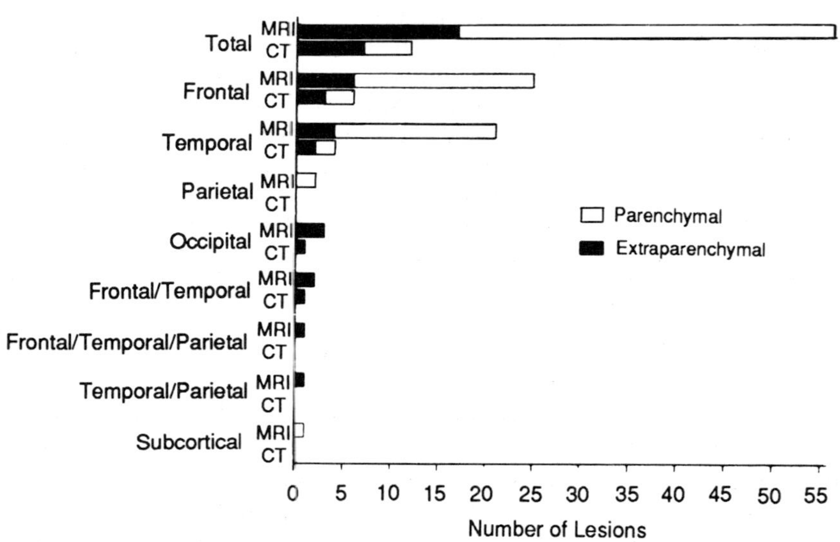

FIGURE 1 Intrahemispheric locus of lesion disclosed by computerized tomography (CT) versus magnetic resonance imaging (MRI) in 20 patients with minor or moderate head injury. (From Ref 8.)

example, Langfitt and colleagues (22) found that PET demonstrated reduced glucose metabolism in the anterior temporal lobes, whereas damage to this region was not noted by CT or MRI.

Deep white matter lesions are related to prolonged cognitive deficits (24,29). Wilson and colleagues (24) observed that patients with deep white matter lesions and ventricular enlargement 5–18 months postinjury had persisting impairments in conceptual reasoning, visuospatial and visuomotor skills, verbal fluency, and memory, when compared with those who had cortical or subcortical white matter lesions. The presence of an interhemispheric disconnection syndrome from lesions within the corpus collosum can similarly contribute to the neuropsychological profile. Levin and co-workers (29) reported that patients with deep white matter lesions displayed an exaggerated right ear advantage for speech under dichotic presentation, indicative of disruption of auditory callosal pathways. Features of impaired transmission between the cerebral hemispheres are typically not examined by clinicians, despite evidence that lesions in the corpus collosum are common after severe CHI (25,30,31).

Finally, the duration of posttraumatic amnesia (32) had been studied in relation to cognitive outcome. Posttraumatic amnesia (PTA) refers to a postinjury period of confusion and memory loss during which the patient is disoriented and unable to register day-to-day information. Relationships have been established between increasing duration of PTA and poor cognitive outcome (4,33–35), although there are discrepancies across studies in its prognostic usefulness (11,36). Inconsistencies may reflect the unreliability of retrospective reports (e.g., asking the patient to estimate when the period of confusion ended) and the variability in PTA duration that is present across the spectrum of head injury. Approximately 10–15% of patients with mild and moderate CHI display a prolonged PTA interval, despite minimal durations of impaired consciousness (37).

Several caveats should be considered in extrapolating from published findings to the clinical situation. First, it is oversimplistic to characterize severity on the basis of one variable because these measures exert a combined influence. Interactive effects are illustrated in a study that compared the neuropsychological performance of two CHI groups (GCS scores of 13–15, with or without a lesion demonstrated by CT) against a moderately injured group (GCS scores of 9–12) (38). Patients who sustained mild impairment of consciousness and had acute intracranial lesions detected by CT exhibited deficits in memory, information processing speed, and word fluency similar to the moderate group. Thus, a GCS score of 13–15 does not necessarily denote a "mild" injury unless other neurological variables are taken into account. In recognition of the interplay among these indices, regression models have been increasingly used to predict recovery.

A second consideration is the role of additional complications or postacute changes on outcome. Raised intracranial pressure, shock, and hypoxia have a detrimental influence on cognitive functioning (18,28) and may be overlooked during the review of records. Ventricular enlargement is related to persistent cognitive deficits, particularly in the area of memory (39,40). This feature, however, is often apparent only in the later stages of recovery (24). Thus, if a patient is seen many months after a head injury, the findings from early scanning may not correlate with performance.

B. Demographic Features and Premorbid Characteristics

In addition to neurological variables, demographic features and premorbid history contribute to recovery. Epidemiological research indicates that there is a rise in mortality from head injury with advancing age (41–43). Figure 2 shows the mortality rate reported by Luerssen and colleagues (44) in over 8500 patients admitted to hospitals in a 4-year period. In this study, mortality decreased until the age of 12 years, followed by a steady increase from 15 years and older.

The effects of age on cognitive outcome have not been investigated systematically enough for firm conclusions to be reached. Brooks (33) reported that paired associate learning was more impaired in patients older than 30 years, as opposed to those who were younger. Alexandre et al. (11)

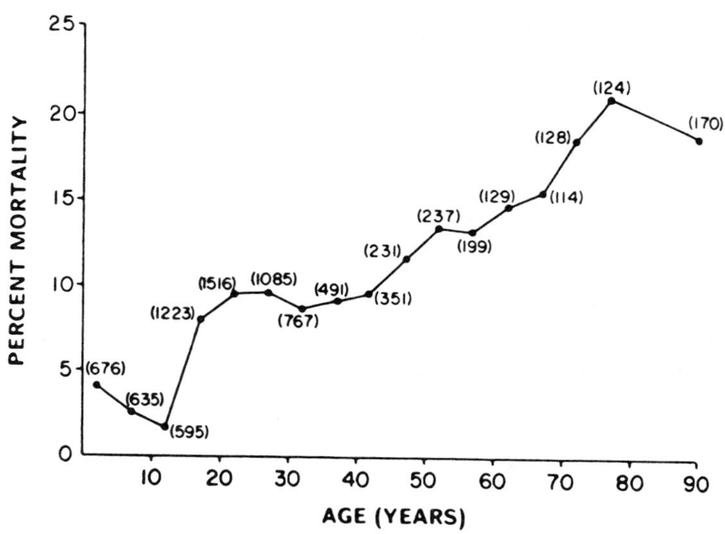

FIGURE 2 Percentage mortality for 8671 patients by 5-year age groups with denominators shown in parentheses. (From Ref. 44.)

also stated that patients older than 30 years had less favorable intellectual or memory outcomes. Other studies have reported that CHI patients 65 years and older have extended hospital stays and require assistance in terms of supportive living environments (45–47). Comparisons between younger versus older adults, however, are complicated by intervening variables in the latter group, including coexisting medical problems, unsupervised home environments (e.g., owing to death of a spouse), and lack of access to head injury programs based on cutoff admission criteria of 55 years. It has been consistently reported that individuals younger than 40 years have a greater likelihood of returning to work (46,48,49). This does not necessarily signify a better cognitive recovery, however, since these persons may be readily accepted by potential employers, motivated to resume work because they have many years left before retirement, and willing to choose alternative positions (50). Questions concerning differential diagnosis of the cognitive sequelae caused by head injury versus other disorders (e.g., Alzheimer's disease), recovery curves, and treatment efficacy in the elderly need to be addressed.

Estimation of premorbid cognitive functioning is important in the context of evaluating neuropsychological peformance and whether further improvement is anticipated. Haas and associates (51) noted a high rate of premorbid learning problems in survivors of severe CHI who were enrolled in rehabilitation. Patients were classified as having academic difficulties based on a diagnosis of learning disability, multiple failed subjects, or dropping out of school. Forty-two percent of the 64 patients exhibited scholastic failure that exceeded state norms. Haas et al. proposed that premorbid academic problems may foster head injuries as a result of features such as impulsivity and distractibility. Conversely, individuals with learning difficulties may adopt a life-style characterized by risk-taking behaviors.

Educational level is one way to gauge premorbid functioning, but interpretation is hindered because many young survivors have their education prematurely disrupted. Regression equations that take into account demographic variables such as age, education, and occupation have been devised to estimate intellectual functioning (52–54). However, these formulas are inaccurate at the lower and higher extremes of intelligence (55,56). Reading performance on the National Adult Reading Test (57) is a means for estimating premorbid functioning, since scores (at least in the United Kingdom) are correlated with Full Scale IQ and are least vulnerable to brain damage. Another strategy has entailed using parental education or occupation as an index of premorbid abilities.

Drug or alcohol use influences the cognitive presentation of patients (36,58). Carlsson et al. (36) found that a history of chronic alcohol abuse was associated with a high number of symptoms reported by survivors.

Brooks and colleagues (58) reported that alcohol consumption at the time of injury was a stronger prognostic indicator of impaired memory performance than a history of habitual drinking. It was proposed that drinking at the time of injury may have a "biologic toxic" effect, thereby potentiating the primary damage. As noted by the authors, their measure of alcohol ingestion was based on an interview with a relative months to years after the injury, rather than objective measures such as blood alcohol levels at admission.

It is necessary to inquire about previous head injuries, since there is evidence that cognitive effects are cumulative (36,59). Table 2 displays data from an investigation by Carlsson et al. (36) examining the influence of the number of accidents on cognitive outcome. Previous accidents resulting in unconsciousness were classified as ranging from none to two or more. As seen, Carlsson and co-workers observed a decrease in motor speed and reaction time as the number of accidents increased. Gronwall and Wrightson (59) found that patients with mild head injuries who also had a prior CHI performed more poorly on an information processing task and had a slower recovery time than a comparable severity group without previous head injuries.

These neurological indices and demographic–social features are only guidelines for generating hypotheses about the nature of cognitive deficits and their potential for recovery. There are numerous "outliers" seen in clinical practice who, despite predictions based on the severity of injury and premorbid characteristics, either perform far below or above expectations. Therefore, statements regarding eventual recovery need to be cautious. In the following sections, we review the salient cognitive sequelae of CHI.

TABLE 2 Relationship Between Test Results and Number of Accidents with Reported Unconsciousness (NARU)

	NARU			
Test	0	1	>2	p Value
Finger-tapping (beats/30 sec)	135.1	131.2	128.1	0.004
Reaction time, single choice (1/100 sec)	39.8	40.6	42.7	0.01
Reaction time, multiple choice (1/100 sec)	43.3	44.3	44.7	0.04
WAIS digit symbol subtest[a]	43.0	42.2	44.0	0.92[b]
Vibration sensitivity	15.6	16.3	17.7	0.60[b]

[a]WAIS, Wechsler Adult Intelligence Scale.
[b]Not statistically significant.
Source: Adapted from Ref. 36.

II. COGNITIVE FEATURES OF HEAD INJURY

A. General Intellectual Functioning

Intellectual recovery is frequently evaluated with the Wechsler Adult Intelligence Test (WAIS) (60,61). This instrument consists of measures assessing verbal abilities (e.g., general knowledge, digit repetition, comprehension of social rules, conceptual reasoning) and visuospatial–visuomotor skills (e.g., arrangement of blocks to form spatial patterns, puzzle completion, speeded transcription of numbers and symbols). Research has indicated a dissociation in the recovery of these two spheres (17,62,63). During the initial 6–12 months after moderate or severe CHI, scores on the Verbal Scale level off, whereas the Performance IQ continues to change. This pattern is hypothesized to reflect the vulnerability of head injury to domains such as visuospatial processing and motor speed as measured by the Performance subtests. In contrast, the Verbal subtests evaluate previously learned facts and material (e.g., comprehension of social conventions, vocabulary). Research has also indicated that the general rate of improvement in intellectual functioning slows after the first year (10,63–65). However, slowing does not imply lack of further recovery, and such statements are constantly modified as investigations extend the injury–test interval.

Relationships have been established between the severity of the acute injury and impaired intellectual functioning using traditional indices, including the degree and length of impaired consciousness (11,17,66), presence and neuroanatomic locus of focal hemispheric injury (10,19), and oculovestibular and pupillary abnormalities (11,17). Wilson and colleagues (24) reported that ventricular enlargement detected on MRI scans 5–18 months after injury was related to impairments on several subtests of the WAIS, including conceptual reasoning (similarities), word definition (vocabulary), visuomotor speed (digit symbol), and construction (block design, object assembly). The presence of acute elevated cerebral blood flow (hyperemia) predicts outcome as well. Uzzell et al. (28) characterized severely injured patients (GCS scores of 6 or less) as manifesting abnormal or normal CBF within 96 h postinjury. As shown in Figure 3, patients with hyperemia consistently performed below the level of the normal flow group, with significant differences involving recall of digits backward, transcription of numbers or symbols, and detection of details missing in pictures.

Although research has examined return to an "average" level of intellectual functioning, the extent to which IQ actually recovers can be appreciated only when compared with premorbid levels. Williams and colleagues (14) employed a formula to estimate premorbid IQ on the WAIS (53) to predict intellectual outcome 11–180 days following CHI. Through use of a regression model, the investigators found that postinjury Full Scale IQ was

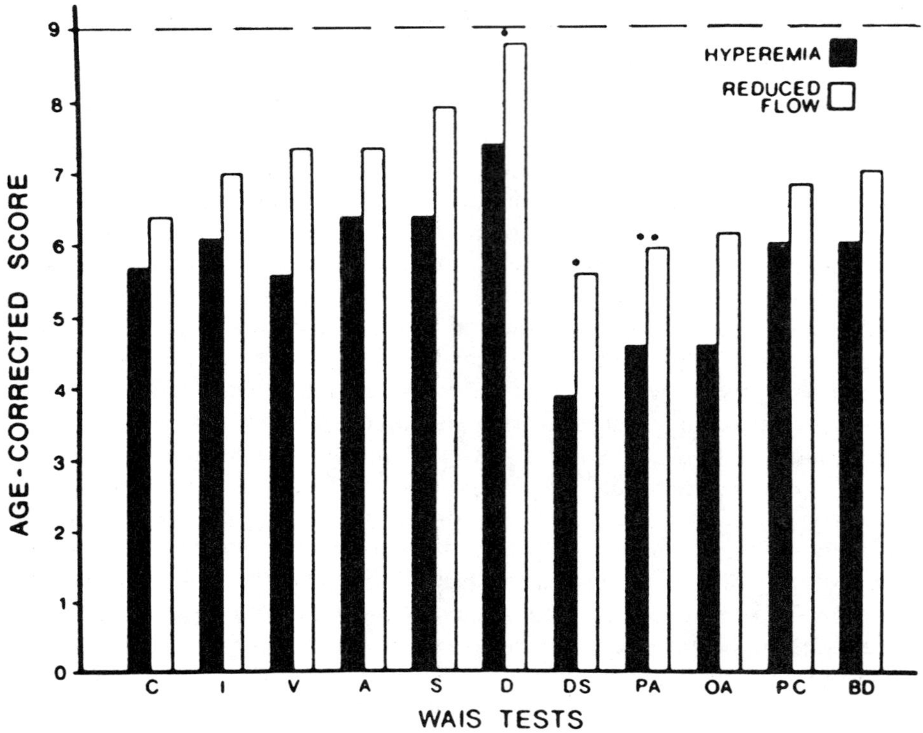

FIGURE 3 Mean Wechsler Adult Intelligence Scale scores for the two cerebral blood flow groups. *p <.03; **p <0.01, one-tailed t-test. C, comprehension; I, information; V, vocabulary; A, arithmetic; S, similarities; D, digit span; DS, digit symbol; PA, picture arrangement; OA, object assembly; PC, picture completion; BD, block design. Dashed line indicates lower limit of average range. (From Ref. 28.)

predicted most accurately by estimated premorbid IQ and coma level. Long-term studies are necessary to fully appreciate the impact of these indices.

It has been increasingly demonstrated that return to a "normal" level of IQ is not sufficient to infer recovery. Numerous areas of impaired functioning have been documented including memory, problem solving, and attention, despite IQs that are within 1 standard deviation of the population mean (12,67,68). This point is illustrated in Figure 4, which indicates the IQ and memory scores of control subjects and moderately or severely injured patients tested 16–42 months postinjury (12). The scores were converted to standard scores to allow comparisons among the measures.

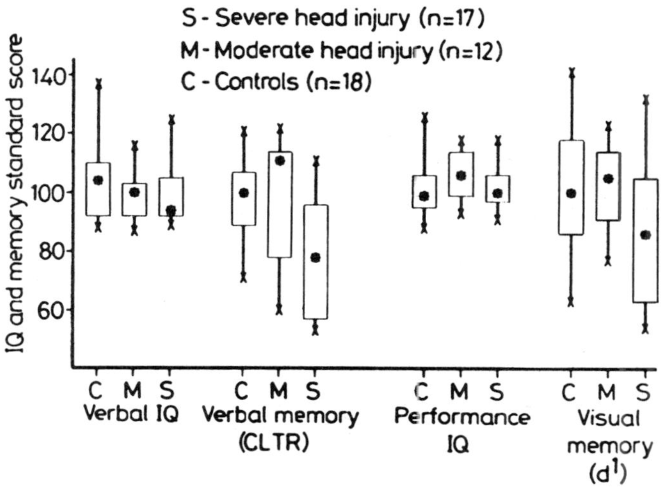

FIGURE 4 Box-plots depicting the distribution of IQ and transformed memory scores for controls, moderate, and severe head-injured patients who obtained IQ scores in the preserved range (> 85) at 16–42 months postinjury. Each asterisk signifies the median, whereas the upper and lower horizontal lines of each bar indicate the 75th and 25th percentile scores. The maximum and minimum scores are depicted by the letter "X". (From Ref. 12.)

Verbal and Performance IQs were similar among the groups, whereas verbal and visual memory were most noticeably depressed for the severe CHI patients. Thus, neuropsychological assessment should be global and include other potential areas of compromise before conclusions concerning the presence and extent of deficits are made.

B. Memory Functioning

Impaired memory functioning is a common manifestation during both the acute and chronic stages of recovery. Over half the survivors of severe CHI display difficulty in learning and retaining new information, as measured by objective techniques and patient or family reports (18,69–71). Mild head injury (i.e., momentary loss of consciousness and no focal neurological deficits or mass lesions) also produces memory deficits that are salient within the first month (8,72,73).

The prominence of memory deficits across the spectrum of severity reflects the vulnerability of the temporal lobes to hematomas and contusions as detected by both neuropathological studies and neuroradiological techniques (8,25,26). In addition, ventricular enlargement and hypoxia contribute to persisting impairments (18,39,40). The GCS score (particularly within 24 h of injury), duration of unconsciousness, and integrity of ocular responses are strongly related to residual memory performance (11–13,17,34,74), with patients who sustain more severe acute injuries exhibiting long-lasting deficits. Goldstein and Levin (75) examined the relationships among these variables in moderately and severely injured patients tested up to 15 months postinjury. Patients either exhibited intact memory for verbal and visual material, deficits for one type of material alone (specific deficit), or memory impairment for both verbal and visual information (global deficit). Longer durations of impaired consciousness and lower GCS scores were characteristic of the globally impaired patients, whereas acute findings of nonreactive pupils–oculovestibular disturbances differentiated memory-impaired groups from patients without deficits.

During the acute stages of recovery, patients may exhibit posttraumatic amnesia (difficulty in acquiring and retrieving new information; 32) accompanied by disorientation and, frequently, agitated and disinhibited behavior, confabulation, and impaired attention. Assessment of this period includes retrospective measures (e.g., asking patients when they first experienced continuous memory after the accident) and prospective techniques (e.g., serial interviews). The Galveston Orientation and Amnesia Test (GOAT; 76) follows the daily recovery of continuous memory by assessing whether orientation is intact and the patient's ability to retrieve information surrounding the head injury. The Westmead PTA Scale (77) specifically measures the ability to exhibit new learning over 3 days, thereby signifying the end of PTA. Ewert and colleagues (78) reported that head-injured patients in PTA demonstrated learning of skills over sessions (e.g., decreased latencies to read words presented as mirror-images), despite lack of memory for the actual training. By extrapolation, rehabilitation therapies during PTA that emphasize physical skills and activities of daily living may be retained (78).

A salient feature of memory after emergence from PTA is an anterograde amnesia characterized by an inability to register or retrieve material. This impairment may manifest as difficulty in retaining information over time, a material-specific deficit (e.g., for verbal as opposed to visual input), and problems in spontaneously using features that enhance recall (e.g., organizing words that belong to categories).

Survivors commonly exhibit relatively preserved immediate but disproportionately impaired delayed recall (33,34,68,79), similar to amnesic patients such as those with Korsakoff's disease. Tests of digit span are particularly sensitive to this dissociation, as seen in relatively preserved recall of digits forward but impaired ability to reverse their order (79). Deficits extend to delayed recall of prose, words, and pictures (33,34,80). One explanation concerns difficulty that survivors have in transferring information from a temporary holding buffer to a long-term store. For example, after the individual reverses the last few digits, memory for the initial digits has dissipated. Another explanation focuses on the heightened vulnerability of memory to interference. Problems in maintaining directed attention over time may account for impairments in delayed recall (68). Finally, CHI patients may exhibit accelerated forgetting owing to underlying temporal lobe lesions (81).

In addition to impaired retention, dissociations have been observed in the recall of particular types of information (e.g., verbal versus visual material). Such dissociations in relation to underlying side or site of lesions are not always striking, however, perhaps due to limitations in neuroimaging techniques or the diffuseness of damage produced by head injury. Goldstein and Levin (75) examined the presence of dissociations encompassing recall of specific types of information (words versus designs), as opposed to global impairments, in survivors of moderate and severe CHI. Although bilateral mass lesions were commonly associated with a global memory deficit, diffuse injuries (e.g., absence of mass lesions) were also characteristic of the groups. Differential recovery of memory for verbal versus visual material has been noted during the first year after head injury (10). The finding of relative strengths is important, since preserved areas can be employed in rehabilitation (e.g., using visual aids to teach a patient to remember the steps needed to transfer from a wheelchair) (82).

The spontaneous use of strategies to aid recall also contributes to memory functioning (74,83). Survivors may fail to take advantage of the categorical nature of a task (e.g., that words belong to hierarchical labels such as fruits or animals) and, therefore, not cluster the words (83). Other inactive retrieval strategies include failing to consistently recall the same words from trial to trial. Although overall capacity may thus improve after head injury, efficiency and organization may remain static (74). Neuropsychological testing needs to include the more effortful aspects of memory that approximate the difficulties patients are likely to have in their everyday environments.

C. Reasoning and Problem Solving

Reasoning and problem-solving behaviors are increasingly recognized as a critical aspect of cognitive functioning following head injury. Deficits in the ability to organize and shift responses, to utilize feedback, and to evaluate final performance have been found across all severity levels (23,73,84), including patients with apparently good recoveries as measured by return to work or intact neurological indices (68). The "executive" processes are conceptualized as the overseer of lower-level functions such as memory and language, modulating the efficiency of these operations. Impairments can result from reduced motivation to apply active strategies, decreases in the productive aspects of thought, and failure to monitor one's actions or to modify behavior based on environmental feedback. Ablation studies have emphasized the role of the frontal lobes in producing these deficits. Although the frequency of frontal lobe contusions or hematomas after head injury is well-established (8,25,26), precise neuroanatomical–neuropsychological links are complicated by the presence of diffuse or multifocal trauma.

One technique to assess deficits in hypothesis testing and ability to benefit from feedback is the Wisconsin (85) and Modified (86) Wisconsin Card-Sorting Tests. These procedures require consecutive sorting on one of three dimensions (color, shape, or number) followed by a shift to another dimension. Feedback is given after each trial concerning the correctness of the sort. Head-injured patients display deficits consisting of generating few correct sorts and making a high percentage of perseverative responses (i.e., staying with an incorrect hypothesis despite negative feedback 23,68,73). Another type of deficit is a reduction in productivity such as the generation of responses under timed conditions. Reduced verbal fluency is a feature of left frontal injury (87), whereas diminished capacity to invent designs occurs with right frontal injury (88).

Lezak (89) has noted that most assessment techniques fail to examine the capacity for self-regulation and hypothesis generation, since they typically require structured, closed-ended responses. In an attempt to evaluate executive dysfunction that eliminated these characteristics, Goldstein and colleagues (90) used a variant of a "twenty questions" procedure (91). Survivors of severe CHI were shown an array of 48 common pictured items that belonged to conceptual categories (e.g., shoe, jacket, dress=clothing), but were presented so that the relationships were not obvious (items from the same category were randomly dispersed). The task was to guess the item the examiner was thinking of in the fewest number of trials. Three conditions were administered with a maximum of 30 attempts per condition. Patients took significantly more trials to guess the correct items (mean, 12.3; SD, 5.7) than demographically matched controls (Mean, 9.0; SD, 4.7). Figure 5 indicates the type of questions that were asked. Survivors asked hypothesis (e.g., "Is it a shoe?") and pseudoconstraint (e.g., "Does it have shoelaces?") questions about the individual pictures, resulting in reduced efficiency of problem solving. In contrast with controls, they were less likely to ask constraint-seeking questions (e.g., "Is it an article of clothing?") that simultaneously eliminated several items.

The impact of executive processing deficits on "apparent" neuropsychological impairments needs to be carefully evaluated during testing.

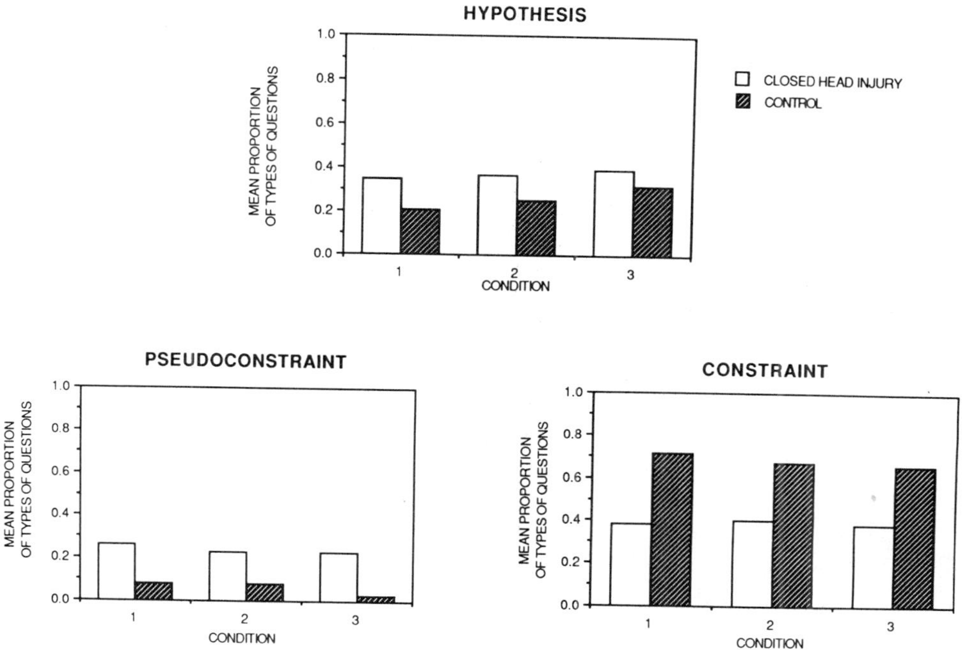

FIGURE 5 Percentage of questions asked as a function of question type for head-injured patients and controls. Hypothesis: asking about a specific item such as, "Is it the shoe?"; Constraint: asking about a category that narrows down several alternatives such as, "Is it an article of clothing?"; Pseudoconstraint: asking about a specific object but in a nondirect fashion such as, "Does it have shoelaces?" (From Ref. 90.)

One may erroneously conclude that there is a core impairment in areas such as memory or language, as opposed to a disruption of higher-order processing abilities. Improved performance under structured conditions (e.g., facilitation of recall when provided with the context of a story as opposed to recall of words; increased word generation when given categories as opposed to letters) may provide clues for underlying deficits in the regulatory executive aspects of behavior.

D. Language

Despite seemingly normal use of language in conversational speech, survivors frequently manifest features of an aphasic disturbance when formal neuropsychological testing is conducted. Sarno (92) recently summarized findings in 125 survivors of severe CHI (coma durations from 10 minutes to

6 months) who were enrolled in rehabilitation. Three profiles of language functioning were observed before testing. Thirty-seven patients exhibited an aphasic deficit characterized by impaired expressive and receptive language in conversational speech; 43 patients displayed dysarthria without obvious aphasia; whereas the remaining 45 survivors had no salient aphasic or dysarthric deficits. Figure 6 displays performance of the groups on subtests of the Neurosensory Center Comprehensive Examination for Aphasia (93) examining confrontation-naming of objects, repetition of sentences, generation of words beginning with different letters under timed conditions, and comprehension of increasingly complex commands. As seen, even those patients who were felt to be spared linguistic deficits performed below control performance on certain measures. Sarno termed these impairments "subclinical," since they were only apparent through formal assessment. Her research stresses the importance of examining language functioning in the clinical setting.

As displayed in Figure 6, and also verified in other studies, anomia or word-finding difficulty is one of the most salient features of acute aphasia following head injury (18,94,95). This deficit may be accompanied by verbal paraphasia (substitution of inappropriate words), perseveration, and circumlocution with relatively preserved comprehension and repetition. Levin et al. (95) reported that almost half of their sample of acutely injured patients displayed defective naming and reduced verbal fluency. Wernicke's aphasia is another clinical syndrome characterized by fluent speech but impaired comprehension for auditory and written information as well as defective repetition (18).

Severity indices are related to the manifestation and prolongation of language difficulties. On the basis of test scores, Levin and colleagues (95) classified patients as exhibiting a specific language deficit (e.g., naming) or a generalized disturbance encompassing both expressive and receptive abilities. Patients with a specific disturbance had less severe injuries, as indicated by shorter durations of impaired consciousness and bilaterally reactive pupils on admission. They were also likely to exhibit recovery of intellectual functioning to the normal range. In contrast, those with pervasive deficits typically had findings on CT of bilateral hematomas and diffuse swelling, and they attained significantly lower scores on an intelligence test. Although one might expect dominant left hemisphere damage to be associated with language disturbance, survivors with diffuse injuries also commonly manifest impairments, representing the widespread nature of head injury.

Apart from characteristics of aphasia, CHI often produces a disruption in the ability to effectively communicate, which may reflect underlying cognitive deficits such as memory, attention, and reasoning. Tangential, irrelevant, and disorganized discourse has been noted by several investiga-

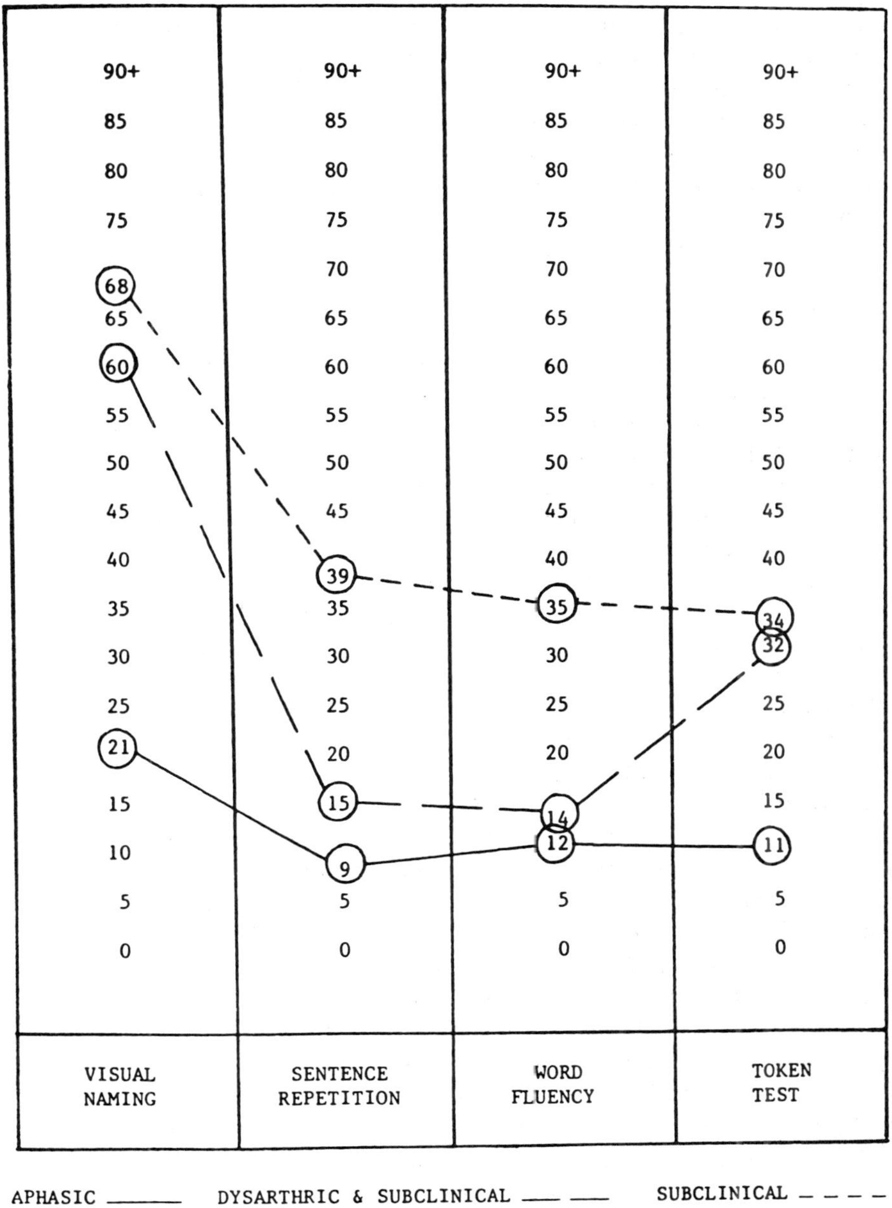

FIGURE 6 Mean percentile ranks of CHI groups on selected subtests of the Neurosensory Center Comprehensive Examination for Aphasia based on the performance of normal adults. (From Ref. 92.)

tors (18,96,97). Lack of cohesiveness (i.e., failure to link words to the appropriate referent such as use of "it" without specifying the noun) has also been identified as a feature of language after head injury (96). These types of impairments are not always appreciated using standardized assessment measures in which structure is provided. Instead, they are more likely captured through informal conversation or assessment techniques emphasizing dyadic interchanges and open-ended responses (e.g., description of the events taking place in a picture; 98).

E. Attention

Mental slowness and difficulty in focusing and maintaining attention are common complaints after head injury. Table 3, adapted from Gronwall (99), summarizes studies examining the frequency of reports of concentration problems according to the severity of injury. As seen, the presence of such complaints exists across the spectrum of patients and abates, but does not entirely disappear, over time. Objective measures including tasks that require controlled, effortful abilities (e.g., vigilance, processing under timed conditions) are particularly vulnerable after head injury (100–105).

Speed of processing has been examined primarily by the Paced Auditory Serial Addition Task (PASAT; 106,107). Numbers are presented at increasing speeds, and the individual adds each digit to the immediately preceding digit without cumulating a sum. Performance is initially impaired in patients with mild head injuries, but scores typically improve to the level of controls within 1 month (73,106). In contrast, patients with severe injuries often demonstrate persistent deficits (23,101). Figure 7 summarizes performance on the PASAT of 15 survivors of severe CHI who were enrolled in rehabilitation and 14 demographically matched controls (101). Information processing rate (correct responses per second) is displayed as a function of presentation speeds (ISI) varying from 2.8 to 1.6 sec between digits. Patients were slower at every ISI relative to controls, and inspection of the individual data indicated only a few violations of this finding. Reaction time tasks, particularly those involving choices between two or more responses depending upon which stimulus is presented, are also sensitive to the effects of slowed decision processes (108,109). Diffuse axonal injury that produces cortical–subcortical disconnection (110) and degeneration of the white matter (111) may reduce the efficiency of information processing under conditions of increasing rates of presentation.

The ability to maintain attention has been examined through tasks requiring prolonged processing demands. Investigators have noted the difficulty that survivors have in focusing and redirecting their attention over time (101,109). Levin and colleagues (101) utilized a 20-min vigilance mea-

TABLE 3 Incidence of Reports of Concentration Problems in Prospective Series of Head-Injury Cases

			Months since injury				
Author	Defined by:	N	1	3	6	12	24
Mild Injuries							
Lidvall et al. (1974)	PTA <24 hr	83	11%	8%			
	Control[a]	83	4%	4%			
McLean et al. (1984)	TOC <24 hr[b]	68	47%				
	Control	102	8%				
Rimel et al. (1981)	GCS >13[c]	424		59%[d]			
Rutherford et al. (1977/79)	PTA <24 hr	145	8%			3%	
Wrightson et al. (1981)	PTA<36 hr	66		16%[d]			6%[d]
Moderate to Severe Injuries							
McLean et al. (1984)	TOC 1–6 d[b]	8	75%				
Rimel et al. (1982)	GCS 9–12[c]	170		90%[d]			
Van Zomeren & Van den Burg (1985)	PTA 1–7 d	18					17%
Severe to Very Severe Injuries							
McKinley et al. (1983)	PTA >2 d C	21		53%	40%	38%	
	NC	21		26%	40%	9%	
McLean et al. (1984)	TOC >7 d[b]	4	75%				
Oddy et al. (1978)	PTA >24 h	48			29%		
Van Zomeren & Van den Burg (1985)	PTA >7 d	39					40%

[a]Postconcussion-like problems, present before injury.
[b]TOC, time to obey commands.
[c]GCS, Glasgow Coma Scale score (7).
C, cases with compensation claims pending; NC, no claims.
[d]Inclusion of memory as well as concentration problems
Source: Adapted from Ref. 99.

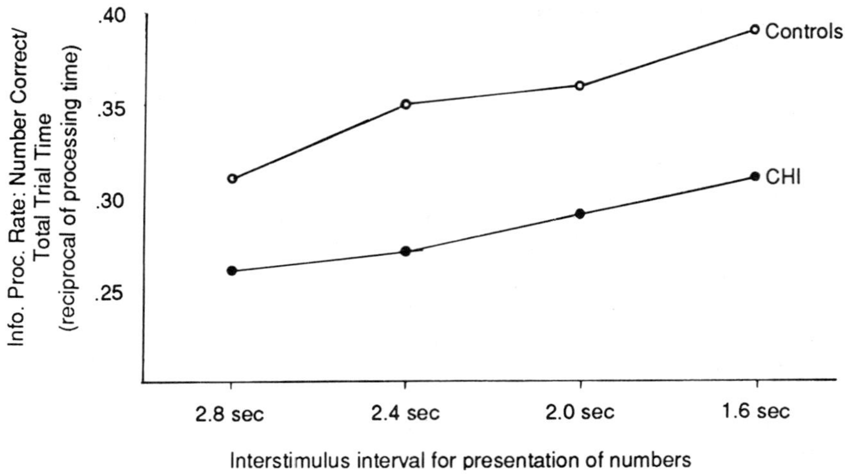

FIGURE 7 PASAT: Information processing rate (correct responses/second) as a function of presentation speed for patients with closed head injuries and controls. (From Ref. 101.)

sure requiring patients to detect long versus short intervals separating digits. After 10 min, controls, who displayed an initial decrement, rebounded to their original high level of performance, whereas the patients' accuracy steadily declined. This same problem in the redirection of attention was noted on a 10-min task requiring the detection of targets in a series of distractors. Detection accuracy improved and was maintained by controls in contrast to a decrease in performance over time for patients. Stuss and colleagues (109) also reported the inconsistency of head-injured patients' attention both within and across test sessions. Neuropsychological assessment needs to include tasks that require effortful processing over extended periods. In addition, scheduling numerous testing sessions may help to detect attentional variability.

Impairments in the simultaneous processing of numerous bits of information have been found to characterize head-injured patients (68,99,101, 105). Divided attention deficits were observed by Stuss and colleagues (109) when patients were required to respond to a target stimulus only if three conditions were present (specified color, shape, and design). Relative to controls, the patients were disproportionately slow on this task. These divided attention problems have been proposed to reflect underlying frontal lobe abnormality and, in particular, disruption of the frontal–limbic–reticular activating system (109).

III. DIRECTIONS FOR REHABILITATION

The preceding sections have delineated a number of compromised cognitive domains after CHI. Although a review of rehabilitation strategies is beyond the scope of this chapter, current trends and findings that hold promise for improving treatment efficacy will be briefly discussed.

It has become increasingly recognized that the motivational level of the patient, including the commitment and energy brought to the training session, plays a major role in the ultimate success of cognitive remediation (112). Reduced or absent motivation (anergia) may stem from factors involving depression, denial of deficits, or lack of awareness of cognitive impairments (anosognosia). Depression is a frequent affective response that occurs across all levels of severity (112–115) and may intensify, rather than diminish, over time (116). Impaired metacognition or knowledge of one's cognitive functioning can also impinge on the willingness of the patient to put forth effort in therapy and to use compensatory techniques (112). In the area of memory, for example, it has been observed that survivors rate their abilities similarly to controls without brain damage. Moreover, there are weak correlations between patients' reports of their memory functioning and objective test data (117,118). Lam and colleagues (119) reported that severe CHI patients who were aware of deficits were judged by their therapists as having more positive treatment performances (e.g., compliance, progress, motivation) than those who denied problems.

The importance of alleviating depression and incorporating awareness training into treatment has thus been emphasized (112,120). Prigatano (112) notes that cognitive remediation without simultaneous instruction in anxiety reduction techniques may produce a catastrophic reaction, leading to further avoidance of therapy. He advocates insight-oriented individual and group psychotherapy to help patients understand their deficits and the effect on daily functioning. Direct training of meta-awareness has also been attempted. For example, Schacter et al. (120) utilized multiple feedback sessions with an amnesic patient who was confronted with his predicted versus actual recall of words and actions. The patient's predictions on these tasks became more realistic. However, he did not apply this increased knowledge to other settings, highlighting the need for a broader-based approach to promote generalization. Behavior modification strategies have been employed to enhance motivational levels in patients who might otherwise not benefit from rehabilitation (121,122). Techniques including positive reinforcement, time out, and token economy systems may decrease dysfunctional and increase appropriate behaviors.

The ultimate success of cognitive remediation depends on variables including the ease of applying the techniques, the theoretical framework on which they are based (e.g., restoration versus substitution of function), maintenance of gains over time, and generalization of these skills to new environments. Computer programs that emphasize rote repetition and exercise, rather than the teaching of abilities, have provided limited success in significantly altering function. These programs typically are "simplistic variations of testing programs already used with brain-injured patients" (123, p. 273). Internal techniques such as visual imagery, semantic elaboration, and ridiculous stories/bizarre images have been attempted in the area of memory, but also are of questionable value because of their artificial nature and difficulty (i.e., they are not used by people without brain damage) (124).

External techniques including environmental aids such as schedule books and wristwatch alarms appear to hold some promise in improving aspects of cognitive functioning, particularly memory. These techniques reduce the burden on memory, since the patient is not required to store or retrieve information. Zencius et al. (125) recently compared the efficacy of an external aid over other cognitive techniques. Survivors of head injury were asked to remember information (employer, job title, experience–education) from two help-wanted advertisements in the newspaper. Training techniques for remembering this information consisted of written rehearsal (writing the information three times), verbal rehearsal (reading the job leads five times), acronym formation (developing code words from the key letters in the job heads) and keeping a notebook log (recording the information and being able to consult it later). Figure 8 depicts the number of memory units recalled (six possible) for each type of technique, including a baseline condition (no training). As seen, all patients demonstrated complete retrieval of the information when they were able to consult their log books. The benefit of remediation strategies that are natural to use and have applicability to a range of settings remains to be examined through future comparative studies.

Pharmacologic treatments to enhance cognitive status have been attempted with survivors of CHI. These studies include administration of cholinergic (126–128) and psychostimulant (129) agents. Levin and colleagues (127) examined the effects of physostigmine and lecithin on memory and attention in 16 survivors of moderate or severe CHI who were enrolled in rehabilitation. In general, comparison of treatment versus placebo conditions did not indicate any significant improvements while patients received the drugs. Goldberg et al. (126) reported the results of a case study involving a patient examined 2 years after sustaining a severe CHI. A significant improvement while receiving physostigmine and lecithin was observed in storage and retrieval of words on a measure of verbal memory. However, no change occurred on a measure of memory for de-

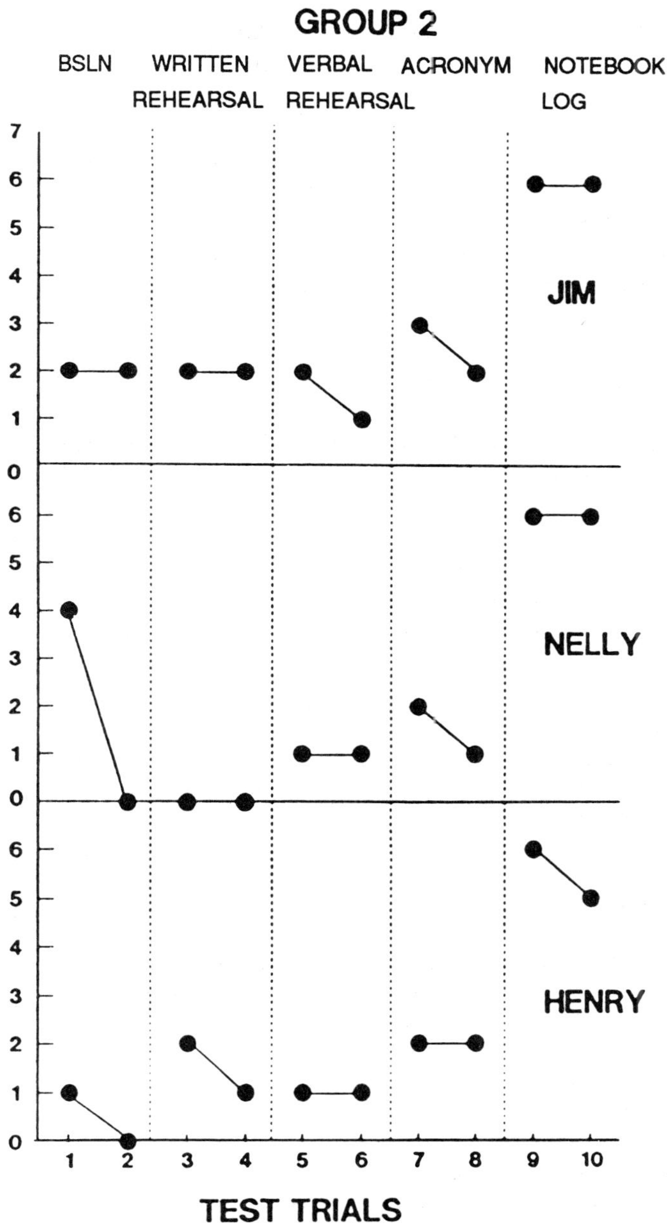

FIGURE 8 Number of memory assignments completed accurately during baseline, written rehearsal, verbal rehearsal, acronym formation, and notebook log, respectively. (From Ref. 125.)

signs. Finally, Evans et al. (129) evaluated the effects of two psychostimulant medications, methylphenidate and dextroamphetamine, on memory and attention in a survivor of severe CHI. Enhancement in the patient's verbal memory was reported, but other functions (e.g., visual memory, fluency, visuospatial processing) were unaffected by the drugs.

Overall, the potential of pharmacologic agents to alter cognitive status in CHI patients has lagged behind the investigations of other clinical groups such as individuals with Alzheimer's disease (see Chaps. 8 and 12). There are few published studies in this area and an overreliance on single case or anectdotal reports. Concentrated research in this area needs to be conducted.

This chapter has focused on cognitive deficits after CHI, while ignoring preserved capabilities that can be used to maximize functioning. The finding by Ewert and colleagues (78) that patients in PTA are able to learn and retain skills suggests the possibility of instituting therapies (e.g., occupational and physical) at an early stage of injury to improve eventual outcome. The research of Schacter and Glisky (130–132) on teaching domain-specific knowledge (knowledge relevant to a particular task) has wide-reaching implications for job training, including data entry positions and everyday activities such as managing household tasks. Evidence for preserved semantic analysis in survivors (e.g., recognition that words belong to categories; 83) could be used to teach strategies such as organizing specific items (e.g., food purchases) on a list into categories before going shopping. One hopes that our ability to devise rehabilitation techniques that significantly improve the quality of life will flourish as we continue to uncover areas of competence in survivors of head injury.

REFERENCES

1. Diller L, Ben-Yishay Y. Outcomes and evidence in neuropsychological rehabilitation in closed head injury. In: Levin HS, Grafman J, Eisenberg HM, eds. Neurobehavioral recovery from head injury. New York: Oxford University Press, 1987:146–165.
2. Lezak MD. Making neuropsychological assessment relevant to head injury. In: Levin HS, Grafman J, Eisenberg HM, eds. Neurobehavioral recovery from head injury. New York: Oxford University Press, 1987:116–128.
3. Brooks DN. Measuring neuropsychological and functional recovery. In: Levin HS, Grafman J, Eisenberg HM, eds. Neurobehavioral recovery from head injury. New York: Oxford University Press, 1987:57–72.
4. Brooks N, McKinlay W, Symington C, Beattie A, Campsie L. Return to work within the first seven years of severe head injury. Brain Injury 1987; 1:5–19.
5. Groswasser Z, Sazbon L. Outcome in 134 patients with prolonged post-

traumatic unawareness: part 2: functional outcome of 72 patients recovering consciousness. J Neurosurg 1990; 72:81–84.
6. Rao N, Rosenthal M, Cronin-Stubbs D, Lambert R, Barnes P, Swanson B. Return to work after rehabilitation following traumatic brain injury. Brain Injury 1990; 4:49–56.
7. Teasdale G, Jennett B. Assessment of coma and impaired consciousness: a practical scale. Lancet 1974; 2:81–84.
8. Levin HS, Amparo E, Eisenberg HM, Williams DH, High WM Jr., McArdle CB, Weiner RL. Magnetic resonance imaging and computerized tomography in relation to the neurobehavioral sequelae of mild and moderate head injuries. J Neurosurg 1987; 66:706–713.
9. Rimel RW, Giordani B, Barth JT, Jane JA. Moderate head injury: completing the clinical spectrum of brain trauma. Neurosurgery 1982; 11:344–351.
10. Tabaddor K, Mattis S, Zazula T. Cognitive sequelae and recovery course after moderate and severe head injury. Neurosurgery 1984; 14:701–708.
11. Alexandre A, Colombo F, Nertempi P, Benedetti A. Cognitive outcome and early indices of severity of head injury. J Neurosurg 1983; 59:751–761.
12. Levin HS, Goldstein FC, High WM Jr, Eisenberg HM. Disproportionately severe memory deficit in relation to normal intellectual functioning after closed head injury. J Neurol Neurosurg Psychiatry 1988; 51:1294–1301.
13. Vilkki J, Poropudas K, Servo A. Memory disorder related to coma duration after head injury. J Neurol Neurosurg Psychiatry 1988; 51:1452–1454.
14. Williams JM, Gomes F, Drudge OW, Kessler M. Predicting outcome from closed head injury by early assessment of trauma severity. J Neurosurg 1984; 61:581–585.
15. Born JD, Albert A, Hans P, Bonnal J. Relative prognostic value of best motor response and brain stem reflexes in patients with severe head injury. Neurosurgery 1985; 16:595–601.
16. Jennett B, Teasdale G, Braakman R, Minderhoud J, Knill-Jones R. Predicting outcome in individual patients after severe head injury. Lancet 1976; 1:1031–1034.
17. Levin HS, Grossman RG, Rose JE, Teasdale G. Long-term neuropsychological outcome of closed head injury. J Neurosurg 1979; 50:412–422.
18. Levin HS, Benton AL, Grossman RG. Neurobehavioral consequences of closed head injury. New York: Oxford University Press, 1982.
19. Uzzell BP, Zimmerman RA, Dolinskas CA, Obrist WD. Lateralized psychological impairment associated with CT lesions in head injured patients. Cortex 1979; 15:391–401.
20. Gandy SE, Snow RB, Zimmerman RD, Deck MDF. Cranial nuclear magnetic resonance imaging in head trauma. Ann Neurol 1986; 16:254–257.
21. Jenkins A, Teasdale G, Hadley MDM, MacPherson P, Rowan JO. Brain lesions detected by magnetic resonance imaging in mild and severe head injuries. Lancet 1986; 2:445–446.
22. Langfitt TW, Obrist WD, Alavi A, Grossman RG, Zimmerman R, Jaggi J, Uzzell B, Reivich M, Patton DR. Computerized tomography, magnetic reso-

nance imaging, and positron emission tomography in the study of brain trauma. J Neurosurg 1986; 64:760–767.
23. Levin HS, Handel SF, Goldman AM, Eisenberg HM, Guinto FC Jr. Magnetic resonance imaging after "diffuse" nonmissile head injury: a neurobehavioral study. Arch Neurol 1985; 42:963–968.
24. Wilson JTL, Wiedmann KD, Hadley DM, Condon B, Teasdale G, Brooks DN. Early and late magnetic resonance imaging and neuropsychological outcome after head injury. J Neurol Neurosurg Psychiatry 1988; 51:391–396.
25. Adams JH, Mitchell DE, Graham DI, Doyle D. Diffuse brain damage of immediate impact type. Brain 1977; 100:489–502.
26. Adams JH, Graham D, Scott G, Parker LS, Doyle D. Brain damage in fatal non-missile head injury. J Clin Pathol 1980; 33:1132–1145.
27. Ruff RM, Buchsbaum MS, Troster AI, Marshall LF, Lottenberg S, Somers LM, Tobias MD. Computerized tomography, neuropsychology, and positron emission tomography in the evaluation of head injury. Neuropsychiatry Neuropsychol Behav Neurol 1989; 2:103–123.
28. Uzzell BP, Obrist WD, Dolinskas CA, Langfitt TW. Relationship of acute CBF and ICP findings to neuropsychological outcome in severe head injury. J Neurosurg 1986; 65:630–635.
29. Levin HS, High WM Jr, Williams DH, Eisenberg HM, Amparo EG, Guinto FC Jr, Ewert J. Dichotic listening and manual performance in relation to magnetic resonance imaging after closed head injury. J Neurol Neurosurg Psychiatry 1989: 52:1162–1169.
30. Lindenberg R, Fisher RS, Durlacher SH, Lovitt WV Jr, Freytag E. Lesions of the corpus callosum following blunt mechanical trauma to the head. Am J Pathol 1955; 31:297–317.
31. Strich SJ. Lesions in the cerebral hemispheres after blunt head injury. In: Sevitt S, Stoner HB, eds. The pathology of trauma. London: BMA, 1970:166–171.
32. Russell WR, Smith A. Post-traumatic amnesia in closed head injury. Arch Neurol 1961; 5:4–17.
33. Brooks DN. Wechsler Memory Scale performance and its relationship to brain damage after severe closed head injury. J Neurol Neurosurg Psychiatry 1976; 39:593–601.
34. Dikmen S, Temkin N, McLean A, Wyler A, Machamer J. Memory and head injury severity. J Neurol Neurosurg Psychiatry 1987; 50:1613–1618.
35. Gronwall D, Wrightson P. Memory and information processing capacity after closed head injury. J Neurol Neurosurg Psychiatry 1981; 44:889–895.
36. Carlsson GS, Svardsudd K, Welin L. Long-term effects of head injuries sustained during life in three male populations. J Neurosurg 1987; 67:197–205.
37. Levin HS, Eisenberg HM. Postconcussional syndrome. In: Current therapy in neurologic disease 2. Philadelphia: BC Decker, 1987:193–196.
38. Williams DH, Levin HS, Eisenberg HM. Mild head injury classification. Neurosurgery 1990; 27:422–428.
39. Cullum CM, Bigler ED. Ventricle size, cortical atrophy and the relationship with neuropsychological status in closed head injury: a quantitative analysis. J Clin Exp Neuropsychol 1986; 8:437–452.

40. Levin HS, Meyers CA, Grossman RG, Sarwar M. Ventricular enlargement after closed head injury. Arch Neurol 1981; 38:623–629.
41. Frankowski RF. Descriptive epidemiologic studies of head injury in the United States: 1974–1984. Adv Psychosom Med 1986; 16:153–172.
42. Kraus J. Epidemiology of head injury. In: Cooper PR, ed. Head injury. Baltimore: Williams & Wilkins, 1987:1–19.
43. Sosin DM, Sacks JJ, Smith SM. Head injury-associated deaths in the United States from 1979 to 1986. JAMA 1989; 262:2251–2255.
44. Luerssen TG, Klauber MR, Marshall LF. Outcome from head injury related to patient's age: a longitudinal prospective study of adult and pediatric head injury. J Neurosurg 1988; 68:409–416.
45. DeMaria EJ, Kenney PR, Merriam MA, Casanova LA, Gann DS. Aggressive trauma care benefits the elderly. J Trauma 1987; 27:1200–1206.
46. Pentland B, Jones PA, Roy CW, Miller JD. Head injury in the elderly. Age Ageing 1986; 15:193–202.
47. Roy CW, Pentland B, Miller JD. The causes and consequences of minor head injury in the elderly. Injury 1986; 17:220–223.
48. McMordie WR, Barker SL, Paolo TM. Return to work (RTW) after head injury. Brain Injury 1990; 4:57–69.
49. Stambrook M, Moore AD, Peters LC, Deviaene C, Hawryluk GA. Effects of mild, moderate and severe closed head injury on long-term vocational status. Brain Injury 1990; 4:183–190.
50. Humphrey M, Oddy M. Return to work after head injury: a review of post-war studies. Injury 1981; 12:107–114.
51. Hass JF, Cope DN, Hall K. Premorbid prevalence of poor academic performance in severe head injury. J Neurol Neurosurg Psychiatry 1987; 50:52–56.
52. Barona A, Reynolds CR, Chastain R. A demographically based index of premorbid intelligence for the WAIS-R. J Consult Clin Psychol 1984; 52: 885–887.
53. Wilson RS, Rosenbaum G, Brown G, Rourke D, Whitman D, Grisell J. An index of premorbid intelligence. J Consult Clin Psychol 1978; 46:1554–1555.
54. Wilson RS, Rosenbaum G, Brown G. The problem of premorbid intelligence in neuropsychological assessment. J Clin Neuropsychol 1979; 1:49–53.
55. Goldstein FC, Gary HE Jr, Levin HS. Assessment of the accuracy of regression equations proposed for estimating premorbid intellectual functioning on the Wechsler adult intelligence scale. J Clin Exp Neuropsychol 1986; 8:405–412.
56. Karzmark P, Heaton RK, Grant I, Matthews CG. Use of demographic variables to predict full scale IQ: a replication and extension. J Clin Exp Neuropsychol 1985; 7:412–420.
57. Nelson HE, O'Connell A. Dementia: the estimation of premorbid intelligence levels using the new adult reading test. Cortex 1978; 14:234–244.
58. Brooks N, Symington C, Beattie A, Campsie L, Bryden J, McKinlay W. Alcohol and other predictors of cognitive recovery after severe head injury. Brain Injury 1990; 3:235–246.
59. Gronwall D, Wrightson P. Cumulative effect of concussion. Lancet 1975; 2:995–997.

60. Wechsler D. The Wechsler adult intelligence scale manual. New York: Psychological Corporation, 1955.
61. Wechsler D. Wechsler adult intelligence scale—revised, manual. New York: Psychological Corporation, 1981.
62. Bond MR, Brooks DN. Understanding the process of recovery as a basis for the investigation of rehabilitation for the brain injured. Scand J Rehabil Med 1976; 8:127–133.
63. Mandleberg IA, Brooks DN. Cognitive recovery after severe head injury. I. Serial testing on the Wechsler adult intelligence scale. J Neurol Neurosurg Psychiatry 1975; 38:1121–1126.
64. Mandleberg IA. Cognitive recovery after severe head injury. 2. Wechsler adult intelligence scale during post-traumatic amnesia. J Neurol Neurosurg Psychiatry 1975; 38:1127–1132.
65. Mandleberg IA. Cognitive recovery after severe head injury. 3. WAIS verbal and performance IQ's as a function of post-traumatic amnesia duration and time from injury. J Neurol Neurosurg Psychiatry 1976; 39:1001–1007.
66. Brooks DN, Aughton ME, Bond MR, Jones P, Rizvi S. Cognitive sequelae in relationship to early indices of severity of brain damage after severe blunt head injury. J Neurol Neurosurg Psychiatry 1980; 43:529–534.
67. McMillan TM, Glucksman EE. The neuropsychology of moderate head injury. J Neurol Neurosurg Psychiatry 1987; 50:393–397.
68. Stuss DT, Ely P, Hugenholtz H, Richard MT, LaRochelle S, Poirier CA, Bell I. Subtle neuropsychological deficits in patients with good recovery after closed head injury. Neurosurgery 1985; 17:41–47.
69. Brooks N, Campsie L, Symington C, Beattie A, McKinlay W. The five year outcome of severe blunt head injury: a relative's view. J Neurol Neurosurg Psychiatry 1986; 49:764–770.
70. Oddy M, Coughlan T, Tyerman A, Jenkins D. Social adjustment after closed head injury: a further follow-up seven years after injury. J Neurol Neurosurg Psychiatry 1985; 48:564–568.
71. Van Zomeren AH, Van Den Burg W. Residual complaints of patients two years after severe head injury. J Neurol Neurosurg Psychiatry 1985; 48:21–28.
72. Binder LM. Persisting symptoms after mild head injury: a review of the postconcussive syndrome. J Clin Exp Neuropsychol 1986; 8:323–346.
73. Levin HS, Mattis S, Ruff RM, Eisenberg HM, Marshall LF, Tabaddor K, High WM Jr, Frankowski RF. Neurobehavioral outcome following minor head injury: a three-center study. J Neurosurg 1987; 66:234–243.
74. Paniak CE, Shore DL, Rourke BP. Recovery of memory after severe closed head injury: dissociations in recovery of memory parameters and predictors of outcome. J Clin Exp Neuropsychol 1989; 11:631–644.
75. Goldstein FC, Levin HS. Memory deficit after closed head injury. Presented at the 96th annual meeting of the American Psychological Association, Atlanta, Georgia, 1988.
76. Levin HS, O'Donnell VM, Grossman RG. The Galveston orientation and amnesia test: a practical scale to assess cognition after head injury. J Nerv Ment Dis 1979; 167:675–684.

77. Shores EA, Marosszeky JE, Sandanam J, Batchelor J. Preliminary validation of a clinical scale for measuring the duration of post-traumatic amnesia. Med J Aust 1986; 144:569–572.
78. Ewert J, Levin HS, Watson MG, Kalisky Z. Procedural memory during posttraumatic amnesia in survivors of severe closed head injury: implications for rehabilitation. Arch Neurol 1989; 46:911–916.
79. Brooks DN. Memory and head injury. J Nerv Ment Dis 1972; 155:350–355.
80. Larsson C, Ronnberg J. Memory disorders as a function of traumatic brain injury. Scand J Rehab Med 1987; 19:99–104.
81. Levin HS, High WM Jr, Eisenberg HM. Learning and forgetting during posttraumatic amnesia in head injured patients. J Neurol Neurosurg Psychiatry 1988; 51:14–20.
82. Wilson B. Memory therapy in practice. In: Wilson BA, Moffat N, eds. Clinical management of memory problems. Rockville, Md: Aspen Systems Corporation, 1984:89–111.
83. Levin HS, Goldstein FC. Organization of verbal memory after severe closed-head injury. J Clin Exp Neuropsychol 1986; 8:643–656.
84. Lenninger BE, Gramling SE, Farrell AD, Kreutzer JS, Peck EA. Neuropsychological deficits in symptomatic minor head injury patients after concussion and mild concussion. J Neurol Neurosurg Psychiatry 1990; 53: 293–296.
85. Grant DA, Berg EA. A behavioral analysis of degree of reinforcement and ease of shifting to new responses in a Weigl-type card-sorting problem. J Exp Psychol 1948; 38:404–411.
86. Nelson HE. A modified card sorting test sensitive to frontal lobe deficits. Cortex 1976; 12:313–324.
87. Benton AL. Differential behavioral effects in frontal lobe disease. Neuropsychologia 1968; 12:557–563.
88. Jones-Gotman M, Milner B. Design fluency: the invention of nonsense designs after focal cortical lesions. Neuropsychologia 1977; 15:653–674.
89. Lezak MD. Neuropsychological assessment. New York: Oxford University Press, 1983.
90. Goldstein FC, Levin HS. Question-asking strategies after severe closed head injury. Brain and Cognition 1991 (in press).
91. Mosher FA, Hornsby JR. On asking questions. In: Bruner JS, Olver RR, Greenfield P, eds. Studies in cognitive growth. New York: John Wiley & Sons, 1966:86–102.
92. Sarno MT. I. Head injury: language and speech defects. Scand J Rehabil Med [Suppl] 1988; 17:55–64.
93. Spreen O, Benton AL. Neurosensory center comprehensive examination for aphasia, revised ed. Victoria, BC: University of Victoria, 1977.
94. Levin HS, Grossman RG, Kelly PJ. Aphasic disorder in patients with closed head injury. J Neurol Neurosurg Psychiatry 1976; 39:1062–1070.
95. Levin HS, Grossman RG, Sarwar M, Meyers CA. Linguistic recovery after closed head injury. Brain Lang 1981; 12:360–374.

96. Mentis M, Prutting CA. Cohesion in the discourse of normal and head-injured adults. J Speech Hearing Res 1987; 30:88–98.
97. Prigatano GP, Roueche JR, Fordyce DJ. Nonaphasic language disturbances after closed head injury. Lang Sci 1985; 1:217–229.
98. Goodglass H, Kaplan E. Boston diagnostic aphasia examination (BDAE), revised ed. Phildelphia: Lea & Febiger, 1983.
99. Gronwall D. Advances in the assessment of attention and information processing after head injury. In: Levin HS, Grafman J, Eisenberg HM, eds. Neurobehavioral recovery from head injury. New York: Oxford University Press, 1987:355–371.
100. Ewing R, McCarthy D, Gronwall D, Wrightson P. Persisting effects of minor head injury observable during hypoxic stress. J Clin Neuropsychol 1980; 2:147–155.
101. Levin HS, High WM Jr, Goldstein FC, Williams DH. Sustained attention and information processing speed in chronic survivors of severe closed head injury. Scand J Rehabil Med [Suppl] 1988; 17:33–40.
102. Gronwall D. Paced auditory serial addition task: a measure of recovery from concussion. Percept Motor Skills 1977; 44:367–373.
103. Miller E. Simple and choice reaction time following severe head injury. Cortex 1970; 6:121–127.
104. Van Zomeren AH. Reaction time and attention after closed head injury. Lisse: Swets & Zeitlinger, 1981.
105. Van Zomeren AH, Deelman BG. Long-term recovery of visual reaction time after closed head injury. J Neurol Neurosurg Psychiatry 1987; 41: 452–457.
106. Gronwall D, Sampson H. The psychological effects of concussion. Auckland: Oxford University Press, 1974.
107. Gronwall D, Wrightson P. Delayed recovery of intellectual function after minor head injury. Lancet 1974; 2:605–609.
108. Van Zomeren AH, Brouwer WH. Head injury and concepts of attention. In: Levin HS, Grafman J, Eisenberg HM, eds. Neurobehavioral recovery from head injury. New York: Oxford University Press, 1987:398–415.
109. Stuss DT, Stethem LL, Hugenholtz H, Picton T, Pivik J, Richard MT. Reaction time after head injury: fatigue, divided and focused attention, and consistency of performance. J Neurol Neurosurg Psychiatry 1989; 52:742–748.
110. Ommaya AK, Gennarelli TA. Cerebral concussion and traumatic unconsciousness: correlation of experimental and clinical observations on blunt head injuries. Brain 1974; 97:633–654.
111. Strich SJ. Diffuse degeneration of the cerebral white matter in severe dementia following head injury. J Neurol Neurosurg Psychiatry 1956; 19:163–185.
112. Prigatano GP. Personality and psychosocial consequences after brain injury. In: Meier MJ, Benton AL, Diller L, eds. Neuropsychological rehabilitation. New York: Churchill-Livingstone, 1987:355–378.
113. Levin HS, High WM Jr, Goethe KE, Sisson RA, Overall JE, Rhoades HM, Eisenberg HM, Kalisky Z, Gary HE Jr. The neurobehavioral rating scale:

assessment of the behavioural sequelae of head injury by the clinician. J Neurol Neurosurg Psychiatry 1987; 50:183–193.
114. Dikmen S, Reitan RM. Emotional sequelae of head injury. Ann Neurol 1977; 2:492–494.
115. Rosenthal M. Behavioral sequelae. In: Rosenthal M, Griffith ER, Bond MB, eds. Rehabilitation of the head injured adult. Philadelphia: FA Davis Co, 1983:197–208.
116. Fordyce DJ, Roueche JR, Prigatano GP. Enhanced emotional reactions in chronic head trauma patients. J Neurol Neurosurg Psychiatry 1983; 46: 620–624.
117. Sunderland A, Harris JE, Baddeley AD. Do laboratory tests predict everyday memory? A neuropsychological study. J Verb Learn Verb Behav 1983; 22:341–357.
118. Sunderland A, Harris JE, Gleave J. Memory failures in everyday life following severe head injury. J Clin Neuropsychol 1984; 6:127–142.
119. Lam CS, McMahon BT, Priddy DA, Gehred-Schultz A. Deficit awareness and treatment performance among traumatic head injury adults. Brain Injury 1988; 2:235–242.
120. Schacter DL, Glisky EL, McGlynn SM. Impact of memory disorder on everyday life: awareness of deficits and return to work. Tupper D, Cicerone K, eds. The neuropsychology of everyday life, vol 1, theories and basic competencies. Boston, Kluwer Academic Publishers, 1990: 231–298.
121. Eames P, Wood R. Rehabilitation after severe brain injury: a follow-up study of a behaviour modification approach. J Neurol Neurosurg Psychiatry 1985; 48:613–619.
122. Newcombe F. The psychological consequences of closed head injury: assessment and rehabilitation. Injury 1982; 14:111–136.
123. O'Connor M, Cermak LS. Rehabilitation of organic memory disorders. In: Meier MJ, Benton AL, Diller L, eds. Neuropsychological rehabilitation. New York: Churchill-Livingstone, 1987:260–279.
124. Harris JE. Memory aids people use: two interview studies. Mem Cogn 1980; 8:31–38.
125. Zencius A, Wesolowski MD, Burke WH. A comparison of four memory strategies with traumatically brain-injured clients. Brain Injury 1990; 4: 33–38.
126. Goldberg E, Gerstman LJ, Mattis S, Hughes JE, Bilder RM Jr, Sirio CA. Effects of cholinergic treatment on posttraumatic anterograde amnesia. Arch Neurol 1982; 39:581.
127. Levin HS, Peters BH, Kalisky Z, High WM Jr, Von Laufen A, Eisenberg HM, Morrison DP, Gary HE Jr. Effects of oral physostigmine and lecithin on memory and attention in closed head injured patients. Central Nervous System Trauma. 1986; 3:333–342.
128. Walton RG. Lecithin and physostigmine for posttraumatic memory and cognitive deficits. Psychosomatics 1982; 23:435–436.
129. Evans RW, Gualtierri CT, Patterson D. Treatment of chronic closed head

injury with psychostimulant drugs: a controlled case study and an appropriate evaluation procedure. J Nerv Ment Dis 1987; 175:106–110.

130. Schacter DL, Glisky EL. Memory remediation: restoration, alleviation, and the acquisition of domain-specific knowledge. In: Uzzell B, Gross Y, eds. Clinical neuropsychology of intervention. Boston: Martinus Nijhoff, 1986.
131. Glisky EL, Schacter DL. Long-term retention of computer learning by patients with memory disorders. Neuropsychologia 1988; 26:173–178.
132. Glisky EL, Schacter DL. Extending the limits of complex learning in organic amnesia: computer training on a vocational domain. Neuropsychologia 1989; 27:107–120.

4

Neuropsychological Aspects of Huntington's Disease

Elsdon Storey* **and M. Flint Beal** *Massachusetts General Hospital, Boston, Massachusetts*

I. INTRODUCTION

Huntington's disease (HD) is an autosomal dominant neurodegenerative disease characterized by disordered movement, intellectual disturbance, and psychiatric illness. Rapid advances in our knowledge of the neurobiology and genetics of HD have been made in the past decade. The genetic defect responsible for the illness has been localized to chromosome 4 (1). In addition, there have been numerous studies examining both neurochemical features of HD as well as animal models (2,3). Symptoms typically develop insidiously in midlife. Although chorea is the most conspicuous symptom, intellectual deterioration and psychiatric disturbances are responsible for most of the functional impairment. A large number of studies have characterized the cognitive impairment present in HD. The present chapter reviews the neuropsychological features of HD, as well as correlative studies using neuroimaging, neuropathology, and neurochemistry. Abnormalities in at-risk individuals are also addressed.

II. NEUROPATHOLOGY AND NEUROCHEMISTRY

The most consistent and probably the earliest pathological changes in HD occur in the caudate and putamen. These changes are first seen in the

**Current affiliation:* The University of Melbourne, Victoria, Australia

medial paraventricular portions of the caudate nucleus, in the tail of the caudate nucleus, and in the dorsal part of the putamen (4). The spiny projection neurons of the striatum are preferentially vulnerable, whereas aspiny interneurons are relatively resistant to degeneration (5).

Consistent with this, neurotransmitters localized to striatal spiny neurons such as γ-aminobutyric acid (GABA), substance P, enkephalin, and dynorphin are preferentially depleted in HD striatum, as well as striatal projection sites. Our own studies have shown that depletions of both GABA and substance P correlate with the pathological grade and estimates of neuronal loss in HD striatum (6,7). In contrast, neurochemical markers for aspiny neurons, such as somatostatin and neuropeptide Y, show approximately threefold increases in HD striatum (5). A histochemical marker for these neurons is the enzyme reduced nicotinamide-adenine dinucleotide phosphate (NADPH)-diaphorase. With this technique we have shown that NADPH-diaphorase neurons are relatively spared by the HD pathological process (8). We have also used acetylcholinesterase staining to show that the large cholinergic aspiny neurons are also spared (9) by the disease process, as are afferent projections to the striatum, such as those containing dopamine.

Whether or not pathological changes occur in cerebral cortex has been a matter of debate. Several authors have noted a loss of neurons in layers 3, 5, and 6 of the cerebral cortex (10–13); however, the implication of these changes is unclear, since anoxia can affect the same neurons, and HD patients frequently die of bronchopneumonia or choking. Most authors have stressed atrophy of the frontal cortex, but others have reported more widespread changes. A recent morphometric study that addressed this issue showed a 60% reduction in the cross-sectional area of the caudate, putamen, and globus pallidus (14). In addition, there was a 20–30% reduction in the area of the cerebral cortex at each of five coronal levels from the anterior frontal to the parietal–occipital fissure. The mean thickness of the cortical ribbon was consistently smaller than in controls, with a maximal 16% reduction at the caudate–putamen–accumbens level. White matter was lost in proportion to the loss of cerebral cortex. The atrophy in cerebral cortex and white matter was similar among patients with differing grades of striatal atrophy, suggesting that these changes occur early in the disease process and are not progressive. There was also evidence of atrophy in the hippocampus.

Although postmortem studies have been equivocal in attempting to demonstrate neuronal loss in HD cerebral cortex, biopsy studies have reported abnormalities (15). Frontal lobe biopsies show neuronal loss, particularly in laminae V and VI, accompanied by gliosis and an accumulation of lipopigment. Cudkowicz and Kowall recently made counts of both neuropeptide Y-containing and pyramidal neurons in the cingulate gyrus and superior frontal cortex of HD brains (16). There were no changes in numbers of neuropeptide Y neurons, but there were significant (25–30%) reductions in the numbers of pyramidal neurons. The loss of pyramidal neurons did not correlate with the pathological grade of striatal atrophy. Consistent with these results, we have found small depletions in glutamate (a marker of pyramidal neurons) in HD cerebral cortex (7). In contrast, there are significant increases in concentrations of somatostatin, neuropeptide Y, cholecystokinin, and to a lesser extent, substance P (5,6,17). These neurochemical changes also do not correlate with the pathological grade of striatal atrophy.

The recent neuropathological and neurochemical studies are, therefore, consistent with early involvement of cerebral cortex in HD, which does not correlate with the striatal pathology. In contrast, subcortical afferent projection systems to cerebral cortex are spared. (18). The pathology in cerebral cortex appears to affect cortical pyramidal projection neurons preferentially, whereas neuropeptide-containing interneurons are spared. The previous failure to find consistent abnormalities in the cerebral cortex of HD patients led to the hypothesis that dementia in HD was subcortical in origin and, therefore, caused by lesions in the neostriatum. The results reviewed in the foregoing suggest, however, that cortical involvement may play a role.

III. NEUROPSYCHOLOGICAL FEATURES OF ESTABLISHED DISEASE

A. General

Since the time of George Huntington's description (19), progressive dementia has been recognized as a hallmark of the disease (20). The memory component of this decline is prominent and will be addressed separately in a later section. Early studies suggested that the pattern of cognitive loss was global on Wechsler Adult Intelligence Scale (WAIS) examination (21,22), with the possible exception of the information subtest (22). In one study, patients were also assessed with the Halstead Neuropsychological Battery and with Reitan's Trail-Making Test, and it was concluded that deficits were seen across a broad spectrum of cognitive activities, including memory, problem solving, concept formation, verbal storage, alertness, and concentration (22). Yet other anecdotal reports (23) and limited studies (24–26) disclosed disproportionate impairment of performance IQ (PIQ) compared with verbal IQ (VIQ) in the WAIS. This disparity was largely attributable to poor performance on the digit–symbol substitution

(DSS) and object assembly subtests (26). Difficulty in changing "mental set" was also revealed on the "trails B" test (26).

The major methodological fault with these early studies was combining patients with different stages of the disease into a single group, since severe cognitive deterioration in advanced disease results in impairment of almost all intellectual functions (27,28). One possible approach to this problem is to separate patients into groups based on duration of disease. A second difficulty was with the use of the WAIS as the principal neuropsychological test. Although it has the advantages of being well-known and relatively easy to administer and score, it is not designed to demarcate accurately a variety of cognitive attributes the assessment of which may be desirable in HD.

These difficulties were partly addressed by Caine et al. (29), who made a lengthy and detailed assessment of 18 patients within 6 years of diagnosis. Mean WAIS full-scale IQ (FSIQ) was 92, indicating only mild impairment on the functions assessed by this test. No significant difference between VIQ and PIQ was found, although some performance subtests were notably impaired (DSS and picture arrangement). Language function was intact, but some elements of a "parietal lobe battery" such as drawing to verbal command and block construction were affected. Of most interest, however, were the qualitative assessments made during their extensive evaluations: "Particular difficulty with organization, planning, and sequential arrangement of information, even when it is presented" was noted. The patients frequently appeared to be "overwhelmed" by too much information. Recall on demand was difficult, although the required items were often successfully recalled at a later time. There was loss of the fine details of remote memory. Many activities could not be initiated spontaneously; but if events were planned and structured, participation was eager and sustained. Irritability and lability of affect were also noted. It was concluded that the syndrome was more like that seen with frontal lobe lesions than that of global dementia.

Another group compared recently diagnosed patients (less than 1 year after diagnosis) with "advanced" patients (3–15 years after diagnosis) (27). The FSIQ was normal (mean 100) in the recently diagnosed group, although significantly different from a large control group matched for age and education (mean 110). The PIQ, but not VIQ, was also significantly reduced in the recently diagnosed group compared with controls; the difference being accounted for by the DSS and picture arrangement subtests. The PIQ was 10 points below VIQ in advanced patients: both these scores and FSIQ (mean 86) were significantly less than those of the recently diagnosed group. The advanced patients were significantly different from controls on all subtests, but from the recently diagnosed groups, only on

DSS and picture arrangement. Memory was strikingly abnormal in the recently diagnosed patients, as assessed by the Wechsler Memory Scale (WMS) and on Petersen short-term memory tests, and did not decline further in advanced disease. The conclusions reached were that advanced disease is "nonfocal," but that early disease is "focal," with differential involvement of verbal, spatial, perceptual, and arithmetic functions.

A wider range of functions was studied by Moses et al. (28), who applied the Luria–Nebraska Neuropsychological Battery to early-, mid-, and late-stage patients (respectively diagnosed for less than 1 year, 3–5½ years, and over 6 years). Early patients differed from controls on the memory and visual scales only: midstage and late-stage patients differed from controls on all 11 primary and 3 secondary scales. Early patients differed significantly from those with midstage disease only on the motor scale, but from the late-stage patients on all scales, except rhythm. These results argued for a pattern of focal problems (memory and visual) emerging early against a background of gradually developing generalized dysfunction. An analogous approach was used by Josiassen et al. (30), who used a wide battery of tests on a group of patients diagnosed for less than a year, a more advanced group diagnosed for over a year (mean 3½ years), and an asymptomatic at-risk group. The results were pooled and subjected to factor analysis, leading to a six factor solution in which visuospatial, followed by verbal, followed by flexibility accounted for over half the variance. Recently diagnosed patients were significantly worse than controls on the visuospatial and motor factors, and were significantly better than the more-advanced patients only on flexibility. There was no significant difference between any of the groups for the verbal factor.

Two other studies have compared "recently diagnosed" patients (mean period since diagnosis 2–3 years) (31), or patients with "mild early-stage symptoms" (mean FSIQ 97) (32), with at-risk and control populations. Both found PIQs more impaired than VIQs in patient populations by about 10 points; with particular deficits in the arithmetic and digit span subtests of VIQ and the DSS test of the PIQ. Information, similarities, vocabulary, and picture completion tasks were all spared. One of these studies also showed disproportionately low memory quotients on the WMS, as well as significant disturbances in visual perception of mosaic discrepancies and in "directionality" on Money's Road Map Test (32).

Two methodological difficulties are encountered with studies that separate patient groups according to the length of the illness. First, although progressive deterioration is inevitable, the actual rate is quite variable (33). In particular, younger patients tend to progress more rapidly, as would be expected if the disease is present ab initio: their age of first clinical manifestation, therefore, would give a rough estimate of the speed of progression to that point. Second, most neurologists diagnose the disorder on the basis of a positive family history, together with the typical movement disorder, although, in all large series, a sizeable proportion of patients have a psychiatric disorder as their first symptom (33–35), and subtle mental and personality changes frequently accompany or precede the chorea or rigidity. The difficulty of pinning down the precise onset of these symptoms retrospectively, combined with the variable propensity of patients to seek medical attention, renders group stratification by duration of symptoms or length of diagnosis rather problematic. Another approach is to subdivide patients on the basis of their degree of functional impairment. At first sight, it may seem tautologous to correlate progressive cognitive decline with progressive functional impairment, but this is only so if the former occurs in a global fashion, and is entirely responsible for the latter.

Such an approach was adumbrated by Brandt et al. (36), who divided their patients into early and late groups on the basis of duration of chorea (less than 1 year and greater than 1 year, respectively) and found the expected disparity between VIQ, PIQ, and MIQ within the groups (increasingly severely affected in that order), with significant declines in only VIQ and PIQ between the two groups. This conventional approach was enhanced by quantitative assessment of chorea and motor impairment, as well as by rating with an activities-of-daily-living (ADL) scale. It was found that duration of chorea or of behavioral symptoms was only weakly correlated with PIQ, VIQ, and MQ scores, but that severity of motor impairment and, to a lesser extent, severity of chorea were strongly correlated with these measures. Interestingly, the ADL score correlated as well with duration of disease as with motor impairment and chorea. No attempt to correlate ADL score with cognitive function was reported, however.

A widely used functional scale was developed by Shoulson and Fahn (37) and, subsequently, slightly adapted (38). It assesses capacity for employment, handling financial affairs, managing domestic duties, and performing ADLs, as well as assessing the most appropriate care facility. One report of a large number of patients followed for several years showed that functional score declined in almost all, although the rate of decline varied considerably (39). Functional decline correlated independently with depression and with a simple semiquantitative measure of cognitive decline (the Mini-Mental State Examination; 40) but not with motor disability. If somatic symptoms of depression were removed, the depressed affect no longer correlated with functional score. Another study compared patients with "early" HD (Shoulson and Fahn stages I and II, mean functional score 8.4) with age and education-matched controls, and with age, education, and disability score-matched multiple sclerosis patients (41). Assessment was with the Boston/Rochester Neuropsychological Screening Test, designed to highlight broad areas of functioning that are not adequately assessed by the WAIS. The HD patients were significantly impaired on confrontational naming, verbal fluency (by letter and category), trails B time, visual immediate recall, verbal delayed recall and recognition, and visual copying. Repetition, reading, narrative content, and long-term memory (US presidents) were intact. The same group (42) later assessed a large group of Shoulson and Fahn stage I and II patients separately, using a different, wide battery of neuropsychological tests condensed by factor analysis of intertest correlations to four factors: complex psychomotor, verbal memory, visuospatial, and general intelligence. Mean functional score was highly correlated with all four factors, especially the first and third, which were also the only two factors to discriminate significantly between stage I and II patients. The authors suggested that verbal memory did not distinguish between the two groups because it is already prominently affected in stage I.

Perceptual–spatial impairment in unstaged HD was investigated by Potegal (43), who found that egocentric spatial localization (requiring pointing to a previously revealed, but now obscured, target after a side-step) was significantly impaired, in the absence of impairment on other apparently equally difficult tasks (such as pointing after a head turn). This was confirmed and extended by Brouwers et al. (44), who investigated unstaged, but presumably mildly affected, HD patients (mean FSIQ, 97) with various visuospatial tests. The patients were significantly impaired on mosaic comparisons (requiring visual discrimination), and on the "toward" section of Money's Road Map Test (which requires an imaginary 180° shift in orientation to predict left and right turns correctly while following a marked route and, therefore, is a test of egocentric spatial judgment). Visuoconstructive ability and route learning were normal. In contrast, a group of Alzheimer's disease patients had no particular difficulty with the toward section of the road map test, but were impaired on all other measures. This double dissociation was similar to that seen with frontal and parietal lesions, respectively (45). That other sensory–perceptual changes may occur early in HD was suggested by a longitudinal study of an at-risk and affected population with various tests from the Halstead–Reitan battery (46). Patients showed significant deficits on the face–hand, fingertip number writing, and speech sounds perception tests. Most at-risk individuals who changed status to affected during the study, and most of those with suspected, but not definite, disease, fell between the rest of the at-risk group and the definitely affected group, suggesting that such impairment does indeed occur early.

In summary, although many studies have been plagued by the methodological difficulties alluded to in the foregoing, it seems that Huntington's disease patients accumulate neuropsychological deficits in a predictable fashion as the disease progresses. Memory (as measured by the WMS) is affected disproportionately early, but then, may tend to stabilize. Visuospatial and sensory–perceptual skills, including egocentric location, are also affected early. They continue to suffer more severely than verbal skills, leading to the almost universal finding of a PIQ diminished in relationship to the VIQ. Particular subtests of the WAIS which contribute to this pattern are DSS and, to a lesser extent, picture arrangement and object assembly (for PIQ), with only arithmetic and sometimes digit span from the VIQ subtests displaying disproportionate declines. As the disease inexorably progresses, the early islands of relatively preserved function tend to disappear, resulting in a rather nonspecific severe and global impairment. The exception to this is language: aphasia is rarely, if ever, seen. Qualitative assessment of patients' behavior in the early and midstages of the disease calls to mind the picture seen with frontal lobe damage.

B. Memory

Memory is not a unitary process. There is now evidence that it operates through several parallel pathways, almost certainly with different anatomical substrates. These may be differentially affected by various disease processes. For HD, therefore, both the nature of the memory disturbance and the temporal pattern of its progression are of interest.

Memory may be divided into procedural and declarative systems (47,48). The former is *implicit,* and can be established only through performance. Skill learning and "priming" (see later discussion) are examples of the operation of this system (48), although some have held these two processes to be distinct (49,50). By contrast, declarative memory is *explicit:* it is available to conscious awareness. Such memories may be retrograde or anterograde, and may be tested using either recognition or free recall paradigms.

Procedural memory is known to be spared in amnesic patients (such as those with Korsakoff's syndrome) with damage to medial temporal/diencephalic structures (47,51). Here, HD patients differ: they are unable to learn skills such as mirror reading (52) or manual rotor pursuit (53) as well as amnesic or Alzheimer's disease (AD) patients, although they retain a better recognition memory for words used repeatedly in the former task (52). The design of the mirror-reading experiment may be criticized on the grounds that eye movements can be affected early in HD, impairing visual scanning. In the rotor experiment, however, target speed is adjusted to compensate for any performance difficulties caused by chorea or bradykinesia. The findings, therefore, appear valid.

In contrast, HD patients perform as well as amnesics, and significantly better than patients with AD, on verbal-priming tasks (54,55). These require either completion of a word from a pluripotent stem after previous "incidental" exposure to the word on a different task (lexical priming), or suggestion of a pairing word in relation to a cue word after previous incidental exposure to word pairs on a previous task (semantic priming). Learning has occurred if the previously suggested word or pair word is chosen more frequently than it is by chance without such previous exposure. Although AD patients do not perform well on this task, they are unimpaired in their ability to produce uncued words and word pairs—the task itself is not beyond them (55).

This double dissociation between AD and HD patients on motor skill learning and priming suggests that different anatomicopathological substrates underlie the procedural memory disorders of the two conditions; furthermore, that neither variety of procedural memory requires an intact medial temporal–diencephalic system, which bears the brunt of injury in amnesic patients (47). It can be hypothesized that motor skill learning requires intact striatal functioning; indeed, there is experimental evidence for this from ablative studies in primates (56), as well as from patients with early Parkinson's disease in some studies (57), but not others (58). Priming, in contrast, may depend on corticocortical associations (53,58).

The pattern of declarative memory loss has been extensively explored, both for anterograde and retrograde deficits. The latter are more difficult to assess, but the approach of Albert et al. (59) appears to be generally accepted. This utilizes a series of famous faces and events from various decades adjusted so that normal controls achieve 80–85% of possible correct answers for each decade, decreasing the likelihood of ceiling effects and of sample bias between the decades. With use of this protocol, HD patients display an equivalent loss for all decades tested ("flat" retrograde amnesia), as distinct from the temporally graded loss (greater for more recent decades) seen with Korsakoff's syndrome (60). Furthermore, early HD patients (within a year of diagnosis) display the same sort of flat retrograde deficit as advanced patients, although to a lesser extent (61). In this respect, HD may differ from AD. Although moderately to severely affected patients with AD display a flat retrograde loss (62), mildly demented AD patients display a graded temporal loss, similar to that seen in Korsakoff's amnesia (63).

The foregoing comments pertain to retrograde episodic memory—that is, the recall of material associated with particular spatial and temporal contexts. Another form of retrograde memory (in the broadest sense) is *semantic memory,* defined by Tulving (64) as "a system for receiving, retaining and transmitting information about the meaning of words, concepts and classification of concepts." This system covers such general knowledge as the rules of grammar, and is activated in tests of verbal fluency, and in the completion of highly structured sentences. In general, amnesic patients do not have severe deficits of semantic memory, in contradistinction to demented patients (65). Butters et al. (66) investigated patients with early (Shoulson and Fahn stages I and II) and advanced (stages III and IV) HD, as well as Korsakoff's patients, with the "F,A,S" test of verbal fluency (67). Normal controls were significantly better than all three patient groups, and amnesic patients were superior to advanced, but not early, HD patients. The amnesic group differed in another way, however: they produced significantly more perseverative errors than the controls or the HD patients. These observations were subsequently extended to include mild AD patients (68). The HD patients (stages II and III) were significantly less fluent on the F,A,S test than amnesics or the AD patients. The latter had the mildest deficit and, in fact, were not significantly different from an elderly control group. They did, however, commit more perseverative errors than the HD group, who were normal in this. When verbal fluency was assessed for semantic categories (animal names), there was no difference among the three patient groups. It has been suggested that this difference arises because AD patients have a preserved syntactical superstructure, with a reduction of the number of exemplars in each group (69), whereas HD patients' memory disorders reflect a generalized retrieval deficit (29,70).

Anterograde episodic memory in HD has received much attention in the literature, where the debate has centered around whether the observed deficits are due to initial difficulties with adequate encoding of the memory (71), with suitable search and retrieval strategies (70,72), or with a generalized motivational defect impairing effortful, but not automatic, recall (73). Normal controls remember high imagery words (such as "house") more readily than those with low imagery (such as "thought") (74), presumably related to ease of encoding; and it was initially reported that HD patients failed to do so (71). Furthermore, when short-term memory tasks are administered to HD and Korsakoff's patients, only the latter benefit from increasing rehearsal time before distraction (75), lengthening intertrial intervals (76), or encouraging visual stimulus analysis (77). These are thought to assist in encoding, and their lack of effect in HD patients was initially thought to be evidence of severely impaired encoding or consolidation (storage). This postulated encoding deficit has been challenged, however: the pictorial memory deficit of HD patients (but not of Korsakoff's or AD patients) improved significantly when they were told a story about the picture during the learning process (78). Furthermore, by using word groups with greater "imageability" difference, Beatty and Butters were able to demonstrate a clear advantage in learning for the high-imagery words (72). More recently, it has been shown that HD patients, like normal controls, remember target words better if a strongly related word is presented for simultaneous learning and then used as a retrieval cue. If a weakly related word is colearned and a (different) strongly related word presented as a cue, recall is worse than if no cue is used at all, as is true for controls (79). Lastly, release from proactive interference has been demonstrated (72,73), although it may be lost in more advanced disease (80). This phenomenon describes the increasing difficulty seen when different lists are learned consecutively from the same semantic category (proactive interference) and the improvement that results if the next list is drawn from a different category (release). Its presence implies semantic encoding. It is possible that the maneuvers to improve encoding (such as prolonging rehearsal time) alluded to earlier were apparently ineffective because minor difficulties with encoding were overshadowed by major retrieval problems.

The postulated search-and-retrieval deficit might also explain another observation: free recall memory is more impaired than recognition memory (66,81). This relative sparing of recognition memory applies to only verbal stimuli, not being evident on testing with spatial, color, pattern, and facial stimuli (82) or olfaction (83). This tends to argue against the suggestion that HD patients perform better on recognition tasks simply because they are less effortful (73), although this explanation cannot be dismissed.

The stability of memory storage in HD after encoding has occurred is demonstrated by the normal rate of pictorial forgetting over a 1-week period, using a recognition paradigm (84). Here, HD patients behave similarly to amnesics associated with diencephalic damage (such as Korsakoff's) and differently from those associated with damage to the hippocampus (85).

Unfortunately, with the exceptions noted in the preceding section, most analyses of memory deficits in HD have been performed on a mixture of patients at varying stages of the disease. Investigations of the temporal pattern of decline in cognition and memory have often utilized the WMS (27,32,36,86) or portions thereof (30). The associative learning, logical memories, and visual reproduction subtests of the WMS are tests of anterograde episodic memory, assessed by recall (70). The memory section of the Luria–Nebraska battery, used by Moses et al. (28), also falls into this category. Such tests, therefore, would be expected to be sensitive to the pattern of memory impairment in HD; and it is not surprising that such studies have uniformly shown "memory impairment" early in the disease, even when the FSIQ was relatively unimpaired. Some reports have noted deterioration in memory (as measured by the WMS) with disease progression (27,28), whereas others report that no significant deterioration has been seen (30,36). It should be noted that striking differences in the pattern of memory impairment have been seen in experiments involving Korsakoff's amnesics, HD patients, and AD patients, for which the subjects have been closely matched for memory quotient as measured by the WMS (68,78).

In summary, it appears that patients with HD develop a problem with retrieval (or at least "effortful" retrieval) of anterograde and retrograde memories at an early stage. Encoding may be impaired, but is certainly still demonstrable. Storage is probably normal. The retrieval deficit results in relative sparing of recognition as opposed to free recall, at least for verbal material. It also results in a flat pattern of retrograde loss and in decreased semantic memory (as assessed by verbal fluency), without increased intrusions or perseverations. Procedural memory (for motor skills only) is also impaired. With disease progression, the memory impairment probably worsens, and may change qualitatively in that encoding may become disrupted (80). Table 1 compares the types of memory deficits found in various cognitive disorders.

C. Language

It has generally been held that language function is relatively preserved during the course of HD (29) (or at any rate during the early stages; 28,30), despite progressive dysarthria and a developing taciturnity that may progress to mutism (87). Exceptions to these findings have been reported lately: a general neuropsychological study by Caine et al. (41) disclosed difficulty with confrontational naming and decreased fluency of narrative language. Several recent studies dealing exclusively with language function in HD have confirmed a significant decrease in syntactic complexity (88–90), verbal fluency (91), and impairment of confrontational naming (89–92). In a small sample, it was found that most misnamings were semantically related, and thus unlikely to be due to impaired visuospatial perception (92), but a more recent and larger study has disputed this and concluded that the deficit is not linguistic (89). Only one of these groups has reported an increased number of paraphasic errors in spontaneous speech (88), and even then, the increase was not significant. Subtle comprehension deficits, as disclosed by the Token Test, have also been reported (89–91), but these have not been out of proportion to the overall degree of dementia (90).

In summary, syntactic complexity and confrontational naming are impaired in HD, the latter possibly on the basis of visuospatial perception difficulties. Language function, as distinct from speech, is otherwise probably unaffected, at least until late in the illness.

TABLE 1 Memory Deficits in Several Cognitive Disorders

	Procedural		Declarative					
			Retrograde		Anterograde			
	Motor	Priming	Episodic	Semantic	Encoding	Storage	Recall	Recognition (verbal)
Korsakoff's amnesia	–	–	Graded	–[a], intrusions	↓	–	↓	↓
Hippocampal damage			Sharply graded			↓		
Alzheimer's disease	–	↓	Graded (flat)[b]	–[a], intrusions	↓	–	↓	↓
Huntington's disease	↓	–	Flat	↓	–, (↓)[b]	–	↓	–

Note: "–" indicates relative, not absolute, preservation.
[a]For letter-cued lists, ↓ for category cued lists.
[b]In more advanced disease.

D. Correlation of Cognitive Deficits with Motor Abnormalities

The topic of correlation is of practical interest for two reasons: First, there may be a particular motor abnormality that correlates strongly with a specific neuropsychological impairment, thus possibly disclosing a common anatomicopathological substrate. Second, particular motor impairments may hinder the performance of those neuropsychological tasks that require a motor output, in the absence of related cognitive impairment.

Considering the first point, an analysis of the literature by Brackenridge revealed that in patients with juvenile-onset (aged 20 or younger), early (progression to) dementia was independently postively correlated both with onset age under 10 years and with rigidity (92). The usefulness of this study is open to question, however, as *early* and *dementia* were not defined. The Johns Hopkins group correlated a chorea score and a (nonchoreic) motor impairment score with WAIS and WMS results (36). The motor impairment score correlated significantly with all the WAIS subtests except information. The chorea score did not add significantly to the explanation of variance beyond that explained by the motor score for any subtest; but did correlate with all PIQ subtests except picture completion, and with the arithmetic and vocabulary subtests of the verbal scale. Both the motor and the chorea scores also correlated, although less strongly, with the memory quotient. The negative correlation of chorea with memory quotient has recently been supported using a mechanical "choreometer" (94). Instrumental measurement of nonchoreic motor abnormalities (reaction time, movement time) was performed by Girotti et al. (95), who also assessed chorea by counting involuntary movements in various body areas. They found no correlation between chorea and the other motor abnormalities, or between chorea and cognitive impairment. Reaction time and movement time did correlate strongly with such tasks as object assembly and a pattern scan–check visuospatial test, however. All in all, it would appear that nonchoreiform motor abnormalities are more strongly related to cognitive impairment than is chorea. The small number of studies and the lack of standardized assessment methods do not allow a more definite statement to be made.

Surprisingly little direct attention has been paid to the second point—whether the motor deficits of HD may result in spuriously bad performances on some "cognitive" tasks in the absence of cognitive impairment. An example might be the DSS subtest of the WAIS, which is often affected early in the course of the disease (discussed earlier) and which, to some extent, requires a rapid motor output. This was addressed by Wexler (96) who noted that a low-performing at-risk group performed poorly on the DSS subtest, despite a normal performance on the more purely motoric Fitts tapping task.

Starkstein et al. (97) administered the similar symbol digit modalities test in written and oral form: HD patients were equally impaired on each. Josiassen et al. (30) used factor analysis to organize an extensive battery of tasks into six factors: motor steadiness (a mechanical measure of chorea) and Reitan's Trails B contributed to the motor (steadiness) factor, but did not contribute to the visuospatial factor under which the DSS subtest was subsumed. From this scanty information, therefore, it would seem likely that even on cognitive tests assessed by motor output, HD patients' deficits cannot be explained solely on the basis of mechanical difficulties.

E. Specificity of the Neuropsychological Profile

Are the neuropsychological deficits of early- to midstage HD specific enough for it to be distinguished from other causes of dementia? In answer to this question, two groups have reported that simple standardized bedside examinations can differentiate between HD and AD in 80–90% of cases. By using the Mini-Mental State examination (40), Brandt et al. (98) found that HD patients performed better on date orientation and recall of three items, and that AD patients performed better on serial 7s, when subgroups within each disease group were matched for total score. Salmon et al. (90) utilized the Dementia Rating Scale (100), and showed that HD patients perform better than AD patients on the recall and orientation (but, surprisingly, not on the recognition) items of the memory subtest. The HD patients did worse than AD patients on the verbal repetition, double-alternating movements, and possible one of the semantic verbal fluency items, of the initiation subtest. In both studies, it was evident that discrimination was less effective in patients with more-advanced cognitive decline. This is not surprising in view of the tendency of the focal deficits of HD to be superceded by a global intellectual decline later in the illness.

Another report compared patients with multiple sclerosis and with HD, matched for (good) functional status (41). The profiles were very similar over an extensive battery of neuropsychological tasks, but the HD patients performed significantly less well on verbal recognition memory, visual recall memory, and arithmetic. Although not dysphasic, they also displayed a poverty of written narrative expression.

These studies lead naturally to consideration of the concept of *subcortical dementia* and *cortical dementia.* The former term was first published by Albert et al. in 1974 with reference to the cognitive decline seen in progressive supranuclear palsy (101) and, subsequently, by McHugh and Folstein for HD (25). The cardinal features of a subcortical dementia are said to be apathy, slowness of information processing, and difficulty with attention, concentration, recall memory, abstraction and categorization, word list generation, and visuospatial tasks. In contrast, cortical dementias have been said to be characterized by aphasia, apraxia, and memory impairment owing to poor encoding with recall and recognition both affected (102). This concept has been extensively reviewed recently (102–105); but has also been attacked (106,107), partly on the grounds that the pathology in representative diseases of each class (such as Alzheimer's and HD) is both cortical *and* subcortical. This is true, but merely argues that the terms are infelicitous. More serious is the assertion that neuropsychological testing cannot reliably distinguish between examples of each category. This point is as yet unsettled, and its resolution will depend on careful testing of large numbers of patients with varying diseases matched, as far as possible, for overall cognitive status. Until such time, the heuristic usefulness of this two-group concept is open to question. It has been useful, however, in reinforcing the idea that patients with different dementias dement in different ways, of which HD and AD diseases are prime examples.

F. Psychiatric Features

A brief mention of the psychiatric manifestations of HD is important, as they are very common, are to some extent treatable, if not recognized may interfere with cognitive assessment, and often limit the ability of relatives to care for the affected patient at home. Huntington himself noted that "the tendency to insanity, and sometimes that form of insanity which leads to suicide, is marked" (19). Although not all reports use currently accepted *DSM-III* criteria, rendering comparisons difficult, affective disorders have usually been held to be predominant. In a community-based series, a major depressive disorder was found in 32%, and a bipolar disorder in 8% (35). Major depressive or dysthymic syndromes were also found in 10 of 30 clinic patients (34) and were the most common single psychiatric syndromes in this population. Episodes of depression may precede other manifestations of the disease by several years (25,94,108) and, indeed, are twice as common before the onset of other symptoms in HD as they are before the onset of AD (109). Such episodes (or at least the associated somatic symptoms; 34) do respond to antidepressant medication (110). The natural inclination to dismiss all depressive symptoms in HD as "reactive" would therefore seem unsupportable.

A schizophreniform psychosis may also occur in HD, but is less common (34,35). Paranoid delusions and even auditory hallucinations may be seen. Response to antipsychotic agents is variable and often incomplete (34,110).

Irritability, aggression, and apathy have been noted frequently in Huntington's disease. The apathy may be "situational" and, therefore, capable of being overcome in a structured setting (29,34). Burns et al. (111) have recently constructed apathy and irritability scales for administration to relatives, which seem to have reasonable validity as well as good interrater and test–retest reliability. Together with a scale for aggression, these were administered to relatives of HD and AD patients. The prevalence of apathy and irritability were similar, although aggression was about twice as common in HD. In a subsample roughly matched for cognitive dysfunction, however, the only significant difference was that the HD patients were more apathetic.

Thus the psychiatric and personality changes in HD are neither rare nor trivial and need to be considered carefully during each patient assessment.

IV. NEUROPSYCHOLOGICAL DEFICITS IN AT-RISK INDIVIDUALS

As the genetic defect in HD is present ab initio, and as the disease itself evolves over 15 or 20 years from an onset that may be very difficult to pinpoint exactly, it is to be expected that subtle neuropsychological abnormalities will occur in gene-carrying at-risk individuals before the onset of overt disease. Three broadly different approaches may be used for their detection: first, a group of at-risk persons may be compared with a control group—any significant differences are assumed to arise as a result of about half the at-risk group being presymptomatic gene carriers. Fedio et al. (32) noted significantly poorer performance by the at-risk group on the digit span subtest of the WAIS, on a visuospatial (mosaic comparison) test, and on the reversed segment of Money's Road Map Test. A similar study in children aged 5–15 at primary risk (50% risk: affected parent) or secondary risk (25% risk: affected grandparent, asymptomatic parent) disclosed significant disparities between subtest scores on the Weschler Intelligence Scale for children—Revised, despite normal overall and individual subtest scores. These disparities were found in 50% of primary at-risk children, 21% of secondary at-risk group, and only 5% of controls (112). Two similar studies have attempted to overcome the dilution of the at-risk group with non-gene-carriers by stratifying the group's total performance and analyzing the strata separately for individual subtests. This potentially involves a circular argument. Wexler (96) found that the low (performance) at-risk group differed from low controls only on the continuous paired-associate memory task, and failed to differ from HD patients only on this test. Of interest is that the DSS subtest and a test of verbal fluency failed to distinguish the low at-risk and low control groups. Another such study utilizing the WAIS, the Halstead–Reitan battery, the Bender Gestalt, the Wisconsin Card-Sorting Test, and an assortment of other tasks, revealed that the tests that separated the low-performance from the high-performance at-risk groups were the DSS subtest, the Tactile Performance Test, and Trails A and B. This pattern of deficits was similar to that seen with symptomatic patients in the same study (30). It should be noted that anxiety about the implications of neuropsychological testing may itself adversely affect the performance of the at-risk group (96).

The second broad approach to recognizing neuropsychological deficits in at-risk individuals is to perform a screening battery of tests and then follow a cohort for a lengthy period, retrospectively seeking differences in those individuals who have developed overt disease. Two reports document a group of 88 at-risk subjects followed for 15–20 years, during which time 28 had developed HD (113,114). Bender Gestalt recall scores (but not clinical ratings) were significantly lower in the 22 "premorbids" for which they were available, than in the 46 other at-risk subjects tested (113). More striking were the Wechsler–Bellvue (later, WAIS) disparities between the still normal at-risk group and the premorbid group (114). The FSIQ, VIQ, and PIQ were all significantly different. If the premorbid subjects who had developed overt symptoms within 2 years of initial testing were removed, 17 premorbids who became symptomatic 6–18 years after first assessment remained. These late-onset premorbids were still significantly different from the asymptomatic at-risk group on FSIQ, VIQ, and especially PIQ and were not significantly different from the 11 early-onset premorbid individuals, although they scored higher than the latter on each of these three measures. Unfortunately, subtest scores were not reported. Nevertheless, despite the significant differences, an attempt at prediction based on these results resulted in a hit/miss ratio of only 3:1, even without cross-validation (114). Another group reported 17 symptomatic and 33 at-risk subjects followed for up to 10 years: 6 of the latter developed overt disease within this time; and 5 more had "suspected early signs." A discriminant function based on sensory–percepetual tests correctly classified 95% of the entire cohort. Although there were too few premorbids to analyze formally, all but 1 had discriminant scores between the two group means (46). The tentative suggestion is that subtle sensory–perceptual deficits may occur in premorbid individuals.

The third approach to detecting abnormalities in premorbid individuals relies on prediction of gene-carrying status using DNA-linkage studies (1). In such studies, subjects should undergo neuropsychological testing before being appraised of their status to avoid confounding psychological variables. Jason et al. studied ten subjects in this fashion, seven of whom had a high probability of being gene carriers by linkage analysis (115). All were at least 12 years younger than the onset age of their affected parents. A comprehensive battery of tests were conducted by neuropsychologists blinded to the result of the linkage studies. Unambiguous clinical impairments were seen in some carriers (but no noncarriers) on the Wisconsin Card-Sorting Test, the visual recall subtest of the WMS, delayed recall of the Rey–Osterreith complex figure, and a free-drawing task. Borderline impairment was seen in some carriers on tests of verbal and design fluency. There was no difference in FSIQ, VIQ, PIQ, or memory quotient (from the WMS) between the groups, although it must be remembered that there were only three non-gene-carrying subjects. The authors concluded that deficits in premorbid individuals were predominantly visuospatial (especially visuospatial memory) and "frontal" (card-sorting test).

In conclusion, there is no doubt that there are statistically significant differences in neuropsychological performance between asymptomatic gene carriers, as a group, and the non-gene-carrying at-risk population. These abnormalities have differed somewhat in different studies, but are obviously reminiscent of the pattern of involvement seen in early disease (discussed earlier). In particular, visuospatial difficulties feature prominently. It is one thing to establish differences between groups, however, and quite another to apply such findings to individual cases. These studies confirm the hypothesis that there is a long presymptomatic period marked by the gradual accumulation of subtle deficits, rather than a sudden onset in middle-age. They do not offer the possibility of confident diagnosis in the (hitherto) presymptomatic phase of the disease.

V. ANCILLARY INVESTIGATIVE TECHNIQUES

A. Positron Emission Tomography, Single Photon Emission Computed Tomography, and Xenon-133 Regional Cerebral Blood Flow

1. Positron Emission Tomography in Established Disease

It has been known for a century that local brain function modulates local brain blood flow and metabolism (116). The advent of positron emission tomgraphy (PET) has enabled regional brain metabolism and blood flow to be studied in numerous disease states, including HD (117). Unlike PET, which is only available in specialized centers, single photon emission computed tomography (SPECT) uses readily available and relatively more stable isotopes, such as ^{99m}Tc and ^{123}I and, therefore, can be performed in most nuclear medicine departments equipped with a tomographic gamma camera. Unfortunately, these isotopes are difficult to incorporate into valid tracers of metabolism, although blood flow can now be imaged reliably (118) Xenon-113 has been used to evaluate total cerebral blood flow for some time, but local cortical perfusion can now be ascertained using radiation dectors applied closely to the head (119)

The PET studies of brain metabolism in HD have utilized 2-[^{18}F]fluoro-2-deoxy-D-glucose ([^{18}F]FDG), which is phosphorylated by brain and subsequently remains trapped in the cell. Such uptake primarily reflects synaptic activity (120). Several such studies have shown caudate hypometabolism in the resting state, even in early cases that have yet to develop caudate atrophy on CT scan (121–124). Furthermore, even in patients with CT findings suggestive of cortical atrophy, there is no evidence of cortical hypometabolism per unit volume (122,123). Young and co-workers (123) found that caudate [^{18}F]FDG uptake decreased over and above the effect of atrophy with progressive functional impairment as measured by the Shoulson and Fahn scale (37), and they noted only putaminal hypometabolism in more advanced cases. They also noted an increase in thalamic uptake (relative to HD cortex, but not to control thalami) such as would be expected as a result of decreased inhibitory input from the pallidum. In contrast, Kuhl et al. (121) found no correlation between disease stage or severity of dementia and the degree of striatal hypometabolism. Neither they nor Hayden et al. (124) noted sparing of the putamen in early disease, or increased thalamic uptake in the patient group. Kuhl et al. (121) did note that the frontal/parietal cortex uptake ratio was reduced in some patients (although absolute values were within normal limits), but this did not correlate with dementia.

Young and co-workers have attempted to correlate various neurological and neuropsychological features of the disease with patterns of hypo- and hypermetabolism (123,125). Total functional capacity (as measured by the Shoulson scale; 38), chorea, bradykinesia, dyskinesia, and slowed saccades all correlated with each other and with the degree of striatal hypometabolism (especially that of the putamen). Dystonia failed to correlate with striatal hypometabolism, but did correlate with increased thalamic uptake (123). In contrast, caudate, but not putaminal, hypometabolism correlated with a verbal subtest from the WMS, although visual memory and WAIS FSIQ failed to correlate with decreased uptake in either area. The PIQ, and its digit–symbol component, correlated with hypometabolism in both areas. Hayden et al. (124) have also shown that caudate hypometabolism does not correlate with chorea. Given the predominantly prefrontal origin of caudate afferents, and the predominantly motor and premotor cortical origin of putaminal afferents, these results are perhaps not unexpected.

2. *Positron Emission Tomography of At-Risk Subjects*

Given the generally accepted presence of caudate hypometabolism in early disease, before evidence of caudate atrophy on CT scanning, the obvious question is whether PET scanning might detect asymptomatic gene carriers. Hayden et al. (126) examined 13 at-risk patients by DNA linkage analysis and PET. Eight were determined to be probable carriers, and 3 of these had caudate metabolic rates more than 2 standard deviations below normal values. One of these subsequently became symptomatic on follow-up. Of the 5 determined to be at low risk of inheriting the genetic defect, 1 had abnormally low caudate metabolism. The authors' contention was that this represented genetic recombination, but this is a circular argument, as the linkage studies were used to evaluate the specificity of the PET scans. Further follow-up of this patient is required.

Mazziotta et al. (127) studied 58 at-risk patients (asymptomatic for motor signs), 34% of whom on age and sex adjustment of affected parent would be expected to be gene carriers. Eighteen (31%) of the at-risk group had caudate metabolic rates of less than the 99.5% confidence limit for the control group. Of the 18, 4 have subsequently become symptomatic, whereas none of the remaining 40 have done so. Of course, some of the asymptomatic at-risk group may have manifested cognitive or psychiatric abnormalities, which may have led to a falsely high "hit rate" compared with other studies. In contrast, Young et al. (128) studied 29 at-risk patients, and failed to discover caudate hypometabolism in any. However, this may have been partly due to technical differences in the method of calculation: the spread of normal values was considerably wider in this report than in the others.

3. Single Photon Emission Computed Tomography

The use of SPECT with ^{99m}Tc-labeled hexamethylpropyleneamine oxime was performed by Smith et al. (129) on six patients with clinically manifest HD and caudate atrophy. All had caudate hypoperfusion out of proportion to the atrophy. One further patient with a positive family history and depression, without other signs of the disease or caudate atrophy, also showed caudate hypometabolism.

4. Xenon-113

Studies by ^{133}Xe regional cerebral blood flow (RCBF) were conducted with eight detectors per hemisphere in 16 patients with mild to moderate HD (130). The RCBF was significantly decreased in frontoparietotemporal regions. This reduction correlated with cognitive impairment as assessed by Mini-Mental State testing (40). No such changes were found in six at-risk individuals, although four of these were 19 or more years younger than the average age of symptom development in their pedigrees.

A more intriguing study measured ^{113}Xe RCBF with 16 detectors per hemisphere in 14 patients with mild to moderate HD in the resting state, as well as during an automated "frontal" neuropsychological task (Wisconsin Card Sorting: WCS), and during an automated digit-matching task (131).

The latter is similar to the WCS in the visual recognition and motor output required, but is unimpaired in HD. No differences between controls and patients were seen in the resting state or during either task, although it was notable that dorsolateral frontal RCBF increased greatly during the WCS, especially when RCBF changes during number matching were subtracted. No correlation between caudate atrophy on CT and RCBF was seen, except during WCS during which increasing atrophy was correlated with *higher* flow. The level of performance on WCS was not correlated with RCBF, although the trend was for increasing flow to be associated with poorer performance. In contrast, there is a strong positive correlation between performance on WCS and prefrontal RCBF in Parkinson's disease (132). The authors postulate that frontal dysfunction may arise through different pathophysiological mechanisms—frontal cortical disease in AD (in which resting prefrontal RCBF may be reduced; 133), frontal deafferentation in Parkinson's disease, and frontal deefferentation ("outflow block") with caudate destruction in HD.

In conclusion, the picture that emerges is one of striatal hypometabolism and decreased blood flow, which precedes caudate atrophy, and may even be present in some premorbid individuals. Most studies have not shown the cortex to be affected per unit volume, even though cortical atrophy is evident later in the disease process. Indeed, there is even a suggestion that prefrontal blood flow may be abnormally increased during frontal tasks.

B. Computed Tomography Scanning

Three ratios are traditionally derived from the CT scan at about the level of the interventricular foramina: CC/OT (the ratio of intercaudate distance to the distance bewteen the outer tables of the skull at the same level), FH/CC (the ratio of the distance between the frontal horn tips to intercaudate distance), and FH/OT (both taken at the level of the frontal horn tips). Such ratios compensate for differences in image magnification. The first is an absolute and the second a relative measure of caudate atrophy (the frontal horns tending to widen during the disease). Both have discriminated successfully between patients and controls (134–137). An FH/CC ratio of less than 2 will be found in 85–90% of patients, but also in 15% of controls (136). Naturally, specificity increases, but sensitivity declines, if a lower figure is used. These CT measurements have been consistently normal in at-risk populations (136,137), a situation not improved with more modern scanners (122–128). As the disease progresses, the initial caudate atrophy steadily worsens and is joined by cortical atrophy (with sulcal widening and ventricular dilatation) that tends to start frontally and spread caudally (86).

Various attempts have been made to correlate the pattern and degree of atrophy with specific features of the disease. Sax et al. (86) performed multiple regression analysis with age, chorea, CC/OT ratio, and FH/OT ratio, against the subtests of the WAIS and the WMS. The CC/OT ratio correlated with (and made a significant contribution to) VIQ, PIQ, and MQ, as well as a number of their component subtests. The FH/OT ratio correlated (less strongly) with the similarities subtest of the WAIS and the mental control subtest of the WMS. Severity of chorea did not correlate with any of the neuropsychological parameters. A similar study (97) reported significant correlations between the CC/OT ratio and cognition; and in particular with visual conceptual tracking, set shifting, and psychomotor speed as revealed by the DSS test and parts A and B of the trail-making test. The CC/OT ratio was also correlated with eye-movement abnormalities (which are common in HD) and with an ADL score, but not with chorea or other motor impairment. The FH/OT ratio correlated only with motor impairment, and frontal cortical atrophy failed to correlate with any of the foregoing variables. In light of the these results, it is interesting to note recent work in primates, for which five segregated corticostriatal "loops" have been described (138). The caudate receives input from dorsolateral frontal, orbitofrontal, and limbic cortices, and from the frontal eyefields. The motor-related cortex, however, connects with the putamen. Another recent study (42) found that the CC/OT ratio was strongly correlated with total functional capacity on the Shoulson scale (38) and with three of four neuropsychological parameters (derived by factor analysis of a large number of tests): complex psychomotor, verbal memory, and visuospatial. The FH/OT ratio correlated only with verbal memory.

In summary, CT scanning may be of ancillary help in confirming the diagnosis in symptomatic patients, but its clinical usefulness is otherwise limited. In contrast, several studies have demonstrated that typical cognitive impairment (but not motor symptoms) correlate with caudate, rather than cortical atrophy, at least in the early and midstages of the disease. These correlations are limited, however, by the inaccuracy of CT scanning in the detection of cortical atrophy.

C. Evoked Potentials

The electrophysiological correlate of dementia that has received most attention recently is the P_{300}. This is a late (300-msec), positive, presumably cortically generated potential related to the conscious recognition of different auditory (or occasionally visual) stimuli randomly interspersed among background stimuli of the same modality (the "oddball paradigm"). Earlier responses (N_{100}, P_{200}) are also elicited in response to the frequent background stimulus.

Rosenberg et al. (139) studied 13 symptomatic HD patients, with a mean illness duration of 4.8 years, using both auditory and visual oddball paradigms. Using a 3 SD (one-tailed) confidence limit, 5 of the 13 had an abnormal auditory P_{300} latency, and 6 an abnormal visual P_{300} latency. Eight had at least one abnormality. There was no correlation between cognitive-evoked potential testing and abnormalities on EEG, CT scanning, or WAIS scores. Another recent report has addressed the question of auditory P_{300} abnormalities in an asymptomatic population at risk for Huntington's disease (140). Unfortunately, there were no significant differences from the control subjects.

Differences in the patterns of cognitive-evoked potential abnormalities between AD and two subcortical dementias (Parkinson's disease and HD) have recently been reported (141). All three dementing processes produced significant P_{300} prolongation, compared with age-matched controls, and the two subcortical dementia groups, but not the AD group, displayed significant prolongation of the N_{100} response to the frequent background stimuli as well. The AD group appeared to be considerably more cognitively impaired than the other two, giving credence to the suggestion that the N_{100} and P_{200} prolongation in the latter groups represent real differences from AD.

In summary, cognitive-evoked potential testing, although interesting, does not appear to be either as sensitive or as specific as clinical evaluation.

VI. NEUROPATHOLOGICAL SUBSTRATE FOR COGNITIVE AND BEHAVIORAL CHANGES: STRIATUM VERSUS CORTEX

The pathology of HD affects the cortex as well as the striatum at an early stage. The question of to what extent, or even whether, the observed neuropsychological deficits might be secondary to striatal damage, therefore, is difficult to answer from studies of the disease in isolation. As has already been pointed out in previous sections, PET and similar studies suggest that caudate hypometabolism is present earlier in the disease than are cortical metabolic changes, and on CT scanning, caudate atrophy correlates with cognitive impairment more closely than does cortical atrophy. Beyond this, the problem is best approached by considering the manifestations of discrete striatal lesions occurring on a different pathological basis. Of course, these do not result in the selective neuronal dropout seen in HD.

The most thorough human study to date has been that by Mendez et al. (142), who reported 12 patients with caudate infarction or abscess. Presenting behavioral changes were apathy, disinhibition, or an apparent psychosis. Extensive neuropsychological testing of 7 disclosed difficulty with verbal fluency, problem solving (WCS and Porteus Mazes), and recall, but not recognition memory. These deficits were not related to the site of the lesion. Other reports of patients with caudate pathology (usually hemorrhage) have disclosed memory problems, language disturbances, and abulia in some cases (143–146). These deficits, apart from the language problems, are obviously reminiscent of those seen in early HD. More precise anatomicobehavioral correlation has been attempted: the dorsolateral caudate head is predominantly connected to the dorsolateral frontal cortex (138), and lesions of either result in apathy (142,147). The ventromedial caudate is principally connected to the orbitofrontal cortex (138), and lesions of either result in disinhibition (142,147). Although the deficits and behavioral changes resulting from unilateral caudate lesions usually resolve fairly rapidly, the two reported patients with bilateral caudate hemorrhages and long-term follow-up both showed persistent abnormalities (145,148). Idiopathic calcification of the basal ganglia can also result in psychosis and dementia (149). Finally, neuropsychological changes, very similar to those of HD, have been reported in choreoacanthocytosis (150), a rare disease in which neuropathological changes are limited to the striatum and pallidum (151).

Studies in primates have borne out the conclusion that the striatum (and especially the caudate) is involved in cognitive as well as in motor functioning. Bilateral lesions are usually required for behavioral changes to be manifest (152,153), probably reflecting the bilateral projection from prefrontal areas to the caudate nuclei (154,155). Features of such lesions in primates have included the alteration of sequential organization of behavior to resemble frontal dysfunction (156), and impaired delayed alternation learning (157,158). In addition, correlations between the site of caudate lesions and subsequent behavior, similar to those already mentioned for humans, have been found (159).

In summary, although there is no doubt that cortical changes do occur in HD, and could clearly account for many of the frontal-type deficits and behavioral alterations seen in the early and midstages of the disease, there is a considerable body of evidence to suggest that similar cognitive and behavioral changes may also occur with isolated striatal lesions. This is especially true of the head of the caudate, which bears the brunt of the pathology in early HD, and which receives strong input from prefrontal regions. The issue must be regarded as unsettled.

VII. DRUG TREATMENT

A. Therapy Based on Neurochemical Analysis

The finding of dopamine depletion in Parkinson's disease, and its rectification with dopaminergic agents, has had enormous influence on the approach to the treatment of neurodegenerative diseases, including HD. The realization that there was a marked depletion of GABA and of its biosynthetic enzyme glutamate decarboxylase in the basal ganglia in HD sparked numerous attempts at replacement therapy. This has been undertaken with a wide variety of agents, including the GABA-mimetic drugs, muscimol (160) and its structural analogue, 4,5,6,7-tetrahydroisoxazolo-(4,5-*c*)-pyridin-3-01 (THIP) (161); direct (acetylenic GABA) (162,163); and indirect (isoniazid) (164–166) inhibitors of GABA transaminase, the principal GABA-metabolizing enzyme. Even though several of these agents were shown to elevate CSF and brain GABA levels (162,164, 167,168), neither clinical improvement nor alteration in the course of the disease was demonstrated. This discouraging finding is hardly surprising when one considers the wide distribution of GABA throughout the brain, in many cases possibly subserving opposite functions in different circuits or even within the same circuit, as has been postulated for the striatopallidothalamic loops (169).

It has recently been reported that somatostatin and neuropeptide Y are increased up to threefold in HD striatum (5). Although this almost certainly reflects preservation of the neurons containing these peptides within the shrunken striatum, it is of interest that somatostatin injected into rat brain produces hyperkinetic and sterotyped movements (170), and that these may arise by stimulation of dopamine release from terminals (171). Systemic cysteamine depletes brain somatostatin (172) and decreases dopamine levels in the striatum (173). Unfortunately, a small controlled trial of cysteamine in HD produced no amelioration of motor deficits (174).

More recently, attention has been focused on the excitotoxin model of HD (175). The anatomical and chemical pathology of HD can be reproduced in animal models with glutamate agonists: specifically those active at *N*-methyl-D-aspartate (NMDA) receptors (3,7). Several NMDA channel blockers exist (such as dizocilpine maleate; MK-801), but psychotomimetic side effects limit their usefulness (phencyclidine also acts at this site) (176). The NMDA receptor also has a coagonist glycine site, which can be blocked by the naturally occurring tryptophan metabolite, kynurenic acid (177). Kynurenic acid has also recently been shown to be decreased in HD, but not in AD or Parkinson's disease (178). Unfortunately, it does not cross the blood–brain barrier, and although its levels within the CNS can be increased by tryptophan loading (179), the recent delineation of the eosinophilic myalgia syndrome (EMS) and its association with tryptophan ingestion (180) has blocked this therapeutic avenue. Nevertheless, such anti-NMDA receptor therapy remains the brightest hope for specific therapy in HD. An indirect attempt to decrease NMDA receptor activation using baclofen (a $GABA_B$ receptor antagonist which may attenuate corticostriatal excitatory neurotransmission) has recently been reported (181). This large, controlled, prolonged trial was unfortunately unsuccessful.

Note, that most of these therapeutic ventures suggested by neurochemical research have addressed the movement disorder of HD. rather than the cognitive changes (although some hope was held for the GABAergic agents and baclofen). This phenomenon is not surprising in view of the lack of agreement of the primary site and nature of the abnormality causing the intellectual decline, and on the relative lack of specific neurochemical changes in the cortex, despite its obvious involvement.

B. Empirically Based Therapy: Symptomatic Treatment

The great importance of recognizing and treating depression in HD has already been mentioned in a previous section. Other than this, drug therapy is most often used to reduce the severity of chorea if it is disabling, and to ameliorate sleeping and behavioral difficulties.

Dopamine receptor antagonists are the usual agents of choice in the United States for damping down chorea (182). Although their effect on this may be disappointing (183), they have been shown to reduce choreic, but not nonchoreic, motor disturbances in another carefully assessed patient population (184). The monoamine-depleting agent tetrabenazine is not generally available in the United States, but is used in Europe and Australia, and provides an alternative to dopamine receptor blockers should the latter prove ineffective or too sedating (185,186). Although hypotensive effects are less marked than with the similarly acting, but less centrally selective, reserpine, depression is a worrisome side effect. It must be emphasized that dopaminergic antagonists should not be unthinkingly prescribed for all HD patients. They do not improve, and may actually worsen, nonchoreic motor disturbances such as bradykinesia, rigidity, dystonia, and gait problems. Although some behavioral disturbances may be improved by these agents, they can equally increase apathy and mental slowing. In those patients for whom such therapy seems warranted (whether for *disabling* chorea or for otherwise unmanageable behavioral disturbances), the dose should be titrated carefully. The treatment of behavioral and sleep disturbance in HD is along the usual symptomatic lines.

On the basis that parkinsonism and chorea appear to be pharmacologic opposites, central cholinergic agents have also been tried in HD. It should be noted that large aspiny cholinergic neurons are spared in HD (9), and the reduction in muscarinic agonist binding probably reflects a loss of target spiny GABAergic projection neurons. Moreover, unlike AD, cholinergic neurons in the basal forebrain are preserved in HD (188), as is cortical choline acetyltransferase (189). With this background, it is not surprising that, despite some initial enthusiasm (190), the results of cholinergic manipulation have generally been disappointing (191).

VIII. CONCLUSION

Huntington's disease produces a particular pattern of cognitive decline. Memory is affected early, and the major deficit seems to be in retrieval. Visuospatial and complex organizational problems are also seen at this stage. As the disease process advances, a more global dementia ensues. Language, however, is relatively spared, although it becomes semantically less complex. Psychiatric manifestations (particularly depression) are common, and they may antedate other symptoms. The overall picture is not unlike that seen with frontal lobe lesions and, clearly, differs from that of AD. Gene carriers, as a group, show neuropsychological abnormalities, but these are insufficiently robust to be of help in individual cases. Neuropathological studies have clearly shown both striatal and cortical involvement at an early stage, despite that most imaging studies have only revealed the former. The cognitive picture could be due to either or (probably) both: this issue must be regarded as unsettled. Treatment at present is purely symptomatic.

ACKNOWLEDGMENT

Partly supported by a grant to E.S. from the Faculty of Medicine, University of Melbourne, Australia, and the Huntington's Disease Center Without Walls—NS16367.

REFERENCES

1. Gusella JF, Wexler NS, Conneally PM, Naylor SL, Anderson MA, Tanzi RE, Watkins PC, Ottina K, Wallace MR, Sakaguchi AY, Young AB, Shoulson I, Bonilla E, Martin JB. A polymorphic DNA marker genetically linked to Huntington's disease. Nature 1983; 306:234–238.
2. Beal MF, Martin JB. Neuropeptides in neurological disease. Ann Neurol 1986; 20:547–565.
3. Beal MF, Kowall NW, Ellison DW, Mazurek MF, Swartz KJ, Martin JB.

Replication of the neurochemical characteristics of Huntington's disease with quinolinic acid. Nature 1986; 321:168–171.
4. Vonsattel J-P, Myers RH, Stevens TJ, Ferrante RJ, Bird ED, Richardson EP. Neuropathological classification of Huntington's disease. J Neuropathol Exp Neurol 1985; 44:559–577.
5. Beal MF, Mazurek MF, Ellison DW, Swartz KJ, McGarvey U, Bird ED, Martin JB. Somatostatin and neuropeptide Y concentrations in pathologically graded cases of Huntington's disease. Ann Neurol 1988; 23:562–569.
6. Beal MF, Ellison DW, Mazurek MF, Swartz KJ, Malloy JR, Bird ED, Martin JB. A detailed examination of substance P in pathologically graded cases of Huntington's disease. J Neurol Sci 1988; 84:51–61.
7. Ellison DW, Beal MF, Mazurek MF, Malloy JR, Bird ED, Martin JB. Amino acid neurotransmitter abnormalities in Huntington's disease and the quinolinic acid model of Huntington's disease. Brain 1987; 110:1657–1673.
8. Ferrante RJ, Kowall NW, Beal MF, Bird ED, Martin JB. Selective sparing of a class of striatal neurons in Huntington's disease. Science 1985; 230:561–563.
9. Ferrante RJ, Beal MF, Kowall NW, Richardson EP, Martin JB. Sparing of acetylcholinesterase-containing neurons in Huntington's disease. Brain Res 1987; 411:162–166.
10. Bruyn GW. Huntington's chorea. Historical, clinical and laboratory synopsis. In: Vinken PJ, Bruyn GW, eds. Handbook of clinical neurology, vol 6. Diseases of the basal ganglia. Amsterdam: North-Holland, 1968:298–378.
11. Forno LS, Jose C. Huntington's chorea: a pathological study. In: Barbeau A, Chase TN, Paulson GW, eds. Huntington's chorea, 1872–1972. New York: Raven Press 1973:453–470.
12. Byers RK, Gilles FH, Fung L. Huntington's disease in children; neuropathological study of four cases. Neurology 1973; 23:561–569.
13. McCaughey WTE. The pathologic spectrum of Huntington's chorea. J Nerv Ment Dis 1961; 133:91–103.
14. Delamonte SM, Vonsattel J-P, Richardson EP. Morphometric demonstration of atrophic changes in the cerebral cortex, white matter, and neostriatum in Huntington's disease. J Neuropathol Exp Neurol 1988; 47:516–525.
15. Tellez-Nagel I, Johnson AB, Terry RD. Studies on brain biopsies of patients with Huntington's chorea. J Neuropathol Exp Neurol 1974; 33:308–332.
16. Cudkowicz M, Kowall NW. Degeneration of pyramidal projection neurons in Huntington's disease cortex. Ann Neurol 1990; 2:200–204.
17. Mazurek MF, Beal MF, Ellison DW, Knowlton SF, Swartz KJ, Martin JB. Cholecystokinin immunoreactivity in Huntington's disease: widespread increases in postmortem cerebral cortex. In: Hughes J, Dockray G, Woodruff G, eds. The neuropeptide cholecystokinin. New York: John Wiley & Sons, 1989:28–32.
18. Mann DMA. Subcortical afferent projection systems in Huntington's chorea. Acta Neuropathol 1989; 78:551–554.
19. Huntington G. On chorea. Med Surg Rep (Philadelphia) 1872; 26:317–321 (reproduced in: Adv Neurol 1973; 1:33–39).

20. Bruyn GW, Went LN. Huntington's chorea. In: Vinken PJ, Bruyn GW, eds. Handbook of clinical neurology, Vol. 49. 1986:267–313.
21. Aminoff MJ, Marshall J, Smith EM, Wyke MA. Pattern of intellectual impairment in Huntington's chorea. Psychol Med 1975; 5:169–172.
22. Boll TJ, Heaton R, Reitan RM. Neuropsychological and emotional correlates of Huntington's chorea. J Nerv Ment Dis 1974; 158:61–69.
23. Brothers CRD, Meadows AW. An investigation of Huntington's chorea in Victoria. J Ment Sci 1955; 101:548–563.
24. Norton JC. Patterns of neuropsychological test performance in Huntington's disease. J Nerv Ment Dis 1975; 161:276–279.
25. McHugh PR, Folstein MF. Psychiatric syndromes of Huntington's chorea: a clinical and phenomonologic study. In: Benson DF, Blumer D, eds. Psychiatric aspects of neurological diseases. New York: Grune & Stratton, 1975:267–286.
26. Taylor HG, Hansotia P. Neuropsychological testing of Huntington's patients: clues to progression. J Nerv Ment Dis 1983; 171:492–496.
27. Butters N, Sax D, Montgomery K, Tarlow S. Comparison of the neuropsychological deficits associated with early and advanced Huntington's disease. Arch Neurol 1978; 35:585–589.
28. Moses JA, Golden CJ, Berger PA, Wisniewski AM. Neuropsychological deficits in early, middle, and late stage Huntington's disease as measured by the Luria–Nebraska neuropsychological battery. Int J Neurosci 1981; 14:95–100.
29. Caine ED, Hunt RD, Weingartner H, Ebert MH. Huntington's dementia: clinical and neuropsychological features. Arch Gen Psychiatry 1978; 35:377–384.
30. Josiassen RC, Curry LM, Mancall EL. Development of neuropsychological deficits in Huntington's disease. Arch Neurol 1983; 40:791–796.
31. Josiassen RC, Curry L, DeBease C. Patterns of intellectual deficits in Huntington's disease. J Clin Neuropsychol 1982; 4:173–183.
32. Fedio P, Cox CS, Neophytides A, Canal-Frederick G, Chase T. Neuropsychological profile of Huntington's disease: patients and those at risk. Adv Neurol 1979; 23:239–255.
33. Hayden MR. Huntington's chorea. New York: Springer-Verlag, 1981.
34. Caine ED, Shoulson I. Psychiatric syndromes in Huntington's disease. Am J Psychiatry 1983; 140:728–733.
35. Folstein SE, Abbot MH, Chase GA, Jensen BA, Folstein MF. The association of affective disorder with Huntington's disease in a case series and in families. Psychol Med 1983; 13:537–542.
36. Brandt J, Strauss ME, Larus J, Jensen B, Folstein SE, Folstein MF. Clinical correlates of dementia and disability in Huntington's disease. J Clin Neuropsychol 1984; 6:401–412.
37. Shoulson I, Fahn S. Huntington's disease: clinical care and evaluation. Neurology 1979; 29:1–3.
38. Shoulson I, Plassche W, Odoroff C. Huntington's disease: caudate atrophy parallels functional impairment. Neurology 1982; 32:A143.
39. Mayeux R, Stern Y, Herman A, Greenbaum L, Fahn S. Correlates of early disability in Huntington's disease. Ann Neurol 1986; 20:727–731.

40. Folstein MF, Folstein SE, McHugh PR. "Mini-mental state." A practical guide for grading the cognitive state of patients for the clinician. J Psychiatr Res 1975; 12:189–198.
41. Caine ED, Bamford KA, Schiffer RB, Shoulson I, Levy S. A controlled neuropsychological comparison of Huntington's disease and multiple sclerosis. Arch Neurol 1986; 43:249–254.
42. Bamford KA, Caine ED, Kido DK, Plassche WM, Shoulson I. Clinical-pathologic correlation in Huntington's disease: a neuropsychological and computed tomography study. Neurology 1989; 39:796–801.
43. Potegal M. A note on spatial–motor deficits in patients with Huntington's disease: a test of a hypothesis. Neuropsychologia 1971; 9:233–235.
44. Brouwers P, Cox C, Martin A, Chase T, Fedio P. Differential perceptual–spatial impairment in Huntington's and Alzheimer's dementias. Arch Neurol 1984; 41:1073–1076.
45. Butters N, Soeldner C, Fedio P. Comparison of parietal and frontal lobe spatial deficits in man: extrapersonal versus personal (ego-centric) space. Percept Mot Skills 1972; 34:27–34.
46. Hayward L, Zubrick SR, Hall W. Early sensory–perceptual changes in Huntington's disease. Aust NZ J Psychiatry 1985; 19:384–389.
47. Cohen NJ, Squire LR. Preserved learning and retention of pattern analyzing skill in amnesia: dissociation of knowing how and knowing that. Science 1980; 210:207–210.
48. Squire LR. Mechanisms of memory. Science 1986; 232:1612–1619.
49. Schacter DL. Priming of old and new knowledge in amnesic patients and normal subjects. Ann NY Acad Sci 1985; 444:41–53.
50. Cermak LS, Talbot N, Chandler K, Wolbarst LR. The perceptual priming phenomenon in amnesia. Neuropsychologia 1985; 23:615–622.
51. Shimamura AP. Priming effects in amnesia: evidence for a dissociable memory function. Q J Exp Psychol 1986; 38A:619–644.
52. Martone M, Butters N, Payne M, Becker JT, Sax DS. Dissociations between skill learning and verbal recognition in amnesia and dementia. Arch Neurol 1984; 41:965–970.
53. Heindel WC, Butters N, Salmon DP. Impaired learning of a motor skill in patients with Huntington's disease. Behav Neurosci 1988; 102:141–147.
54. Shimamura AP, Salmon DP, Squire LR, Butters N. Memory dysfunction and word priming in dementia and amnesia. Behav Neurosci 1987; 101:347–351.
55. Salmon DP, Shimamura AP, Butters N, Smith S. Lexical and semantic priming deficits in patients with Alzheimer's disease. J Clin Exp Neuropsychol 1988; 10:477–494.
56. Mishkin M, Malamut B, Bachevalier J. Memories and habits: two neural systems. In: Lynch G, McGaugh JL, Weinberger NM, eds. Neurobiology of learning and memory. New York: Guilford Press, 1984:287–296.
57. Saint-Cyr JA, Taylor AE, Lang AE. Procedural learning and neostriatal dysfunction in man. Brain 1988; 111:941–959.
58. Heindel WC, Salmon DP, Shults CW, Walicke PA, Butters N. Neuropsychological evidence for multiple implicit memory systems: a comparison of

Alzheimer's, Huntington's and Parkinson's disease patients. J Neurosci 1989; 9:582–587.
59. Albert MS, Butters N, Levin J. Temporal gradients in the retrograde amnesia of patients with alcoholic Korsakoff's disease. Arch Neurol 1979; 36:211–216.
60. Albert MS, Butters N, Brandt J. Patterns of remote memory in amnesic and demented patients. Arch Neurol 1981; 38:495–500.
61. Albert MS, Butters N, Brandt J. Development of remote memory loss in patients with Huntington's disease. J Clin Neuropsychol 1981; 3:1–12.
62. Wilson RS, Kaszniak AW, Fox JH. Remote memory in senile dementia. Cortex 1981; 17:41–48.
63. Beatty WW, Salmon DP, Butters N, Heindel WC, Granholm EL. Retrograde amnesia in patients with Alzheimer's disease or Huntington's disease. Neurobiol Aging 1988; 9:181–186.
64. Tulving E. Episodic and semantic memory. In: Tulving E, Donaldson W, eds. Organization of memory. New York: Academic Press, 1972:383–403.
65. Weingartner H, Grafman J, Boutelle W, Kaye W, Martin PR. Forms of memory failure. Science 1983; 221:380–382.
66. Butters N, Wolfe J, Granholm E, Martone M. An assessment of verbal recall, recognition and fluency abilities in patients with Huntington's disease. Cortex 1986; 221:11–32.
67. Benton AL. Differential behavioral effects in frontal lobe disease. Neuropsychologia 1968; 6:53–60.
68. Butters N, Granholm E, Salmon DP, Grant I. Episodic and semantic memory: a comparison of amnesic and demented patients. J Clin Exp Neuropsychol 1987; 9:479–497.
69. Martin A, Fedio P. Word production and comprehension in Alzheimer's disease: the breakdown of semantic knowledge. Brain Lang 1983; 19:124–141.
70. Butters N. The clinical aspects of memory disorders: contributions from experimental studies of amnesia and dementia. J Clin Neuropsychol 1984; 6:17–36.
71. Weingartner H, Caine ED, Ebert MH. Imagery, encoding, and retrieval of information from memory: some specific encoding-retrieval changes in Huntington's disease. J Abnorm Psychol 1979; 88:52–58.
72. Beatty WW, Butters N. Further analysis of encoding of patients with Huntington's disease. Brain Cogn 1986; 5:387–398.
73. Wilson RS, Como PG, Garron DC, Klawans HL, Barr A, Klawans D. Memory failure in Huntington's disease. J Clin Exp Neuropsychol 1987; 9:147–154.
74. Paivio A. Imagery and verbal processes. New York: Holt, Rinehart and Wilson, 1971.
75. Butters N, Grady M. Effect of predistractor delays on the short-term memory performance of patients with Korsakoff's and Huntington's disease. Neuropsychologia 1977; 15:701–706.
76. Butters N, Tarlow S, Cermak LS, Sax D. A comparison of the information processing deficits of patients with Huntington's disease and Korsakoff's syndrome. Cortex 1976; 12:134–144.
77. Biber C, Butters N, Rosen J, Gerstman L, Mattis S. Encoding strategies and

recognition of faces by alcoholic Korsakoff and other brain damaged patients. J Clin Neuropsychol 1981; 3:315–330.
78. Butters N, Albert MS, Sax DS, Miliotis P, Nagode J, Sterste A. The effect of verbal mediators on the pictorial memory of brain damaged patients. Neuropsychologia 1983; 21:307–323.
79. Granholm E, Butters N. Associative encoding and retrieval in Alzheimer's and Huntington's disease. Brain Cogn 1988; 7:335–347.
80. Huber SJ, Paulson GW. Memory impairment associated with progression of Huntington's disease, Cortex 1987; 23:275–283.
81. Butters N, Wolfe J, Martone M, Granholm E, Cermak LS. Memory disorders associated with Huntington's disease: verbal recall recognition, and procedural memory. Neuropsychologia 1985; 23:729–743.
82. Moss MB, Albert MS, Butters N, Payne M. Differential patterns of memory loss among patients with Alzheimer's disease, Huntington's disease, and alcoholic Korsakoff's syndrome. Arch Neurol 1986; 43:239–246.
83. Moberg PJ, Pearlson GD, Speedie LJ, Lipsey JR. Olfactory recognition: differential impairments in early and late Huntington's and Alzheimer's diseases. J Clin Exp Neuropsychol 1987; 9:650–664.
84. Martone M, Butters N. Some analyses of forgetting of pictorial material in amnesic and demented patients. J Clin Exp Neuropsychol 1986; 8: 161–178.
85. Squire LR. Two forms of human amnesia: an analysis of forgetting. J Neurosci 1981; 1:635–640.
86. Sax DS, O'Donnell B, Butters N, Menzer L, Montgomery K, Kayne HL. Computed tomographic, neurologic, and neuropsychological correlates of Huntington's disease. Int J Neurosci 1983; 18:21–36.
87. Folstein MF, McHugh PR. The neuropsychiatry of some specific brain disorders. In: Lader MH, ed. Mental disorders and somatic illness. Handbook of pyschiatry, vol. 2 Cambridge: Cambridge University Press, 1983:107–118.
88. Gordon WP, Illes J. Neurolinguistic characteristics of language production in Huntington's disease: a preliminary report. Brain Lang 1987; 31:1–10.
89. Podoll K, Caspary P, Lange HW, Noth J. Language functions in Huntington's disease. Brain 1988; 111:1475–1503.
90. Wallesch CW, Fehrenbach RA. On the neurolinguistic nature of language abnormalities in Huntington's disease. J Neurol Neurosurg Psychiatry 1988; 51:367–373.
91. Kennedy J, Fisher J, Shoulson I, Caine E. Language impairment in Huntington's disease. Neurology 1981; 31(suppl):81–82.
92. Bayles K, Tomoeda DK. Confrontation naming impairment in dementia. Brain Lang 1983; 19:98–114.
93. Brackenridge CJ. Factors influencing dementia and epilepsy in Huntington's disease of early onset. Acta Neurol Scand 1980; 62:305–311.
94. Webb M, Trzepacz PT. Huntington's disease: correlations of mental status with chorea. Biol Psychiatry 1987; 22:751–761.
95. Girotti F, Marano R, Soliveri P, Geminiani G, Scigliano G. Relationship

between motor and cognitive disorders in Huntington's disease. J Neurol 1988; 235:454–457.
96. Wexler NS. Perceptual–motor, cognitive, and emotional characteristics of persons at risk for Huntington's disease. Adv Neurol 1979; 23:257–271.
97. Starkstein SE, Brandt J, Folstein S, Strauss M, Berthier ML, Pearlson GD, Wong D, McDonnell A, Folstein M. Neuropsychological and neuroradiological correlates in Huntington's disease. J Neurol Neurosurg Psychiatry 1988; 51:1259–1263.
98. Brandt J, Folstein SE, Folstein MF. Differential cognitive impairment in Alzheimer's disease and Huntington's disease. Ann Neurol 1988; 23:555–561.
99. Salmon DP, Kwo-On-Yuen PF, Heindel WC, Butters N, Thal L. Differentiation of Alzheimer's disease and Huntington's disease with the dementia rating scale. Arch Neurol 1989; 46:1204–1208.
100. Mattis S. Mental status examination for organic mental syndrome in the elderly patient. In: Bellak L, Karasu TB, eds. Geriatric psychiatry: a handbook for psychiatrists and primary care physicians. New York: Grune & Stratton, 1976:77–121.
101. Albert ML, Feldman RG, Willis AL. The "subcortical dementia" of progressive supranuclear palsy. J Neurol Neurosurg Psychiatry 1974; 37:121–130.
102. Cummings JL. Subcortical dementia: neuropsychology, neuropsychiatry, and pathophysiology. Br J Psychiatry 1986; 149:682–697.
103. Cummings JL, Benson DF. Subcortical dementia: review of an emerging concept. Arch Neurol 1984; 41:874–879.
104. Huber SJ, Paulson GW. The concept of subcortical dementia. Am J Psychiatry 1985; 142:1312–1317.
105. Cummings JL, Benson DF. Psychological dysfunction accompanying subcortical dementias. Annu Rev Med 1988; 39:53–61.
106. Mayeux R, Stern Y, Rosen J, Benson DF. Is "subcortical dementia" a recognizable clinical entity? Ann Neurol 1983; 14:278–283.
107. Whitehouse PJ. The concept of subcortical and cortical dementia: another look. Ann Neurol 1986; 19:1–6.
108. Bolt JM. Huntington's chorea in the west of Scotland. Br J Psychiatry 1970; 116:259–270.
109. Mindham RHS, Steele C, Folstein MF, Lucas J. A comparison of the frequency of major affective disorder in Huntington's disease and Alzheimer's disease. J Neurol Neurosurg Psychiatry 1985; 48:1172–1174.
110. Folstein SE, Folstein MF, McHugh PR. Psychiatric syndromes in Huntington's disease. Adv Neurol 1979; 23:281–289.
111. Burns A, Folstein S, Brandt J, Folstein M. Clinical assessment of irritability, aggression, and apathy in Huntington and Alzheimer disease. J Nerv Ment Dis 1990; 178:20–26.
112. Catona MC, Lazzarini AM, McCormack MK. A psychometric study of children at-risk for Huntington disease. Clin Genet 1985; 28:307–316.
113. Lyle O, Quast W. The Bender Gestalt: use of clinical judgement versus recall scores in prediction of Huntington's disease. J Consult Clin Psychol 1976; 44:229–232.

114. Lyle OE, Gottesman II. Premorbid psychometric indicators of the gene for Huntington's disease. J Consult Clin Psychol 1977; 45:1011–1022.
115. Jason GW, Pajurkova EM, Suchowersky O, Hewitt J, Hilbert C, Reed J, Hayden MR. Presymptomatic neuropsychological impairment in Huntington's disease. Arch Neurol 1988; 45:769–773.
116. Roy CS, Sherrington CS. On the regulation of the blood supply of the brain. J Physiol (Lond) 1890; 11:85–108.
117. Kuhl DE. Imaging local brain function with emission computed tomography. Radiology 1984; 150:625–631.
118. Sharp PF, Smith FW, Gemmell HG, Lyall D, Evans NTS, Gvozdanovic D, Davidson J, Tyrell DA, Pickett RD, Neirinckx RD. Technetium-99m-HM-PAO stereoisomers as potential agents for imaging regional cerebral blood flow: human volunteer studies. J Nucl Med 1986; 27:171–177.
119. Obrist WD, Thompson HK, Wang HS, Wilkinson WE. Regional cerebral blood flow estimated by ^{133}xenon inhalation. Stroke 1975; 6:245–256.
120. Sokoloff L. The relationship between function and energy metabolism: its use in the localization of functional activity in the nervous system. Neurosci Res Prog Bull 1981:19:159–210.
121. Kuhl DE, Phelps ME, Markham CH, Metter EJ, Riege WH, Winter J. Cerebral metabolism and atrophy in Huntington's disease determined by ^{18}FDG and computed tomographic scan. Ann Neurol 1982; 12:425–434.
122. Kuhl DE, Metter EJ, Riege WH, Markham CH. Patterns of cerebral glucose utilization in Parkinson's disease and Huntington's disease. Ann Neurol 1984; 15(suppl):S119–S125.
123. Young AB, Penney JB, Starosta-Rubinstein S, Markel DS, Berent S, Giordani B, Ehrenkaufer R, Jewett D, Hichwa R. PET scan investigations of Huntington's disease: cerebral metabolic correlates of neurological features and functional decline. Ann Neurol 1986; 20:296–303.
124. Hayden MR, Martin WRW, Stoessl AJ, Clark C, Hollenberg S, Adam MJ, Ammann W, Harrop R, Rogers J, Ruth T, Sayre C, Pate BD. Positron emission tomography in the early diagnosis of Huntington's disease. Neurology 1986; 36:888–894.
125. Berent S, Giordani B, Lehtinen S, Markel D, Penney JB, Buchtel HA, Starosta-Rubinstein S, Hichwa R, Young AB. Positron emission tomographic scan investigations of Huntington's disease: cerebral metabolic correlates of cognitive function. Ann Neurol 1988; 23:541–546.
126. Hayden MR, Hewitt J, Stoessl AJ, Clark C, Ammann W, Martin WRW. The combined use of positron emission tomography and DNA polymorphisms for preclinical detection of Huntington's disease. Neurology 1987; 37:1441–1447.
127. Mazziotta JC, Phelps ME, Pahl JJ, Huang S-C, Baxter LR, Riege WH, Hoffman JM, Kuhl DE, Lanto AB, Wapenski JA, Markham CH. Reduced cerebral glucose metabolism in asymptomatic subjects at risk for Huntington's disease. N Eng J Med 1987; 316:357–362.
128. Young AB, Penney JB, Starosta-Rubinstein S, Markel D, Berent S, Rothley J, Betley A, Hichwa R. Normal caudate glucose metabolism in persons at risk for Huntington's disease. Arch Neurol 1987; 44:254–257.

129. Smith FW, Besson JAO, Gemmell HG, Sharp PF. The use of technetium-99m-HM-PAO in the assessment of patients with dementia and other neuropsychiatric conditions. J Cereb Blood Flow Metab 1988; 8:S116–S122.
130. Tanahashi N, Meyer JS, Ishikawa Y, Kandula P, Mortel KF, Rogers RL, Gandhi S, Walker M. Cerebral blood flow and cognitive testing correlate in Huntington's disease. Arch Neurol 1985; 42:1169–1175.
131. Weinberger DR, Berman KF, Iadarola M, Driesen N, Zec RF. Prefrontal cortical blood flow and cognitive function in Huntington's disease. J Neurol Neurosurg Psychiatry 1988; 51:94–104.
132. Weinberger DR, Berman KF, Chase TN. Prefrontal cortex physiological activation: effect of L-DOPA in Parkinson's disease. Neurology 1986; 36(suppl 1):170.
133. Foster NL, Chase TN, Mansi L, Brooks R, Fedio P, Patronas NJ, DiChiro G. Cortical abnormalities in Alzheimer's disease. Ann Neurol 1984; 16:649–654.
134. Sax DS, Menzer L. Computerized tomography in Huntington's disease. Neurology 1977; 27:388.
135. Barr AN, Heinze WJ, Dobben GD, Valvassori GE, Sugar O. Bicaudate index in computerized tomography of Huntington's disease and cerebral atrophy. Neurology 1978; 28:1196–1200.
136. Neophytides AN, DiChiro G, Barron SA, Chase TN. Computed axial tomography in Huntington's disease and persons at-risk for Huntington's disease. Adv Neurol 1979; 23:185–191.
137. Oepen G, Ostertag C. Diagnostic value of CT in patients with Huntington's chorea and their offspring. J Neurol 1981; 225:189–196.
138. Alexander GE, DeLong MR, Strick PL. Parallel organization of functionally segregated circuits linking basal ganglia and cortex. Annu Rev Neurosci 1986; 9:357–381.
139. Rosenberg C, Nudleman K, Starr A. Cognitive evoked potentials (P_{300}) in early Huntington's disease. Arch Neurol 1985; 42:984–987.
140. Lawson EA, Barrett G, Kriss A, Halliday AM. P_{300} and VEPs in Huntington's chorea. Ann NY Acad Sci 1984; 425:592–597.
141. Goodin DS, Aminoff MJ. Electrophysiological differences between subtypes of dementia. Brain 1986; 109:1103–1113.
142. Mendez MF, Adams NL, Lewandowski KS. Neurobehavioral changes associated with caudate lesions. Neurology 1989; 39:349–354.
143. Cambier J, Elghozi D, Strube E. Hemorragie de la tête du noyau caudé gauche: désorganisation du discours et de l'expression graphique, peturbations des séries gestuelles. Rev Neurol 1979; 135:763–774.
144. Stein RW, Kase CS, Hier DB, Caplan LR, Mohr JP, Hemmati M, Henderson K. Caudate hemorrhage. Neurology 1984; 34:1549–1554.
145. Fernández Pardal MM, Micheli F, Asconapé J, Paradiso G. Neurobehavioral symptoms in caudate hemorrhage: two cases. Neurology 1985; 35:1806–1807.
146. Pozzilli C, Passafiume D, Bastianello S, D'Antona R, Lenzi GL. Remote effects of caudate hemorrhage: a clinical and functional study. Cortex 1987; 23:341–349.

147. Stuss DT, Benson DF. Neuropsychological studies of the frontal lobes. Psychol Bull 1984; 95:3–28.
148. Richfield EK, Twyman R, Berent S. Neurological syndrome following bilateral damage to the heads of the caudate nuclei. Ann Neurol 1987; 22:768–771.
149. Cummings JL, Gosenfeld LF, Houlihan JP, McCaffrey T. Neuropsychiatric disturbances associated with idiopathic calcification of the basal ganglia. Biol Psychiatry 1983; 18:591–601.
150. Medalia A, Merriam A, Sandberg M. Neuropsychological deficits in choreoacanthocytosis. Arch Neurol 1989; 46:573–575.
151. Bird TD, Cederbaum S, Valpey RW, Stahl WL. Familial degeneration of the basal ganglia with acanthocytosis: a clinical, neuropathological, and neurochemical study. Ann Neurol 1978; 3:253–258.
152. Iverson SD. Behaviour after neostriatal lesions in animals. In: Divac I, Oberg RGE, eds. The neostriatum. New York: Pergamon Press, 1979.
153. Villablanca JR, Olmstead CR. The striatum: a fine tuner of the brain. Acta Neurobiol Exp 1982; 42:227–299.
154. Royce GJ. Laminar origin of cortical neurons which project upon the caudate nucleus: a horseradish peroxidase investigation in the cat. J Comp Neurol 1982; 205:8–29.
155. Arikuni T, Kubota K. The organization of prefrontocaudate projections and their laminar origin in the macaque monkey: a retrograde study using HRP-gel. J Comp Neurol 1986; 244:492–510.
156. Van Der Bercken JHL, Cools AR. Evidence for a role of the caudate nucleus in the sequential organization of behavior. Behav Brain Res 1982; 4:319–337.
157. Battig K, Rosvold HE, Mishkin M. Comparison of the effects of frontal and caudate lesions on delayed response and alternation in monkeys. J Comp Physiol Psychol 1960; 53:400–404.
158. Butters N, Rosvold HE. Effects of caudate and septal nucleus lesions on resistance to extinction and delayed-alternation. J Comp Physiol Psychol 1968; 65:397–403.
159. Divac I, Rosvold HE, Szwarcbart MK. Behavioral effects of selective ablation of the caudate nucleus. J Comp Physiol Psychol 1967; 63:184–190.
160. Shoulson I, Goldblatt D, Charlton M, Joynt RJ. Huntington's disease: treatment with muscimol, a GABA-mimetic drug. Ann Neurol 1978; 4:279–284.
161. Foster NL, Chase TN, Denaro A, Hare TA, Tamminga CA. THIP treatment of Huntington's disease. Neurology 1983; 33:637–639.
162. Tell G, Bohlen P, Schechter PJ, Koch-Weser J, Agid Y, Bonnet AM, Coquillat G, Chazot G, Fischer C. Treatment of Huntington's disease with gamma-acetylenic GABA, an irreversible inhibitor of GABA-transaminase: increased CSF GABA and homocarnosine without clinical amelioration. Neurology 1981; 31:207–211.
163. Scigliano G, Giovannini P, Girotti F, Grassi MP, Caraceni T, Schechter PJ. gamma-Vinyl GABA treatment of Huntington's disease. Neurology 1984; 34:94–96.
164. Manyam BV, Katz L, Hare TA, Kaniefski K, Tremblay RD. Isoniazid-

induced elevation of CSF GABA levels and effects on chorea in Huntington's disease. Ann Neurol 1981; 10:35–37.

165. Perry TL, Wright JM, Hansen S, Baker Thomas SM, Allan BM, Baird PA, Diewold PA. A double-blind clinical trial of isoniazid in Huntington disease. Neurology 1982; 32:354–358.
166. McLean DR. Failure of isoniazid therapy in Huntington's disease. Neurology 1982; 32:1189–1191.
167. Manyam BV, Tremblay RD. Free and conjugated GABA in human cerebrospinal fluid: effect of degenerative neurologic diseases and isoniazid. Brain Res 1984; 307:217–223.
168. Perry TL, Wall RA, Hansen S. Brain amino compounds in a Huntington's disease patient on isoniazid therapy. Neurology 1985; 35:755–758.
169. Albin RL, Young AB, Penney JB. The functional anatomy of basal ganglia disorders. Trends Neurosci 1989; 12:366–375.
170. Rezek M, Havlicek V, Leybin L, Pinsky C, Kroeger EA, Hughes KR, Friesen H. Neostriatal administration of somatostatin: differential effect of small and large doses on behavior and motor control. Can J Physiol Pharmacol 1977; 55:234–242.
171. Chesselet M-F, Reisine TD. Somatostatin regulated dopamine release in rat striatal slices and cat caudate nuclei. J Neurosci 1983; 3:232–236.
172. Sagar SM, Landry D, Millard WJ, Badger TM, Arnold MA, Martin JB. Depletion of somatostatin-like immunoreactivity in the rat central nervous system by cysteamine. J Neurosci 1982; 2:225–231.
173. Vécsei L, Kovács GL, Faludi M, Bollók I, Telegdy G. Dose-related effects of cysteamine treatment on hypothalamic and striatal dopamine, noradrenaline and serotonin neurotransmission. Acta Physiol Hung 1985; 66:213–217.
174. Shults C, Steardo L, Barone P, Mohr E, Juncos J, Serrati C, Fedio P, Tamminga CA, Chase TN. Huntington's disease: effect of cysteamine, a somatostatin-depleting agent. Neurology 1986; 36:1099–1102.
175. Choi DW. Glutamate neurotoxicity and diseases of the nervous system. Neuron 1988; 1:623–634.
176. Koek W, Colpaert FC. Selective blockade of *N*-methyl-D-aspartate (NMDA)-induced convulsions by NMDA antagonists and putative glycine antagonists: relationship with phencyclidine-like behavioural effects. J Pharm Exp Ther 1990: 252:349–357.
177. Danysz W, Fadda E, Wroblewski JT, Costa E. Kynurenate and 2-amino-5-phosphonovalerate interact with multiple binding sites of the *N*-methyl-D-aspartate-sensitive glutamate receptor domain. Neurosci Lett 1989; 96:340–344.
178. Beal MF, Matson WR, Swartz KJ, Gamache PH, Bird ED. Kynurenine pathway measurements in Huntington's disease striatum: evidence for reduced formation of kynurenic acid. J Neurochem 1990; (in press).
179. Swartz KJ, During MJ, Freese A, Beal MF. Cerebral synthesis and release of kynurenic acid: an endogenous antagonist of excitatory amino acid receptors. J Neurosci 1990; (in press).

180. Klibourne EM, Swygert LA, Philen RM, Sun RK, Auerbach SB, Miler L, Nelson DE, Falk H. Interim guidance on the eosinophilia–myalgia syndrome. Ann Intern Med 1990; 112:85–87.
181. Shoulson I, Odoroff C, Oakes D, Behr J, Goldblatt D, Caine E, Kennedy J, Miller C, Bamford K, Rubin A, Plumb S, Kurlan R. A controlled clinical trial of baclofen as protective therapy in early Huntington's disease. Ann Neurol 1989; 25:252–259.
182. Klawans HL, Weiner WJ. The pharmacology of choreatic movement disorders. Prog Neurobiol 1976; 6:49–80.
183. Shoulson I. Huntington disease: functional capacities in patients treated with neuroleptic and antidepressant drugs. Neurology 1981; 31:1333–1335.
184. Girotti F, Carella F, Scigliano G, Grassi MP, Soliveri P, Giovannini P, Parati E, Caraceni T. Effect of neuroleptic treatment on involuntary movements and motor performances in Huntington's disease. J Neurol Neurosurg Psychiatry 1984; 47:848–852.
185. Asher SW, Aminoff MJ. Tetrabenazine and movement disorders. Neurology 1981; 31:1051–1054.
186. Jankovic J. Treatment of hyperkinetic movement disorders with tetrabenazine: a double-blind crossover study. Ann Neurol 1982; 11:41–47.
187. Enna SJ, Bird ED, Bennet JP, Bylund DB, Yamamura HI, Iversen LL, Snyder SH. Huntington's chorea: changes in neurotransmitter receptors in the brain. N Engl J Med 1976; 294:1305–1309.
188. Mann DMA. Subcortical afferent projection systems in Huntington's chorea. Acta Neuropathol 1989; 78:551–554.
189. Spokes EGS. Neurochemical alterations in Huntington's chorea: a study of post-mortem brain tissue. Brain 1980; 103:179–210.
190. Davis L, Holister LE, Barchas JD, Berger PA. Choline in tardive dyskinesia and Huntington's disease. Life Sci 1976; 19:1507–1515.
191. Nutt JG. Effect of cholinergic agents in Huntington's disease: a reappraisal. Neurology 1983; 33:932–935.

5

Cognitive Disorders Associated with Psychiatric Illnesses

John S. Kennedy and John T. Kenny *University Hospitals of Cleveland, Case Western Reserve University, Cleveland, Ohio*

I. INTRODUCTION

Disturbance of cognitive function is an established feature of the major psychiatric disorders of middle age: schizophrenia and mood disorders. Patients frequently complain of problems in concentration and memory and manifest difficulty completing activities of daily living. This chapter reviews the reported disturbances in attention, memory, executive, language, and visuospatial functions in these common disorders. The emphasis on cognitive disorders in the middle-aged adult has precluded review of the pseudodementia syndromes, as these syndromes are predominantly disorders of older adults aged 55 and above.

II. SCHIZOPHRENIA

A. Clinical Features

Although schizophrenia, a disorder of brain function, may manifest prior to age 15 and after age 45, its peak age of onset is around age 20 (1). It is therefore appropriately considered here with the disorders of the middle years.

The major symptomatic features of schizophrenia include: delusions, auditory, visual, and tactile hallucinations, and disturbances in thinking (including loose associations, tangentiality, incoherence, circumstantiality, and illogicality). These symptoms are generally referred to as positive symptoms to distinguish them from negative symptoms such as withdrawal and inattentiveness, blunted and inappropriate affect, anergia, anhedonia (difficulties in experiencing interest and pleasure), and poverty of both the amount and content of speech (2). Positive symptoms usually coexist with negative symptoms and are most prominent during acute, episodic exacerbations of schizophrenia. Negative symptoms may be more disabling to daily functioning than positive symptoms and typically are most prominent during the nonacute phases of the disorder. Patients who present with the cluster of negative symptoms characterizing a "deficit syndrome" (3) (which includes poverty of speech, blunted affect, and impaired sense of purpose) are thought to exhibit the greatest degree of persistent social dysfunction. The symptoms that often emerge in schizophrenia patients during their course of illness include mood disturbance, anxiety, and cognitive dysfunction. Mood symptoms, when prominent and persistent, may warrant consideration of the diagnosis schizoaffective disorder. In addition to the features of cognitive dysfunction reviewed below, cognitive impairment may arise independently of the schizophrenia disorder itself as a consequence of treatment (4,5) or of other diseases causing dementia, such as Alzheimer's disease (6).

Natural history studies as well as cognition studies of schizophrenia are confounded by the influence of formal and informal diagnostic criteria used over the years and by the changes made in official nosologies over time. The absence of definitive biological markers for schizophrenia and its differentiation from similar disorders forces diagnosis based solely on symptomatology, course, and exclusion characteristics (7,8). Earlier use of broad diagnostic criteria in most instances resulted in the inclusion of mood disorders and schizotypal/borderline personality-disordered individuals.

The prevalence of schizophrenia worldwide is approximately 1% (9). It is somewhat more common and severe in males than females and has an earlier onset in males (10). Because of changes in diagnostic criteria, incidence data remains uncertain, as does evidence for a declining occurrence of the disorder (11). The absence of adequate incidence data has limited assessment of the environmental factors that may interact with genetic vulnerability to produce the disorder.

Research data support the presence of a strong genetic relationship in the development of schizophrenia. Concordance rates in monozygotic twin pairs of 30–70% and dizygotic rates of 10–20% have been reported (12). Molecular genetic research has recently focused on the search for chromosomal regions linked to the disorder. In addition to advances in technology, this effort was initiated by a case report associating a partial trisomy of chromosome 5 in an Asian Canadian uncle-nephew schizophrenia dyad (13). One group studying several Icelander and British family pedigrees found a schizophrenia susceptibility linkage to chromosome 5 (14); another group did not find this linkage in a large isolated Swedish kindred (15). Such difference may reflect an underlying heterogeneity in schizophrenia (16).

B. Pathogenesis

The etiology of schizophrenia remains unknown, but an abnormal neurodevelopmental process is currently suspected. Many patients with schizophrenia have neuropathological abnormalities in the cortex (17–20) and temporal/hippocampal complex (21,22). The presence of neuropathological abnormalities is also supported by physiological evidence of dysfunction of the prefrontal cortex (23). Unqualified acceptance of these structural changes awaits new controlled studies. Changes in neurotransmitter systems have also been proposed, including alterations in dopamine (24), serotonin (25), noradrenergic (26), and peptidergic systems (27). The relationship between these proposed abnormalities and manifestation of schizophrenia psychopathology remains poorly understood. This is particularly true for less obvious symptoms such as deficits in the schizophrenia patient's attentional, memory, and executive abilities.

C. Cognitive Dysfunction

Recalling that schizophrenia was once termed dementia praecox, cognitive function in this disorder has long been of interest (28). Alterations in attention, memory, and executive function have received the most attention.

1. Attention

Attention has been defined as the voluntary direction of the mind upon an object, with the intention of fully apprehending it (29). It is a composite function of the brain which in schizophrenia research has been extensively evaluated under four distinct constructs: sensory memory, evaluated by span of apprehension (30,31) and backward masking (32,33); vigilance, evaluated by the Continuous Performance Test (CPT) (34,35) and simple reaction time/reaction time crossover (36,37); selective attention, evaluated by digit or word span with use of distraction (38,39) and the Stroop Color Word Interference Test (40,41); divided attention, evaluated by techniques such as auditory shadowing (42,43).

a. Sensory Memory. Schizophrenia patients have a reduced span of apprehension—sometimes as much as 50% (44). The extent to which the deficit is a nonspecific result of psychoses (45) or due to high dosages of neuroleptics remains unclear (46,47). Employing the backward masking paradigm, patients with schizophrenia have been shown to require a longer interval between termination of the target stimuli and onset of the masking stimuli to correctly identify the target (48–50). The extent to which this deficit is remedied by reduction in psychosis or the effects of neuroleptics remains unclear (51,52).

b. Vigilance. Under distracting conditions, many patients produce an abnormally low number of target identifications in the Continuous Performance Test (53). Test performance improves with appropriate neuroleptic medication therapy and is worsened in the presence of psychosis (54–56).

Reaction time crossover has been perhaps the most studied paradigm of attentional dysfunction in schizophrenia research. Schizophrenia patients show a distinct pattern in reaction time studies, responding faster to irregular compared to regular preparatory intervals that intervene between a warning signal and presented stimuli (57). Although not specific to schizophrenia, this finding is more prevalent in this population than in other mental disorders (58). Forty-seven to seventy-two percent of patients with schizophrenia exhibit this phenomenon (59). This paradigm appears to be insensitive to neuroleptic therapy (37).

c. Selective Attention. Patients with schizophrenia demonstrate a different response to distraction while attending to a series of digits or words than normal individuals. While normals demonstrate decrements in attending to items in the middle of the series, schizophrenic patients do poorly on both the first and middle items (60). This paradigm is sensitive to the effects of psychoses (61) and probably also to neuroleptic therapy (37). Unlike the digit/word span distraction tasks, the Stroop appears to be insensitive to neuroleptic therapy (62,63).

d. Divided Attention. Only one study of divided attentional ability employing "shadowing" in patients with schizophrenia was found and no differences were reported (64).

2. Memory

Memory has two major dimensions (capacity and time) and two basic functional processes (input and retrieval of information).

a. Short-Term Memory. Short-term memory's chief function is to acquire and briefly retain information for subsequent transfer to long-term memory. Short-term memory is considered to be of limited capacity and persists for 15–30 sec (65). Because short-term storage capacity is limited, information is only briefly retained before being rapidly displaced by subsequent information. Information may therefore be permanently lost. Two types of short-term memory are reviewed here: recognition memory and free recall.

Short-Term Recognition Memory Recognition memory is evaluated by requiring the individual to correctly identify those items they have been previously exposed to, as well as those they have not previously seen, among a list of presented test items.

The Sternberg task of short-term recognition memory (66) relies on varying the size (number of items) of a set to be memorized and a calculated reaction time slope (67). In normal individuals, the mean reaction time increases linearly with the number of items in the set (67). Several studies of patients with schizophrenia indicate that this type of memory function is unaltered in this disorder (68–70).

Short-Term Free Recall Memory Free recall memory requires the individual to remember items in any order, on request, without the assistance of any cues or prompts. Patients with schizophrenia have been evaluated most commonly with one of three short-term memory free recall procedures: Brown-Peterson (71), nondistraction memory span (71), and evaluation of the recency component of the serial position effect (65).

Results of studies using the Brown-Peterson memory task to assess patients with schizophrenia are unclear. One study noted no difference between normal controls and nonparanoid chronic patients, but found that paranoid chronic patients performed more poorly (70). Another study found that both these schizophrenia groups performed more poorly than normal controls (72). Both studies varied in diagnostic criteria, and patients were medicated (70,72). Others have found the performance of neuroleptic-free schizophrenia patients impaired relative to normal controls (73). The extent to which this paradigm is influenced by psychoses and neuroleptics is uncertain; we have found it to be unaffected by clozapine (74).

Nondistraction span tasks include procedures such as the WAIS digit span forward (75), as well as other digit span forward procedures which use a longer string of numbers (69), and the supraspan task (71). Procedures such as the digit span forward which use a relatively short string of digits likely evaluate passive storage ability, while the reverse procedure may evaluate the short-term capacity for information being actively processed (67). The supraspan task evaluates the effect of extending the load capacity of the digit span forward procedure. Digit span forward and reverse have been suggested to be unaffected by neuroleptics (76) and are not different in patients with schizophrenia compared to controls (77,78). Patients with schizophrenia may demonstrate differences from normal controls as the number of digits is increased, thereby producing an increased processing load. However, theoretical conclusions from these data are at best limited (79).

When an individual is given a series of stimuli such as words to recall, the likelihood of recalling any word presented is to some extent dependent on the position of the stimuli in the list. Stimuli at the beginning and end of the presented list are better recalled than stimuli in the middle. Recency refers to the enhanced recall of stimuli at the end of the list (67). In the only identified study, recency was intact in schizophrenic patients who were medicated (80).

b. Long-Term Memory. There are many classifications of the components of long-term memory (81,82). We restrict our discussion to episodic-semantic memory dichotomy.

Episodic Memory Episodic memory is memory for details contained in an episode of personal experience. It is believed that requiring a person to recall a list of words is similar to asking a person to recount what he or she bought at a store (67). Episodic memory has both free recall and recognition elements. Patients with schizophrenia have been shown to have free recall deficits in this form of memory (83–85).

This apparent deficit has been argued to be due to faulty memory organizational strategies, giving rise to the retrieval deficit. Studies have attempted to evaluate this hypothesis by having the patient structure the material to be freely recalled using semantic orienting procedures. Schizophrenia patients who are early in the course of illness and only mildly disturbed may be able to utilize such organizational techniques to normalize this deficit. This may not be the case for more chronic patients (86).

Similarly, when semantic orienting procedures are used, episodic recognition memory appears to be intact early in the course of illness in mildly impaired patients, but is impaired in the more chronic patients. This is apparent even when the difficulty level of free recall and recognition memory tasks are equated (87).

Semantic Memory Semantic memory requires the patient to recall previously learned (remote) information. Using methods such as the Information subtest of the WAIS-R (71), the controlled word association test (oral production of spoken words beginning with a designated letter, also called the FAS) (71), and the set test (name as many items as possible from several categories, i.e., fruits) (71), several studies of patients with schizophrenia have found that, as the effortful processing requirements increase, performance on semantic memory tasks deteriorates in patients compared to controls (73,88).

3. *Executive/Frontal Functions*

Integration of the attentional, memory, and organizational systems of the brain depends on the integrity of the brain's executive functions, which control the directing and sustaining of attention and provide the organizational mechanism to enhance subsequent retrieval (89). Executive functions have been conceptualized as being responsible for several observed human phenomena, including goal formulation, planning, implementation of goal-directed plans, as well as monitoring performance and flexibly shifting problem-solving strategies. These complex cognitive functions are presumed to be mediated by the frontal brain (90).

Clinically, schizophrenia patients frequently present with symptoms that appear similar to those shown by patients with frontal lobe lesions. Such symptoms include deficits in planning, organization, behavioral regulation, and judgment. Patients with schizophrenia, particularly those with negative symptoms, have been suggested to resemble individuals with lesions involving the dorsolateral aspect of the frontal lobes (90).

Several hypotheses focusing on the nature of the deficit in schizophrenia have been proposed. Weinberger (91) has postulated a neurodevelopmental model of schizophrenia which suggests that dorsolateral prefrontal dysfunction in schizophrenia mediates a complex interaction between the mesolimbic and mesocortical dopamine system. The model implicates frontal dysfunction in negative symptoms and subcortical mechanisms in positive symptoms. Firth and Done (92) have suggested that negative symptoms of schizophrenia are reflective of a defect in the initiation of spontaneous action, which depends on the integrity of connections between prefrontal cortex and basal ganglia. Positive symptoms are conceptualized as being a result of changes in mechanisms that link the prefrontal and hippocampal areas. On the basis of eye movement and psychomotor/reaction time studies, Levin (93) has proposed that attentional deficits in schizophrenia may be reflective of subtle functional disturbance of the frontal lobes and their connections to the limbic system, cortical-sensory, and association cortex. Levin (93) further proposed that this attentional matrix (characterized by an inability to focus attention, distractibility, slowed initiation of goal-directed behavior, perseveration, poorly modulated motivation, and arousal) may be related to a disturbance in the mesocortical dopamine projections to the dorsolateral and orbital frontal cortex.

Frontal lobe cognitive processing in schizophrenia has been evaluated with the Wisconsin Card Scoring Test (WCST). Using Xenon inhalation–based positron emission tomography (PET), Weinberger et al. (94) compared regional cerebral blood flow (RCBF) during rest and activation with results from the WCST and a simple number matching procedure. Increased RCBF during activation distinguished 25 normal control subjects from 20 medication-free subjects who showed no activation in RCBF. Subsequently (23,95,96), this finding was replicated in an additional 16 patients. These findings may indicate that dorsolateral prefrontal cortex dysfunction results from a regionally specific defect. This defect is most apparent when the prefrontal cortex is activated. Weinberger's conclusions should not be overinterpreted to imply that WCST is specific to dorsolateral frontal dysfunction. There is evidence from examination of patients with focal frontal lesions that the ability to perform well on the WCST also involves functions attributable to the medial frontal lobe (97). It has also been suggested that orbital-frontal pathology, resulting in failure to maintain a learning set, may contribute to impaired WCST performance in patients with schizophrenia (98). Linking neurochemical pathology and physiological findings, Weinberger et al. proposed that schizophrenia involves prefrontal cortical hypoactivity and limbic dopamine hyperactivity caused by a prefrontal cortical deafferentation lesion (94).

4. *Other Functions*

a. Visual-Spatial Functions. A number of studies have reported intact visual-spatial functions that are presumed to be subserved by the parietal cortex (71) in schizophrenia patients. Schizophrenia patients are unimpaired in simple visual-spatial tasks such as copying a complex design (99,100) or judging the angular orientation of lines (105). As the degree of difficulty of the task is increased by employing more complex visual-spatial tasks such as the Block Design (62,100), Object Assembly (62,100), and Picture Completion (62) subtests of the WAIS, patients with schizophrenia frequently encounter difficulty. These findings suggest visual-spatial ability tends to be impaired on more complex tasks.

b. Language. In contrast to patients with aphasia, the schizophrenia patient does not exhibit disturbances in basic language functions (71). Naming-to-confrontation (101,102) and repetition (102) have been found to be unimpaired in schizophrenic patients, as are basic language functions and simple syntactic processing (103,104). Where language deficits have been shown, they are believed to be secondary to disturbances in cognitive functions such as attention or executive abilities subserved by frontal subcortical systems (105). These disturbances include complex syntactic processing (105), coherence of discourse structure (106), and comprehension (107).

III. DEPRESSION

The major disorders of mood states outlined in DSM-III-R (7) include mania (severely elevated, expansive, or irritable mood with or without psychosis), hypomania (less severely elevated, expansive, or irritable mood; delusions are never present), and major depression (requiring either depressed mood or loss of interest or pleasure). The classification and nosology of mood disorders remains controversial. A massive synthesis of the literature on manic-depressive illness has recently been published, and the reader seeking an in-depth discussion of the current understanding of the mood disorders is referred to this superb work (108). We will discuss cognition in the disordered mood states from the simple dichotomy of major depression and the manic phase of bipolar disorder.

A. Clinical Features

Major depression may occur as an isolated single episode during life or recurrently as a component state in either unipolar depression or bipolar disorder, depressed phase. Major depression has an overall peak onset age of about 45–55. The major features of the depressed state typically include depressed mood or loss of interest or pleasure as principal defining features. These cardinal symptoms are present almost all day, every day, and, for an episode to be considered major, must last longer than 2 weeks. Other features may include increased or decreased weight, increased or decreased sleep, increased or decreased psychomotor activity; fatigue/loss of energy; reduced feelings of sense of self-worth or excessive or inappropriate guilt; very often recurrent thoughts of death or suicidal ideation; and diminished ability to think or concentrate, or indecisiveness. Some patients may develop delusions or hallucinations, which may or may not be thematically congruent with the presence of the depressed state.

Suicide is a significant potential risk during depression. Suicidal ideation should never be minimized. Attempts should never be thought of as simple attention seeking. Particularly in the depressed phase of bipolar disorder, rates of suicidal ideation may be as high as 82% (109); 25–50% of such patients attempt suicide at least once (108), and in one study, 90% of attempts were judged to be sufficiently severe to warrant hospitalization (110).

The natural history of a treated episode of depression is that treatment with medication or electroshock therapy will, within several weeks, induce a significant remission in most patients. Frequently a patient will demonstrate a preferential response to one medication and not others. Today, it is not possible to predict which medication will benefit specific patients. Untreated episodes often remit spontaneously but frequently only after extended periods of many months to years. Characterization of the natural history of recurrent illness has been complicated by the heterogeneity of the population subsumed by diagnostic criteria such as DSM-III-R (7). Most patients who have had an episode of major (unipolar or bipolar) depression will experience a recurrence at some point in their life (108). At least one study has found that increasing age of onset of the initial episode is correlated with an increased probability of recurrence within the subsequent 2 years (111). Later age of onset has also been suggested to be associated with a longer-lasting initial episode (112). A current controversy is whether antidepressant medication alters the cyclicity of the disorders which are recurrent, by increasing the recurrence frequency. This concern has been most focused on the bipolar-disordered patient where evidence is accumulating suggesting the recurrence rate may be seriously increased by agents such as the tricyclic antidepressants (113). Some recurrent patients when treated with tricyclic antidepressants may enter a state of "ultrarapid cycling." In this phenomenon, the frequency of mood cycling may alternate over hours and persist unabated in a mood state that could be thought of as being akin to status epilepticus. The phenomenon of "rapid cycling," defined as four or more recurrences in a year, is believed to most likely occur in females (114) and to arise later in the course of illness (108). This possible complication of therapy reaffirms the physician's need to carefully characterize the patient's history of illness before initiating antidepressant therapy and supports the need to follow the patient after therapy is initiated. The depressed patient who cycles frequently is thought to be best treated prophylactically with lithium, Tegretol®, or possibly valproate therapy, in conjunction with a tricyclic antidepressant.

Major depression as defined by DSM-III affects approximately 3% of the population (4% of women and 1.7% of men) during any 6-month period in the United States (115), and 4.4% of the population during any 1 year (116). The prevalance of major depression is believed to be increasing (117).

The genetics underlying mood disorders has long been of interest. Twin studies suggest a concordance rate of 59% for depression in monozygotic twins when a criterion of three or more episodes is used as the diagnostic threshold. Inheritance of bipolar disorder has a reported monozygotic concordance rate of 80% (118). A recent review of chromosomal linkage mapping studies examined the inconsistent evidence of reported linkage of manic-depressive disorder to chromosome X markers (color blindness, glucose-6-phosphate dehydrogenase, Xq28), chromosome 11 (insulin-RAS oncogene region, Harvey-ras-1), and HLA linkages (188). The conclusions were that no consistent marker has been identified, and that failure to identify a consistent marker may be a result of illness heterogeneity.

B. Pathogenesis

Many studies have focused on clarifying the underlying pathophysiology of depression and mania. The volume of findings and contradictory findings preclude a concise summary. We therefore restrict ourselves to a brief overview of the neurochemical hypotheses being evaluated. The interested reader is directed to several recent reviews of neuroanatomical, electrophysiological, and functional imaging studies indicating the presence of abnormal frontal brain function in the disordered mood states (108,119,120).

Neurochemical hypotheses concerned with mood disorder etiology emerged in the early 1960s with the amine hypothesis. This hypothesis was based on the observed effects of central aminergic neurotransmitter-depleting drugs, such as reserpine, which induced depression in some susceptible individuals. More recent hypotheses have proposed interactional changes in neurotransmitter systems such as the serotonin-norepinephrine permissive hypothesis (121,122). This hypothesis proposes that low levels of serotonin permit instability in other transmitter systems to arise and manifest as altered mood states. Thus, serotonin is seen to dampen fluctuations in the tone of other neurotransmitter systems. Others have proposed involvement of the cholinergic system (123), dopamine (124), GABA (125), and other systems. A large amount of information is available supportive of consistent neurotransmitter system changes within subgroups of individuals with mood problems including results of endocrine studies (126).

C. Cognitive Dysfunction in Depression

The examination of cognitive function in depression in the middle aged has been less extensively undertaken than in the older adult or schizophrenia patient. Because the literature is so limited, we will discuss results of research in depression in both unipolar and bipolar depressed populations as a single entity while acknowledging that this may not be a precise characterization of the depressed patient population. Changes in diagnostic criteria over time have limited conclusions that can be derived from earlier studies. While less studied than schizophrenia, cognitive deficits evident in depressed patients are believed to resolve with antidepressant therapy (127).

1. Attention

While clinicians frequently suggest that depressed patients are inattentive, there are few systematic investigations of attentional abilities in the young depressed population.

The span of apprehension test has been examined in depressed (bipolar) patients, with no deficit in performance noted (128). Backward masking evaluation of depressed patients in several studies has produced unclear results. One study noted no significant difference in the performance of depressed patients compared to normal controls (49), while several other studies, which compared depressives to other psychiatric patient groups, found depressive patient performance to be better than that of patients with schizophrenia. These latter studies did not include normal controls, therefore limiting conclusions about the presence or absence of a sensory memory deficit in depression (129–131).

The Continuous Performance Test has been evaluated in at least one study of depressed patients, and the results suggested that visual vigilance is reduced in depressed persons compared to normal controls (132). Vigilance impairment has also been demonstrated employing an auditory task, and the deficit may be correlated to self-reported mood (133). Vigilance evaluated by simple reaction time has also been shown to be reduced in depression.

Selective attention evaluated by digit span with distraction is impaired in depression (134). At least two studies employing the Stroop test have found performance decrements in depressed patients compared to normal controls, particularly in the interference component (62,135).

A single study of divided attention performance by depressives employed an auditory shadowing task and found no differences compared to normal controls (64).

In general, attentional measures demonstrating performance decrements in depressed patients also reveal impaired performance in patients with schizophrenia and mania. The degree of impairment in these other patient populations is more severe than is seen in simple depression.

2. *Memory*

Depressed patients often complain of difficulties with remembering. Memory complaints are most clearly expressed in relation to the period of depression, and this is often of most concern to the patient after the depressive symptoms have remitted. An early study demonstrated that depressed patients manifest a deficit in registering information. This study also demonstrated that once information had been learned, it was retained (136). The extent to which information is retained and retrieved, as well as the factors that negatively influence retrieval, remains only minimally explored in young depressives.

a. Short-Term Memory

Recognition Memory Recognition memory has been examined employing the Sternberg paradigm in at least one study of depressed patients. Compared to normal control subjects, no significant differences were observed (137).

Free Recall Memory In the only identified study of the Brown-Peterson paradigm, it was reported that medication-free depressed patients performed more poorly than normal control subjects (138). In a recently completed study comparing unmedicated depressives and normal controls, we found no group differences in performance employing a task similar to that employed by the authors of the above study (101). The reasons for the different results in these two studies of short-term free recall are unclear but could be due to differences in severity of depressive symptoms in the two populations. The evaluation of nondistraction span abilities, employing either digit span or supraspan tasks in depressed patients, suggests that short-term memory is not impaired (78).

The recency component of the serial position effect has been evaluated in at least one study of depressed patients, compared to normal control subjects. This study found no performance differences between the patient and normal subject control group (80).

b. Long-Term Memory

Episodic Memory Depressed patients report episodic memory impairments. Several studies support this finding. Stromgreen (139) has demonstrated that the degree of depression is inversely related to performance on both verbal (logical memory/paragraph recall) and nonverbal (design recall) subtests of the Wechsler Memory Scale (at both immediate and delayed [30 min] recall). In a series of studies reviewed by Weingartner and Silberman (140), important underlying aspects of the memory disturbance in depression have been delineated. These investigators demonstrated that depressed patients generate fewer categories when presented with unrelated words than nondepressed control subjects. When presented with words from well-defined categories, performance of depressed individuals is equal to that of nondepressed control subjects. Caine reviewed the available literature on cognitive function in young depressives and suggested that memory deficits in depressed patients arise because of attentional impairment and difficulty in the initial acquisition of information. He argued that the acquisition problem is a result of the presence of a deficient organizational capacity associated with the mood state. Caine reported that when organizational structure is provided, depressed patients perform normally (141).

Semantic Memory In addition to difficulties with episodic memory, depressed patients have also been shown in some, but not all, studies to manifest deficits in retrieval of information from semantic memory. The controlled word association test has been evaluated in three studies of depressed patients. Two studies found that depressed patients are impaired relative to controls when asked to generate words beginning with specific letters of the alphabet (142,143). We found no performance differences using this memory evaluation paradigm in depressed patients compared to normal controls (101). Wolfe et al. (142) noted that the bipolar depressed population manifested impairment, while unipolar depressives did not. Our sample included primarily unipolar depressives and may not be inconsistent with the other reports. Calev et al. (143) reported that the performance of depressed patients on the set test was better than on the controlled word association test. This supports the view that the controlled word association test is more difficult than the set test, as discussed in the section on schizophrenia.

3. *Executive Function*

Executive function, assessed by the WCST, has been found to be unimpaired in one study that utilized unmedicated, mixed, (unspecified) depressed patients (144). A more recent study utilizing unipolar depressed patients showed that the degree of impairment on the categories achieved measure of the WCST varied with the extent of overall cognitive disturbance. Depressed subjects with minimal cognitive disturbance were found to be unimpaired on this measure, whereas those with global cognitive deficits were substantially impaired. Patients with the least degree of cognitive impairment rated themselves as more depressed, and following ECT treatment, a number of patients were able to improve performance on the WCST (145). A recent study has demonstrated that, at least in schizophrenia, a major covariate of WCST performance is attention (73). The study reporting improved WCST performance with ECT treatment of depressed patients (145) may possibly be explained by improved attentional abilities in treatment-responsive patients.

4. *Other Functions*

a. Visual-Spatial Functions. Two studies of depressed patients reported no deficits in performance on the Bender-Gestalt test of visual-spatial ability (144,146). The latter study limited its findings of no deficit to the bipolar depressed population, as the unipolar depressives in their study manifested deficits. Performance on the Block Design test has been reported to be impaired in one study (144) but not in another study of a mixed group of unspecified depressed patients (147). As with schizophrenia, deficits in visual-spatial functions in depression appear to be made more prominent as tasks are made more complex and make greater demands for effortful processing.

b. Language. Depressed patients are well known to demonstrate increased speech latency, but no consistent findings of formal language impairment have been reported. One study (148) found that patients with mixed unspecified depression were unimpaired in the aphasia screening test, whereas another study (149) reported deficits on this measure in a similar patient group. Two studies (49,150) found impaired expressive vocabulary in depressed patients, although at least one study showed no such impairments (148). Caine et al. (151) reported story comprehension deficits in unmedicated endogenously depressed patients compared to normal controls.

IV. MANIA

A. Clinical Features

Bipolar disorder has a peak onset period of age 15–24 and may present with either depression or hypomania/mania. The overall mean onset age for the disorder is 30 (108). Because initial episodes vary in their intensity and patients frequently do not initially seek help, the manic patient not infrequently presents to the physician at a later age.

The major features of the manic syndrome, in addition to abnormal and persistent mood elevation, may include: excessive involvement in pleasurable but potentially painful activities (such as spending excessive money or impulsive sexual indiscretions), inflated or grandiose self-esteem, decreased need for sleep, subjectively experienced racing thoughts, flight of ideas, distractibility, excessive or pressured talkativeness, increased activity which is often goal directed (cleaning house, studying for school, being sexually demanding), and increased psychomotor behavior (7). The distinction between mania and hypomania is the relative absence of impairment in occupational or social functioning and the absence of psychosis in hypomania. Symptoms of psychosis may be present in either mania or major depression and are often identical to those seen in schizophrenia. This symptom overlap makes the differentiation of the mood disorders from schizophrenia difficult at times.

Bipolar disorder (defined as a manic episode) has a 6-month prevalence in the United States of 0.9%, a 1-year prevalence of approximately 1% (116), and is believed to occur equally in men and women.

B. Pathogenesis

As with depression, the pathophysiology of mania has been proposed to involve dysregulation of various neurotransmitter systems. The interested reader may refer to those references outlined in the discussion of the pathophysiology of depression for an in-depth review of the pathophysiology of mania.

C. Cognitive Dysfunction in Mania

Cognitive function during the mood-elevated phase of bipolar disorder (hypomania and, during the psychotic phase, mania) has been less studied than cognitive changes in patients with either schizophrenia or depression. Reasons for this include the lower prevalence of this disorder as well as difficulties related to patient cooperation with assessment. The major body of literature in bipolar mania is focused on the differentiation of patients with this disorder from similarly psychotic patients with schizophrenia. As with depression, reported cognitive deficits are believed to resolve with mood-stabilizing therapy (127).

1. Attention

Two studies have examined bipolar-manic patients using the span of apprehension test. Performance deficits are similar to that seen in the schizophrenia patient (45). Backward masking studies have not definitively established the response pattern of mood-elevated bipolar disorder patients. Three backward masking studies have demonstrated psychotic bipolar patient performance as being equivalent to that of patients with schizophrenia (49,129,152). One study has suggested that bipolar-manic patients do not perform significantly differently than normal controls (50); another study reached the same conclusion about bipolar-hypomanic patients (49).

Evaluation of the Continuous Performance Test disclosed similar, but less severe, errors in patients with mania compared to patients with schizophrenia (59). The reaction time crossover phenomenon has also been observed in patients with mania but is believed to occur less frequently than in schizophrenia (58).

Digit span and word span with distraction have been assessed in several studies that included bipolar-manic patients. A consistent finding has been the presence of a performance deficit but one which is less severe than is observed in schizophrenia (60,153–155). Our literature review for this chapter revealed no studies of the Stroop test in the mania population.

Divided attention employing auditory shadowing has been examined in at least one study of bipolar-manic patients. This study found no performance differences in bipolar-manic patients compared to a group of normal control subjects (64).

2. Memory

a. Short-Term Memory. We were unable to identify any studies of either recognition or free recall short-term memory in bipolar-mania patients, the exception being a single study of digit span forward. This study found no differences in patients with bipolar disorder compared to normal control subjects (61).

b. Long-Term Memory. Episodic long-term memory has been little studied in the bipolar mania patient population. Deficits in the recall of verbal (list learning) and nonverbal (Graham-Kendall designs) material have been reported for bipolar-manic patients (149). The recall performance of bipolar manic patients has been suggested to be correlated with the level of disorganization and severity of mania (156).

Semantic Memory Bipolar-manic patients have been found to exhibit impaired performance when assessed by the controlled word association test as well as on the set test (143). It is unclear whether semantic memory performance deficits are related to the degree of disorganization and severity of the mania state.

3. *Executive Ability*

Manic patients have been shown (157) to exhibit a fewer number of categories achieved and a greater number of perseverative errors on the WCST compared to controls. In the same study, the performance of manics was also compared to that of schizophrenia patients. Both patient groups were medicated. The patients with mania and those with schizophrenia performed comparably.

4. *Other Functions*

a. Visual-Spatial Functions. Visual-spatial functions have been minimally studied in bipolar mania patients. One study suggested that this patient group is impaired in performance assessed by the Hooper Visual Organization test (158). Two other studies, using different methods to evaluate visual-spatial functions, found no evidence of impairment (149,159). The meager literature allows for no conclusions to be drawn.

b. Language. Formal disorders of language are not a reported feature of mania. Speech is altered in hypomania/mania with usually observed pressured speech; often, in more severe mood elevation, speech incoherence is present, and features such as punning and rhyming, which are believed to reflect changes in the patient's cognitive associations, are often evident.

V. CONCLUSIONS

Cognitive dysfunction is frequently identified in objective testing of the patient with either schizophrenia or a major mood disorder. Demonstration of deficits in attention in both groups depends on the type of attention assessed, the use of medications, and the sensitivity of the test. Short-term free recall memory tasks, which introduce interpolated activities and delay procedures, consistently reveal deficits in schizophrenia that may not be present in depression. Such procedures may not have been assessed in the manic patient population. Short-term recognition memory is unaffected in schizophrenia or depression and also may not have been studied in mania. In both groups, evaluation of long-term memory and visual-spatial functions frequently reveals impairment when the requirement for effortful processing is increased. Basic language functions appear to be intact in both patient groups. Assessment of executive functions employing techniques such as the WCST in schizophrenia consistently reveals impairment believed to result from prefrontal lobe dysfunction. Depressed patients also manifest deficits in WCST performance. This deficit may be most evident in depressed patients with global cognitive deficits. Patients with mania may not be distinguishable from patients with schizophrenia on this measure of executive function. While the presence of psychosis may confound differentiation of schizophrenia from the bipolar manic group, impairment in cognitive functions is not simply a result of psychoses. Most patients with depression and mania, when successfully treated, respond with reversal of cognitive disturbance. This is unfortunately not the case in patients with schizophrenia, in whom deficits in memory and executive abilities are particularly refractory to treatment.

ACKNOWLEDGEMENT

The preparation of this manuscript was supported in part by USPHS MH 41684 and a grant from the Elizabeth Severance Prentiss Foundation. The authors are grateful to Dr. Herbert Meltzer for his many discussions regarding this manuscript. The secretarial assistance of Mrs. Diane Mack is greatly appreciated.

REFERENCES

1. Lewis MS. Age incidence and schizophrenia: Part II. Beyond age incidence. Schizophrenia Bull 1989; 15:75–80.
2. Andreasen NC, Olsen, S. Negative vs positive schizophrenia: definition and validation, Arch Gen Psychiatry 1982; 39:789–94.
3. Wagman AMI, Heinrich DW, Carpenter WT Jr. Deficit and nondeficit forms of schizophrenia: neuropsychological evaluation. Psychiatr Res 1987; 22:319–30.
4. Ganguli R, Raghu U. Tardive dyskinesia, impaired recall and informed consent. J Clin Psychiatry 1985; 46:434–5.
5. Famuyiwa OO, Eccleston D, Donaldson AA, Garside RS. Tardive dyskinesia and dementia. Br J Psychiatry 1979; 135:500–4.
6. Harvey PD, Davidson M, Ponchik P, Parella M, Losonczy M, Katz S, Mons RC. Assessment of dementia in elderly schizophrenic patients. Poster presentation, American College of Neuropharmacology, Puerto Rico, December 1990.
7. American Psychiatric Association. Diagnostic and statistical manual of mental disorders. 3rd ed, revised, Washington, DC: APA, 1988.
8. Endicott J, Spitzer RL. A diagnostic interview: the schedule for affective disorders and schizophrenia. Arch Gen Psychiatry 1978; 35:837–44.
9. Torrey EF. Prevalence studies in schizophrenia. Br J Psychiatry 1987; 598–608.
10. Lewine R, Strauss JS, Gift TE. Sex differences in age at first admission for schizophrenia. Am J Psychiatry 1981; 138:440–4.
11. Saugstad LF. Social class, marriage and fertility in schizophrenia. Schizophrenia Bull 1989; 15:9–43.

12. Kendler KS. The genetics of schizophrenia and related disorders: a review. In: Dunner DL, Gershon ES, Barrett JE, eds. Relatives at risk for mental disorder. New York: Raven Press, 1988.
13. Bassett AS, McGillivray BC, Jones B, Pantzar JR. Partial trisomy chromosome 5 cosegregating with schizophrenia. Lancet 1988; 1:799–801.
14. Sherrington R, Brynjolfsson J, Petursson H, et al. Location of a susceptibility locus for schizophrenia on chromosome 5. Nature 1988; 336:164–7.
15. Kennedy JL, Giuffra LA, Moises HW, et al. Evidence against linkage of schizophrenia to markers on chromosome 5 in a northern Swedish pedigree. Nature 1988; 336:167–70.
16. Garver DL, Reich T, Isenberg KE, Cloninger CR. Schizophrenia and the question of genetic heterogeneity. Schizophrenia Bull 1989; 15:421–30.
17. Weinberger DR, Torrey EF, Neophytides AN, Wyatt RJ. Structural abnormalities in the cerebral cortex of chronic schizophrenic patients. Arch Gen Psychiatry 1979; 36:935–9.
18. Weinberger DR, Wagner RL, Wyatt RJ. Neuropathological studies of schizophrenia: a selective review. Schizophrenia Bull 1983; 9:193–212.
19. Benes FM, Davidson J, Bird ED. Quantitative cytoarchitectonic studies of the cerebral cortex in schizophrenia. Arch Gen Psychiatry 1986; 43:31–5.
20. Shelton RC, Karson CN, Doran AR, Pickar D, Bigelow LB, Weinberger DR. Cerebral structural pathology in schizophrenia: evidence for a selective prefrontal cortical defect. Am J Psychiatry 1988; 145:154–63.
21. Scheibel AB, Kovelman JA. Disorientation of the hippocampal pyramidal cell and its processes in the schizophrenic patient. Biol Psychiatry 1981; 16:101–2.
22. Suddath RL, Christison GW, Torrey EF, Casanova MF, Weinberger DR. Anatomical abnormalities in the brains of monozygotic twins discordant for schizophrenia N Engl J Med 1990; 322:789–94.
23. Berman KF, Zec RF, Weinberger DR. Physiologic dysfunction of dorsolateral prefrontal cortex in schizophrenia. II. Role of neuroleptic treatment, attention and mental effort, Arch Gen Psychiatry 1986; 43:126–35.
24. Losmczy MF, Davidson M, Davis KL. The dopamine hypothesis of schizophrenia. In: Meltzer HY, ed. Psychopharmacology: the third generation of progress. New York: Raven Press, 1987.
25. vanKammen DP, Gelernter J. Biochemical instability in schizophrenia. II. The serotonin and gaba-aminobutyric acid system. In: Meltzer HY, ed. Psychopharmacology: the third generation of progress. New York: Raven Press, 1987.
26. vanKammen DP, Gelernter J. Biochemical instability in schizophrenia. I. The norepinephrine system. In: Meltzer HY, ed. Psychopharmacology: the third generation of progress. New York: Raven Press, 1987.
27. Nemeroff CB, Berger PA, Bissette G. Peptides in schizophrenia. In: Meltzer HY, ed. Psychopharmacology: the third generation of progress. New York: Raven Press, 1987.
28. Kraeplin E. Dementia praecox and paraphrenia. Edinburgh: Livingstone, 1919.
29. The compact edition of the Oxford English dictionary. Vol. I. 1971: 550.

30. Estes WK, Taylor HA. A detection method and probabilistic models for assessing information processing from brief visual displays, Proc Natl Acad Sci USA 1964; 52:446–54.
31. Strauss ME. Cognitive markers for schizophrenia: an appraisal. In: Schultz SC, Tamminga CA, eds. Schizophrenia: scientific progress. New York: Oxford University Press, 1989:103–9.
32. Exner S. Uber die zu einer gesichts wahrnehmung Nothige Zeit. Wiener Sitzungsbericht der mathematisch - Natur Wissensch aft Lichen classe der Kaiser-Lichen Akademie der Wissenschaften 58; Part 2, 601–32. In: Breitmeyer BJ, ed. Visual masking: an integrative approach. A history of visual masking. New York: Oxford University Press, 1984:17.
33. Schuck JR, Lee RC. Backward masking, information processing and schizophrenia. Schizophrenia Bull 1989; 15:491–500.
34. Kornetsky C, Orzack MA. Physiological and behavioral correlates of attention dysfunction in schizophrenic patients. In: Wynne LC, Cromwell RL, Matthysse S, eds. The nature of schizophrenia: new approaches to research and treatment. New York: Wiley, 1978.
35. Nuechterlein KH. Signal detection in vigilance tasks and behavioral attributes among offspring of schizophrenic mothers and among hyperactive children. J Abnorm Psychol 1983; 92:4–28.
36. Neuchterlein KH. Reaction time and attention in schizophrenia: a critical evaluation of the data and theories, Schizophrenia Bull 1977; 3:373–428.
37. Spohn HE, Strauss ME. Relation of neuroleptic and anticholinergic medication to cognitive functioning in schizophrenia. J Abnorm Psychol 1989; 98:367–80.
38. Oltmanns TF, Neale JF. Schizophrenic performance when distractions are present: attentional deficit or differential task difficulty, J Abnorm Psychol 1975; 84:205–9.
39. Oltmanns TF. Selective attention in schizophrenic and manic psychoses: the effect of distraction on information processing. J Abnorm Psychol 1978; 87:212–25.
40. Otteson MH, Holzman PS. Cognitive controls and psychopathology. J Abnorm Psychol 1976; 85:125–35.
41. McGhie A, Chapman J, Lawson JS. The effect of distraction on schizophrenic performance. I perception and immediate memory. Br J Psychiatry 1965; 111:383–90.
42. Posner MI, Early TS, Reiman E, Pardo PJ, Dhawan M. Asymmetries in hemispheric control of attention in schizophrenia. Arch Gen Psychiatry 1988; 45:814–21.
43. Madden DJ. Adult age differences in visual word recognition: semantic encoding and episodic retention. Exp Aging Res 1986; 12:71–8.
44. Neale JM, McIntyre CW, Fox R, Cromwell RL. Span of apprehension in acute schizophrenia. J Abnorm Psychol 1969; 74:593–6.
45. Strauss ME, Prescott CA, Gutterman DF, Tune LE. Span of apprehension deficits in schizophrenia and mania. Schizophrenia Bull 1987; 13:699–704.

46. Pearl D. Phenothiazine effects in chronic schizophrenia. J Clin Psychol 1962; 18:86–9.
47. Spohn HE, Coyne L. Lacoursiere R, Mazur D, Hayes K. Relation of neuroleptic dose and tardive dyskinesia to attention, information processing and psychophysiology in medicated schizophrenics. Arch Gen Psychiatry 1985; 42:849–59.
48. Sacazzo DP, Miller S. Critical interstimulus intervals in delusional schizophrenics and normals. J Abnorm Psychol 1977; 86:261–6.
49. Sacuzzo DP, Braff DL. Early information processing deficits in schizophrenia. Arch Gen Psychiatry 1981; 38:175–9.
50. Green M, Walker E. Symptom correlates of vulnerability to backward masking in schizophrenia. Am J Psychiatry 1986; 143:181–6.
51. Braff DL, Sacazzo DP. The effects of antipsychotic medication on speed of information processing in schizophrenic patients. Am J Psychiatry 1982; 139:1127–30.
52. Harvey PD, Keefe RSE, Moskowitz K, Mohs RL, Davis KL. Attentional markers of vulnerability to schizophrenia: performance of medicated and unmedicated patients and normals. Psychiatry Res 1990; 33:179–88.
53. Asarnow RF, MacCrimmon DJ. Residual performance deficit in clinically remitted schizophrenics: a marker of schizophrenia. J Abnorm Psychol 1978; 87:597–608.
54. Orzack MH, Kornetsky C, Freeman H. The effect of daily administration of carphenazine on attention in the schizophrenic patient. Psychopharmacologia 1967; 11:31–8.
55. Cornblatt BA, Lenzenweger MF, Erlenmeyer-Kimling L. The continuous performance test identical pairs version. II. Contrasting attentional profiles in schizophrenic and depressed patients. J Psychiatr Res 1984; 29:66–85.
56. Walker E. Attentional and neuromotor functions of schizophrenics, schizoaffectives and patients with other affective disorders. Arch Gen Psychiatry 1981; 38:1355–8.
57. Cromwell RL, DeAmicis L, Hayes T, Briggs D. Reaction time crossover, a vulnerability index: mean reaction time, a symptom severity index, Psychopharmacol Bull 1979; 15:24–5.
58. Bohannon WE, Strauss ME. Reaction time crossover in psychiatric outpatients. Psychiatr Res 1983; 9:17–22.
59. Neuchterlein KH, Dawson ME. Information processing and attentional functioning in the developmental course of schizophrenia. Schizophrenia Bull 1984; 10:160–203.
60. Oltmanns TF. Selective attention in schizophrenic and manic psychoses: the effect of distraction on information processing. J Abnorm Psychol 1978; 87:212–25.
61. Harvey PD, Earle-Beyer MA, Levinson BA. Distractibility and discourse failure: their association in mania and schizophrenia. J Nerv Men Dis 1986; 174:274–9.
62. Killiam GA, Holzman PS, Davis JM, Gibbons R. Effect of psychotropic

medication on selected cognitive and perceptual measures. J Abnorm Psychol 1984; 93:58–70.

63. Serafetinides EA, Collins S, Clark ML. Haloperidol, clopenthixol and chlorpromazine in chronic schizophrenia, J Nerv Ment Dis 1972; 154:31–42.
64. Pogue-Geile MF, Oltmanns TF. Sentence perception and distractibility in schizophrenic, manic and depressed patients. J Abnorm Psychol 1980; 2: 115–24.
65. Morris RG, Baddely AD. Primary and working memory functioning in Alzheimer-type dementia. J Clin Exp Neuropsychol 1988; 10:279–96.
66. Sternberg S. High-speed scanning in human memory. Science 1966; 153: 652–4.
67. Kausler DH. Experimental psychology, cognition and human aging, 2nd ed. New York: Springer-Verlag, 1991.
68. Koh SD, Szoc R, Peterson RA. Short-term memory scanning in schizophrenic young adults. J Abnorm Psychol 1977; 86:451–60.
69. Marusarz TZ, Koh SD. Contextual effects on the short-term memory retrieval of schizophrenic young adults. J Abnorm Psychol 1980; 89:683–96.
70. Broga MI, Neufeld RWJ. Multivariate cognitive performance levels and response styles among paranoid and nonparanoid schizophrenics. J Abnorm Psychol 1981; 90:495–509.
71. Lezak MD. Neuropsychological assessment. 2nd ed. New York: Oxford University Press, 1983:416–9.
72. Weinberger E, Cermak LS. Short-term retention in acute and chronic paranoid schizophrenics. J Abnorm Psychol 1973; 82:220–5.
73. Kenny JT, Meltzer HY. The effect of attention on higher cortical functions in schizophrenia. J Neuropsychiatry Clin Neurosci 1991; 3:269–275.
74. Kenny JT. Freidman L, Ubody D, Meltzer HY. The effect of clozapine on neuropsychological functions in schizophrenia, Arch Gen Psychiatry 1991 (in press).
75. Wechsler D. Wechsler Adult Intelligence Scale manual. New York: Psychological Corporation, 1955.
76. Cassens G, Inglis A, Appelbaum PS, Gutheil TG. Neuroleptics: effects on neuropsychological function in chronic schizophrenic patients. Schizophrenia Bull 1990; 16:477–99.
77. Gilgash CA. Effects of Thorazine on Wechsler scores of adult catatonic schizophrenics. Psychol Rep 1957; 3:561–4.
78. Small IF, Small JG, Millstein V, Moore JE. Neuropsychological observations with psychosis and somatic treatment: neuropsychological examinations of psychiatric patients. J Nerv Ment Dis 1972; 155:6–13.
79. Weiss KM, Vrtunski PG, Simpson DM. Information overload disrupts digit recall performance in schizophrenics. Schizophrenia Res 1988; 1:299–303.
80. Frame CL, Oltmanns TF. Serial recall by schizophrenic and affective patients during and after psychotic episodes. J Abnorm Psychol 1982; 91:311–8.
81. Tulving E. Episodic and semantic memory. In: Tulving E, Donaldson W, eds. Organization of memory. New York: Academic Press, 1972.
82. Winograd T. Understanding natural language. In: Bobrow D, Collens A, eds. Representation and understanding. New York: Academic Press, 1975.

83. Neale JM, Oltmanns TF. Schizophrenia. New York: Wiley, 1980.
84. Calev A. Memory in schizophrenia. In: Weller M, ed., International perspectives in schizophrenia: biological, social and epidemiological findings. London: John Libbey, 1990:29–41.
85. Koh SD. Remembering of verbal materials by schizophrenic young adults. In: Schwartz S, ed. Language and cognition in schizophrenia. Hillsdale, NJ: Lawrence Erlbaum, 1978:55–99.
86. Calev A. Memory in schizophrenia. In: Weller M, ed. International perspectives in schizophrenia: biological, social and epidemiological findings. London: John Libbey, 1990:29–41.
87. Calev A. Recall and recognition in mildly disturbed schizophrenics: the use of matched tasks. Psychol Med 1984; 14:425–9.
88. Rosen WG. Verbal fluency in aging and dementia. J Clin Neuropsychol 2:135–146.
89. Goldberg TE, Weinberger DR, Pushkin NH, Berman KF, Podd MH. Recall memory deficit in schizophrenia: a possible manifestation of prefrontal dysfunction. Schizophrenia Res 1989; 2:251–7.
90. Stuss DT, Benson DF. Frontal lobe lesions and behavior. In: Kertesz A, ed. Localization in neuropsychology. New York: Academic Press, 1983.
91. Weinberger DR. Implications of normal brain development for the pathogenesis of schizophrenia. Arch Gen Psychiatry 1987; 44:660–9.
92. Firth CD, Done DJ. Towards a neuropsychology of schizophrenia. Brit J Psychiatry 1988; 153:437–43.
93. Levin S. Frontal lobe dysfunction in schizophrenia. II. Impairments of psychological and brain functions. J Psychiatr Res 1984; 18:57–72.
94. Weinberger DR, Berman KF, Zec RF. Physiologic dysfunction of dorsolateral prefrontal cortex in schizophrenia. I. Regional cerebral blood flow (CBF) evidence. Arch Gen Psychiatry 1986; 43:114–24.
95. Weinberger DR, Berman KS, Illowsky BP. Physiologic dysfunction of dorsolateral prefrontal cortex in schizophrenia. III. A new cohort of evidence for monoaminergic mechanism. Arch Gen Psychiatry 1988; 45:609–15.
96. Berman KF, Illowsky BP, Weinberger DR. Physiological dysfunction of dorsolateral prefrontal cortex in schizophrenia. IV. Further evidence for regional and behavioral specificity. Arch Gen Psychiatry 1988; 45:616–22.
97. Drewe EA. The effect of type and area of brain lesions on Wisconsin Card Sorting test performance. Cortex 1974; 10:159–70.
98. Stuss DT, Benson DF. Frontal lobe lesions and behavior. In: Kertesz A, ed. Localization in neuropsychology. New York: Academic Press, 1983: 429–54.
99. Kolb B, Whishaw IQ. Performance of schizophrenic patients on test sensitive to left or right frontal, temporal or parietal function in neurological patients. Nerv Ment Dis 1983; 171(7):435–43.
100. Stuss DT, Benson DF, Kaplan EF, Della Malva CL, Weir WS. The effect of prefrontal leucotomy on visuoperceptice and visuoconstructive tests. Bull Clin Neurosci 1984; 49:43–51.
101. Kenny J, Meltzer HY. Unpublished observations.

102. Morice RD, McNicol D. Language changes in schizophrenia: a limited replication. Schizophrenia Bull 1986; 12:239–51.
103. Andreasen NC, Grove W. The relationship between schizophrenic language, manic language and aphasia. In: Gruzelier J, Flor-Henry P, eds. Hemispheric asymmetries of function in psychopathology. New York: Elsevier/North Holland, 1979:373–90.
104. Schwartz S. Is there a schizophrenic language? Behav Brain Sci 1982; 5:579–626.
105. Levin S, Yurgelun-Todd D, Craft S. Contributions of clinical neuropsychology to the study of schizophrenia. J Abnorm Psychol 1989; 98:341–56.
106. Hoffman RE. Verbal hallucinations and language production processes in schizophrenia. Behav Brain Sci 1986; 9:503–17.
107. Green M. Walker E. Neuropsychological performance and positive and negative symptoms in schizophrenia. J Abnorm Psychol 1985; 94:460–9.
108. Goodwin FK, Redfield Jamison K. Manic-depressive illness. New York: Oxford University Press, 1990.
109. Winokur G, Clayton PJ, Reich T. Manic depressive illness. St. Louis: CV Mosby, 1969.
110. Johnson GF, Hunt G. Suicidal behavior in bipolar manic-depressive patients and their families. Compr Psychiatry 1979; 20:159–64.
111. Zis AP, Grof P, Webster M, Goodwin FK. Prediction of relapse in recurrent affective disorder. Psychopharmacol Bull 1980; 16:47–9.
112. Roy-Byrne P, Post RM, Uhde TW, Porcu T, Davis D. The longitudinal course of recurrent affective illness: life chart data from research patients at the NIMH. Acta Psychiatr Scand 1985; 71 (Suppl 317):1–34.
113. Wehr TA, Goodwin FK. Rapid cycling in manic-depressives induced by tricyclic antidepressants. Arch Gen Psychiatry 1979; 36:555–9.
114. Parry BL. Reproductive factors affecting the course of affective illness in women. Psychiatr Clin North Am 1989; 12:207–20.
115. Weissman MM, Myers JK, Leaf PJ, Tischler GL, Holzer CE. The affective disorders: results from the Epidemiologic Catchment Area Study (ECA). In: Hippilis H, Kierman GL, Matussek N, eds. New results in depression research. Berlin, Heidelberg: Springer-Verlag, 1986.
116. Weissman MM, Leaf PJ, Tischler GL, Blazer DG, Karno M, Bruce ML, Fiorio LP. Affective disorders in five United States communities. Psychol Med. 1988; 18:141–53.
117. Klerman GL. Evidence for increase in rates of depression in North America and Western Europe in recent decades. In: Hippilis H, Klerman GL, Matussek N, eds. New results in depression research. Berlin, Heidelberg: Springer-Verlag, 1986.
118. Gershon ES. Genetics. In: Goodwin FK, Redfield Jamison K, eds. Manic depressive illness. New York: Oxford University Press, 1990:373–401.
119. Potter WZ, Rudorfer MV, Goodwin FK: Biological findings in bipolar disorders. In: Hales RE, Frances AJ, eds. American Psychiatric Association annual review. Vol 6. Washington, DC: American Psychiatric Press, 1987:32–60.
120. Post RM, Ballenger JC, eds. Neurobiology of mood disorders. Baltimore: Williams & Wilkins, 1984.

121. Kety SS. Brain amines and affective disorders. In: Ho BT, McIsaac WM, eds. Brain chemistry and mental disease. New York: Plenum Press, 1971.
122. Prange AJ Jr, Wilson IC, Lynn CW, Alltop LB, Stikeleather RA. L-tryptophan in mania: contribution to a permissive hypothesis of affective disorders. Arch Gen Psychiatry 1974; 30:56–62.
123. Risch SC, Janowsky DS. Cholinergic-adrenergic balance in affective illness, In: Post RM, Ballenger JC, eds. Neurobiolody of mood disorders. Baltimore: Williams & Wilkins, 1984.
124. Antelman JP, Caggiula AR. Norepinephrine-dopamine interactions and behavior. Science 1977; 195:646–53.
125. Lloyd KG, Zivkovic B, Scatton B, Monselli PL, Bartholini G, The GABA-ergic hypothesis of depression. Prog Neuropsychopharmacol Biol Psychiatry 1989; 13:341–51.
126. Meltzer HY, Umberkoman-Wiita B, Robertson A, Tricon BJ, Lowy M, Perline R. Effect of 5-hydroxytryptophan on serum cortisol levels in major affective disorders. I. Enhanced response in depression and mania. Arch Gen Psychiatry 1984; 41:366–74.
127. Johnson MH, Magaro PA. Effects of mood and severity on memory processes in depression and mania. Psychol Bull 1987; 104:28–40.
128. Strauss ME, Bohannon WE, Stephens JG, Parker NE. Perceptual span in schizophrenia and affective disorders. J Nerv Ment Dis 1984; 172:431–5.
129. Schubert DL, Sacuzzo DP, Braff DL. Information processing in borderline patients, J Nerv Ment Dis 1985; 173:26–31.
130. Sacuzzo DP, Braff DL. Information processing abnormalities: trait- and state-dependent components. Schizophrenia Bull 1986; 12:447–59.
131. Braff DL, Sacuzzo DP. The time course of information-processing deficits in schizophrenia. Am J Psychiatry 1985; 88:170–4.
132. Cornblatt BA, Lenzenweger MJ, Erlenmeyer-Kimling L. The continuous performance test, identical pairs version: contrasting attentional profiles in schizophrenic and depressed patients. J Psychiatr Res 1984; 29:66–85.
133. Byrne DC. Affect and vigilance performance in depressive illness. J Psychiatr Res 1977; 13:185–91.
134. Pogue-Geile MF, Oltmanns TF. Sentence perception and distractibility in schizophrenic, manic and depressed patients. J Abnorm Psychol 1980; 89:115–24.
135. Raskin A, Friedman AS, DiMascio A. Cognitive and performance deficits in depression. Psychopharmacol Bull 1982; 18:196–202.
136. Cronholm B, Ottosson JO. Memory functions in endogenous depression. Arch Gen Psychiatry 1961; 5:101–7.
137. Koh SD, Wolpert EA. Memory scanning and retrieval in affective disorders, Psychiatr Res 1983; 8:289–97.
138. Cohen RM, Weingartner H, Smallberg SA, Murphy DL. Effort and cognition in depression. Arch Gen Psychiatry 1982; 39:593–7.
139. Stromgreen LS. The influence of depression on memory. Acta Psychiatr Scand 1977; 56:109–28.

140. Weingartner H, Silberman E. Models of cognitive impairment in depression. Psychopharmacol Bull 1982; 18:27–42.
141. Caine ED. The neuropsychology of depression: the pseudodementia syndrome. In: Grant I, Adams KM, eds. Neuropsychological assessment of neuropsychological disorders. New York: Oxford University Press, 1986.
142. Wolfe J, Granholm E, Butters N, Saunders E, Janowsky D. Verbal memory deficits associated with major affective disorders: a comparison of unipolar and bipolar patients, J Affect Dis 1987; 13:83–92.
143. Calev A, Negal D, Chazan S. Retrieval from semantic memory using meaningful and meaningless constructs by depressed, stable bipolar and manic patients. Br J Clin Psychol 1989; 28:67–73.
144. Hart RP, Kwentus JA, Taylor JR, Harbins ST. Rate of forgetting in dementia and depression. J Consult Clin Psychol 1987; 55:101–5.
145. Cassens G, Wolfe L, Zola, M. The neuropsychology of depression. J Neuropsychiatry Clin Neurosci 1990; 2(2):202–13.
146. Donnely EF, Murphy DL, Goodwin FK, Waldman IN. Intellectual function in primary affective disorder. Br J Psychiatry 1982; 140:633–6.
147. Johansen AM, Gustafson L, Risbery J. Psychological evaluation in dementia and depression. Danish Med Bull 1985; 32:60–2.
148. Gray JW, Dean RS, Rattan G, Cramer KM. Neuropsychological aspects of primary affective depression. Int J Neurosci 1987; 32:911–8.
149. Flor-Henry P, Yendoll LT. Neuropsychological investigation of schizophrenia and manic depressive psychosis. In: Gruzelier J, Flor-Henry P, eds. Hemisphere asymmetries of function in psychopathology. Amsterdam: Elsevier-North Holland, 1979.
150. Crawford JR, Besson JA, Parker DM, Sutherland KM, Keen PL. Estimation of premorbid intellectual status in depression. Br J Clin Psychol 1987; 26:313–4.
151. Caine ED, Yerevanian BI, Bamford KA. Cognitive function and the dexamethasone suppression test in depression. Am J Psychiatry 1984; 141:116–8.
152. Knight RA, Elliott DS, Freedman EG. Short-term visual memory in schizophrenics. J Abnorm Psychol 1985; 94:427–42.
153. Green M, Walker F. Attentional performance in positive- and negative-symptom schizophrenia. J Nerv Ment Dis 1986; 174:208–13.
154. Harvey PD, Earle-Beyer MA, Levinson BA. Distractibility and discourse failure. Their association in mania and schizophrenia. J Nerv Ment Dis 1986; 174:274–9.
155. Malone JRL, Hemsley DR. Lowered responsiveness and auditory signal detectability during depression. Psychol Med 1977; 7:717–22.
156. Henry G, Weingartner H, Murphy D. Idiosyncratic patterns of learning and association during mania. Am J Psychiatry 1971; 128:564–73.
157. Morice R. Cognitive inflexibility and pre-frontal dysfunction in schizophrenia and mania. Br J Psychiatry 1990; 157:50–4.
158. Taylor MA, Redfield J, Abrams R. Neuropsychological dysfunction in schizophrenia and affective disease. Biol Psychiatry 1981; 16:467–78.
159. Blackburn IM. Mental and psychomotor speed in depression and mania. Br J Psychiatry 1975; 126:329–33.

6

Consequences of Drug and Ethanol Use on Cognitive Function

David N. Stephens, Frank Dahlke, and Theodora Duka
Schering AG, Berlin, Germany

I. INTRODUCTION

Over the last 50 years the development of chemical agents for the treatment of psychiatric conditions has emptied the hospitals for the mentally ill and offered a return to more-or-less normal life for millions of patients. The availability of such agents has also led to the treatment with psychoactive agents, especially benzodiazepines, of a large population of patients with only mild disorders. In addition to these patients, an even larger population makes use of more traditional and readily available psychoactive substances, such as alcohol, nicotine, caffeine, marijuana, and opiates. This latter group ranges from occasional users to those suffering from different levels of addiction to these agents. This chapter will review the negative cognitive effects observed after use of some of these substances, especially the central nervous system (CNS) depressants, and ignore the possible abilities of stimulants, such as caffeine, to improve performance on certain cognitive tasks.

The effects of agents in the patient population for which they are prescribed will not be considered; hence, for instance, the abilities of neuroleptics to treat the cognitive disturbances of schizophrenia will not be discussed. There are several reasons for this approach. In patients, the mental disorder itself may produce cognitive effects that are difficult to dissociate from drug effects or from an interaction of the drug with that state. Thus the present review will concentrate on the effects of drugs in otherwise normal subjects, although the long-term effects of misuse of alcohol will also be considered in some detail.

A further problem that we have faced is the heterogeneity of technical terms used in cognitive research. In general, investigators of drug effects on cognitive function have not concerned themselves unduly with the subtleties of different theories of learning and memory and have only seldom specified the theoretical framework in which their experiments have been carried out. Consequently, different terms may have been used to mean the same thing, or even more confusingly, the same term may mean different things to different people. This chapter is not the appropriate place, nor are we particularly competent, to clear this particular Augean stable, but the result is that the terminology used here may not always be consistent. For a useful introduction to theories of memory, the reader is referred to Squire (1).

II. BENZODIAZEPINE EFFECTS ON COGNITIVE FUNCTIONS

Over the past decades, benzodiazepines have become a popular class of drug for the treatment of various emotional and physical disorders. The widespread use of benzodiazepines is attributable to their effectiveness not only as anxiolytics and hypnotics, but also as muscle relaxants and anticonvulsants. Although generally very safe drugs, the benzodiazepines do give rise to a range of side effects, including a wide array of cognitive impairments. The business man who takes a benzodiazepine to help him sleep on a long flight, and later cannot recall either the flight or what he did on arrival, is a familiar figure in talks on benzodiazepines and may not be purely anecdotal. In the clinic, use has been made of this phenomenon in using benzodiazepines to induce amnesia for unpleasant preoperative or minor surgical procedures, but it is not only clinicians who are able to exploit scientific observations: prostitutes in Paris have been reported as slipping their clients a benzodiazepine before persuading them to sign checks for large sums; under the influence of the drug, the client remembers nothing of his adventures and only later wonders at the hole in his bank account (2)!

A. Acute Effects on Cognitive Function

In more formal settings, the main cognitive effect of benzodiazepines is memory impairment. The limited clinical data are supported by studies in healthy subjects suggesting that the primary effect is an anterograde amnesia (i.e., a loss of memory for events occurring after drug administration). In exploring these effects, most investigators have employed information-processing models, dividing memory into steps of sensory input, encoding, storage, and retrieval (3). Such studies consistently document the benzodiazepines' ability to impair the learning of new material, while leaving retrieval of previously learned material intact. Typically, tasks such as digit span or repeating short lists of words that require only short-term memory, are unaffected (4,5). If, however, the list of digits or words to be remembered is lengthened beyond the capacity of the short-term store, then benzodiazepines induce marked impairments. Because remembering lists longer than those that can be accommodated in the short-term store implies transfer to a longer-term store, the effects of benzodiazepines suggest an impairment in consolidation processes involved in the transfer, or encoding, of information into long-term memories (e.g., 6; see Refs. 7,8 for reviews). This interpretation is strengthened by studies involving the later recall or recognition of material learned under benzodiazepine treatment; such recall or recognition tests, carried out several hours following acquisition, consistently reveal marked memory deficits, irrespective of the sensory modality of presentation (e.g., 5).

In contrast with the marked effects of benzodiazepines on encoding, they appear to have no deleterious effects on retention (9) or retrieval. A curious effect of benzodiazepines on human memory is their ability to enhance the recall of information presented immediately before drug administration. Typically, these effects have been seen in experiments in which the subjects received drug following the presentation of the initial items of word or picture lists. Memory for material presented after drug administration shows the normal impairment, but recall of material presented before drug administration is superior to that seen in a parallel placebo group (10). The probable explanation of this phenomenon is that by blocking the storage of material presented after drug administration, benzodiazepines reduce competition with the material presented before the drug was taken, thereby improving storage of these items (11). Similar effects have also been observed with alcohol (e.g., 12).

In addition to their effects on memory, it should not be forgotten that at high enough doses, benzodiazepines severely impair attentional processes and psychomotor performance. These effects are easily assessed in digit–symbol substitution (DSST), letter cancellation tasks, and other tests requiring sustained attention or distribution between parallel tasks (e.g., 13,14). Not surprisingly, the benzodiazepines have their most profound disruptive effects in the more difficult tasks, or when more than one task has to be performed simultaneously, and simple clerical type tasks such as letter cancellation are impaired only by high doses (15). These laboratory measures find their everyday counterpart in drowsiness and impairments in driving and operation of machinery.

An important question is whether the amnesia induced by benzodiazepines is a consequence of their sedative effects, or whether it occurs independently of sedation. This possibility has been addressed in some detail elsewhere (8). Although some authors (e.g., 16) suggest that the amnesia cannot be wholly attributed to sedation, lack of clarity about a definition of sedation (subjective or objective; motor sedation or reduced vigilance) and other methodological problems mean that an equally convincing case can be made for the opposite argument.

B. Long-Term Use of Benzodiazepines and Cognitive Impairments

Only a few studies have evaluated the long-term effects of benzodiazepines on psychological performance. Questions to be asked in long-term treatment are whether a tolerance to the cognitive impairment is induced or whether the cognitive impairment is progressive. Although the disruptive effects of benzodiazepines on certain aspects of cognitive performance do appear to undergo tolerance, the generality of this effect is not clear, and several possible confounding factors make interpretation problematic. First, substantial practice effects are seen with a number of the tests used to demonstrate cognitive impairments; thus, the benzodiazepine effects may simply be overcome by more practice. Second, tolerance to benzodiazepines may develop differently for different measurements. Third, anxious patients perform poorly on several cognitive and psychomotor tasks; hence, the antianxiety effect of the drug may result in differential effects in different tests. Accordingly, both Lader and Petursson (17) and Sakol and Power (18) found that the impairments induced by benzodiazepines in certain tests continued for the duration of treatment, whereas performance in other tests returned to predrug levels.

The data discussed in the foregoing are especially relevant for longer-term continuous treatment of generalized anxiety with benzodiazepines. Benzodiazepines are also used widely as hypnotics; accordingly, not only the marked amnestic effects of single, short-term doses, but also daytime performance following a single administration the night before need attention. Disruption of memory has also been reported for events occurring the morning after nighttime administration of several benzodiazepines, including lorazepam, flunitrazepam, flurazepam, and triazolam, and negative effects on psychomotor performance are also routinely reported (see Ref. 19 for a review). However, it is also conceivable that, at least in insomniacs, daytime performance may even improve after a good night's sleep. A wide range of tasks have been used to assess daytime functioning following hypnotic medication the previous night; although psychomotor speed tests and tests of higher cognitive functioning can be impaired the morning after clinically relevant doses of some benzodiazepine hypnotics, such effects are not consistently observed.

III. ALCOHOL EFFECTS ON COGNITIVE FUNCTIONS

A second area of clinical interest for studying impairment of cognitive function is the area of alcohol abuse. As with the benzodiazepines, the most prominent cognitive disruption in acute intoxication with alcohol is impairment of memory. This can be detected in laboratory tests as a decrement of performance, but it can also be recognized as a circumscribed transient amnesia, the so-called blackout. Although the immediate effects of alcohol have been studied in the laboratory, in clinical terms, the *chronic* effects of alcohol are more important. Nevertheless, most neuropsychological studies of acute alcohol effects focus on subjects who are normal in their clinical and neurological assessment and, in such subjects, the effects are transient and reversible; the question remains open about how these acute effects develop into the profound incapacitating impairment of memory that was first described by Korsakoff.

A. Acute Alcohol Effects on Cognitive Functions

What is the nature of alcohol-induced amnesia in the laboratory setting under brief administration of alcohol? The phenomenon of blackout is characterized by an amnesia that is clearly circumscribed and in which memory loss for significant events results in a sense of lost time. The memory loss is total and seemingly permanent (20). When alcohol plasma levels were measured during high consumption of alcohol, a relation was found between the occurrence of blackout and a rapid increase of plasma levels (21).

In the laboratory, most early studies indicated that the effect of alcohol is on short-term processing and retention of information. Thus, Moskowitz and Murray (22), using a technique to evaluate the transfer of information from initial sensory stores to a short-term memory, found that alcohol increased the time required to perform the transfer. Furthermore, in tests of recall of word lists presented a short time previously, alcohol impaired recall only for early and middle list items (23,24). These effects suggest an impairment in encoding or storage under alcohol (24–26) and are reminiscent of the benzodiazepine effects described earlier.

As with the benzodiazepines, there is little evidence that alcohol is able to induce forgetting of already-learned material. One apparent exception to this rule is a study of Maylor and Rabbitt (27) in which rates of forgetting were investigated by using a continuous recognition paradigm in which speed of response as well as accuracy were measured. Words were introduced on a screen sequentially, and subjects asked to respond with one key to words that had been presented previously and with a second key to new words. The number of items intervening between the first and second presentation varied, allowing an evaluation of forgetting curves. The results suggested that alcohol increased the rate of forgetting (27). Importantly, however, in the Maylor and Rabbitt experiment, the interval between initial word presentation and recognition varied from 2 secs to 1 min, so that the "forgetting" most probably reflects loss of material from working memory. Studies of the effects of alcohol on the rate of forgetting of already-encoded material (presentation–recognition intervals of minutes to days) have failed to demonstrate alcohol effects (21,28). Thus, the Maylor and Rabbitt data appear to be more consistent with alcohol reducing the capacity in working memory.

Craik (29) has argued that the effects of alcohol on memory are due to failure to process deeply at the encoding stage, as a result of a reduction in processing resources. This view entails two separate hypotheses: first, that encoding resources are limited under alcohol; and second, that depth of processing is impaired. These two factors are not necessarily identical, and the first closely resembles explanations of the effects of benzodiazepines on information processing (8).

Three experiments suggest that alcohol does not, in fact, influence depth of processing. First, in tests of word categorization, Maylor et al. (25) did not find that alcohol-induced decrements differentiated between words that could be processed using surface cues (like simple digits) and those that required semantic processing (based on knowledge). Although alcohol increased the time needed to perform the categorization, there was no clear difference in the level of processing required. This is reminiscent of the study of Curran et al. (30), who found no differential effects of benzodiazepines on tasks requiring differing depths of processing.

Second, Maylor et al. (31) examined the extent to which alcohol has an influence on the efficiency of access to information already in long-term memory. In a computerized version of the Mill–Hill vocabulary test, subjects were required to define words by making multiple-choice responses as quickly as possible. Decision time for correct responses increased with item difficulty (i.e., if the presented words were unusual, it was more difficult to decide on the correct definition). Although the time required to respond tended to increase under the influence of alcohol, this was not dependent on word difficulty.

Similarly, in a lexical decision task in which nonsense words were presented together with real words of low, medium, and high frequency of occurrence in everyday speech, and subjects were required to decide as quickly as possible whether the presented word was real or not, alcohol increased the time to respond, but this effect did not vary with word difficulty (31). Thus, alcohol may have a general effect on speed of retrieval, irrespective of the depth of processing. There is also some evidence that alcohol induces a delay in selection of the necessary response, rather than influencing stimulus recognition (32,33).

Comparison of the effects of alcohol and benzodiazepines suggests a considerable resemblance, but, whereas both affect acquisition by impairing encoding, alcohol may additionally influence response selection and, hence, performance during retrieval. However, it should be noted that investigations of the effects of benzodiazepines and those of alcohol have often been carried out within different theoretical frameworks, and differences in their effects may be more apparent than real. Direct comparative studies do not exist, and it is our contention that such comparative studies would reveal more similarities than differences (Table 1).

B. Cognitive Impairments in Chronic Alcohol Abuse

Studies of the acute effects of alcohol have taken place largely in the laboratory setting, using a variety of neuropsychological tests to measure performance. Studies of the chronic effects of alcohol, on the other hand, concentrate mainly on clinical aspects and have used different test batteries. The parallels, if any, between the precise psychological deficits observed under brief and extended alcohol intake, therefore are not clear. Furthermore, it must be stressed that, whereas the effects described in the foregoing are pharmacologic and reversible, the chronic effects of alcohol are likely to be partially or entirely related to structural brain damage, resulting from alcohol toxicity, or to nutritional (especially vitamin B_1) deficiencies, resulting from prolonged alcohol intake, and are mostly permanent. Nevertheless, it is noteworthy that the main features of Korsakoff's dementia, as well as of acute alcohol-induced amnesia and of benzodiazepine-induced amnesia, are an anterograde impairment of episodic memory (34).

1. Nonamnestic Alcoholics

In 50–70% of patients with long-term alcohol abuse, but without organic mental syndromes, neuropsychological assessments uncover signs of mild

TABLE 1 Effects of Benzodiazepines and Alcohol on Cognitive Function

	Clinical cognitive symptomatology	Cognitive impairments	Sensitive tests (examples)
Acute benzodiazepines	Anterograde amnesia	Impairment of acquisition of new information	Long-term recall of visually or verbally acquired information (short-term recall remains intact)
		Impairment of working memory	Tasks involving attending to and manipulating information
	Sedation	Impairment of attentional processes	Tasks of divided attention; tasks of continuous attention
	Lack of motor coordination	Impairment of psychomotor performance (motor skill performance)	DSST; driving simulator
Chronic benzodiazepines	Anterograde amnesia (?)	Impairment of acquisition (?)	Long-term recall
	Sedation (not always found)	Impairment of attentional processes (not always found)	Divided/continuous attention tasks
	Lack of motor coordination (not always found)	Impairment of psychomotor performance (not always found)	DSST; driving simulator
Acute alcohol	Anterograde amnesia	Impairment of acquisition of new information	Long-term recall
		Impairment of transfer from sensory memory to short-term storage (working memory)	Continuous recognition paradigm
		Impairment of transfer from storage to conscious awareness	Delayed resonse during semantic retrieval (semantic memory remains intact)
	Sedation	Impairment of attention	Divided/continuous attention tasks
	Lack of motor coordination	Impairment of psychomotor performance	DSST; driving simulator

Long-term alcohol abuse	Not readily detectable without cognitive testing	Impairment of visuospatial and perceptual functions Slight impairment of frontal lobe functions Slight anterograde memory deficits Prolonged sobriety may attenuate symptoms	WAIS/HRNB overall scores normal: Block design (WAIS) Trail-making test (HRNB) Wisconsin card-sorting task Paired associate learning (complex stimuli)
Korsakoff's syndrome	Amnestic syndrome with:		
	Severe anterograde amnesia		
	Retrograde amnesia with better preservation of remote events	Episodic memory more affected than semantic memory	WMS severely impaired Word lists: recall and recognition impaired
	Disorientation in time and place Normal consciousness No delirium	Impairment of visuospatial and perceptual functions	WAIS overall score almost normal, but impairments in: Block design (WAIS) Trail-making test (HRNB) Wisconsin card-sorting task
	Lack of drive and interest	Impairment of frontal lobe functions Proactive interference	
	Other intellectual and higher cortical functions unaffected or less affected	Ability to learn and retain motor skills	e.g., tracking tasks unaffected
		Immediate recall preserved	e.g., digit span unaffected
Alcohol dementia	Dementia syndrome with impairment of Short- and long-term memory Other cognitive or higher cortical functions Personality Severe enough to interfere with social and occupational life	Impairment of short- and long-term memory Frontal dysfunction Impairment of judgment and abstract thinking Impairment of visuospatial relations	Standard clinical tests of dementia including mini-mental state examination; Blessed test; also tasks as for Korsakoff's syndrome when feasible

brain dysfunction, even when the patients are tested while sober (35,36). Subtests of standard assessment instruments, such as the Wechsler Adult Intelligence Scale (WAIS; 37) or the Halstead–Reitan Neuropsychological Battery (HRNB), reveal deficits in such patients, despite overall scores being within normal limits (e.g., 38,39). Thus, the WAIS subtests block design, object assembly, and digit-symbol substitution test (DSST), and the category- and trail-making-test, part B form of the HRNB can be regarded as standard tools for the assessment of the selective cognitive deficits of chronic alcoholics (39–41). The common feature of these observations is a deficit in visuospatial and perceptive functions, which is usually regarded as evidence for cortical dysfunction in the temporal and parietal association areas or the prefrontal region (e.g., 42,43). Frontal lobe pathology is also suggested by deficiencies in planning and problem solving, or perseverative tendencies in measures such as the Wisconsin Card-Sorting Task.

It must be remembered, however, that these tests also require attentional and limited memory capacities, as well as psychomotor speed for their optimal performance. Furthermore, although the tests are sensitive to alcohol-induced cognitive impairments, performance is also influenced by concomitant variables such as age, socioeconomic status, and education, as well as by the medical and nutritional status of the patient (40). Thus, the attribution of impairments directly to alcohol is uncertain. It is interesting that prolonged sobriety over a period of 1 or 2 weeks attenuates some cognitive symptoms in these patients (44,45).

Although it has sometimes proved difficult to distinguish nonamnestic (non-Korsakoff) alcoholics from normal controls in standard assessments of memory deficit, such as the Wechsler Memory Scale (WMS) (46,47), an anterograde memory deficit of non-Korsakoff alcoholics can be found when they are tested with more complex verbal and nonverbal stimuli on short-term memory and paired associated-learning tasks (48).

2. *Alcohol-Induced Organic Mental Syndrome*

Chronic alcohol abuse may also lead to severe organic mental syndromes, with memory or global intellectual failure and personality disturbance, in about 10% of patients (49). These patients can be further subdivided into those suffering from alcohol amnestic disorder (Korsakoff's syndrome) or from dementia associated with alcoholism (50).

a. Korsakoff's Syndrome. The psychopathological characteristics of the alcohol amnestic disorder, or Korsakoff's syndrome, are severe memory disorders in the form of both anterograde and retrograde amnesia, with a preponderance of the former. Patients with Korsakoff's syndrome are unable to learn and retain new verbal or nonverbal information (e.g., their doctor's name or the location of their room on the ward); they are disoriented in time and place, but there are no signs of clouded consciousness or delirium, and they are still able to recall very recent information, as long as they are not distracted. This suggests they are able to retain information in short-term memory. This deficit can be formally demonstrated in the Brown–Peterson task (51).

Patients who have Korsakoff's syndrome also exhibit considerable difficulties in retrieving information about the period just before disease onset, with a tendency for memories of the more remote past to be better preserved (52,53). On the other hand, other intellectual functions, typically assessed by subscales of intelligence tests, such as the WAIS, seem unaffected in comparison with nonamnestic alcoholics (54) and normal controls matched for age and education (55). Clinical experience suggests that severe impairments of language functions, writing, and simple calculating skills do not occur.

On the level of neuropsychological evaluation, performance deficits of patients with Korsakoff's syndrome on the visuoperceptual and visuospatial subscales of WAIS or the HRNB are similar to those of nonamnestic alcoholics or patients with the alcohol dementia syndrome (53), suggesting a common underlying etiology for the two deficits. A further comparison of the two syndromes on visual and verbal tasks sensitive to frontal lobe function suggests a common frontal lobe deficit (56). Further evidence for frontal lobe deficits can be adduced from the Wisconsin Card-Sorting Task (51), and similarly to nonamnestic alcoholics, Korsakoff patients also exhibit perseverative response tendencies during neuropsychological experiments (e.g., 38,52,54) and demonstrate a considerable lack of drive and disinterest, a personality change typically seen in patients with a frontal lobe disorder (57).

Differences between nonamnestic alcoholics and alcoholics with Korsakoff's syndrome are more distinct in the memory field; in contrast with the slight impairment in nonamnestic alcoholics, Korsakoff patients are severely impaired on the Wechsler Memory Scale (WMS), and their diverging test performances on the WMS and the WAIS tend to be so stable that a 15-point difference between the scores has been used to identify amnestic patients (e.g., 58). Korsakoff's syndrome patients show severely impaired episodic memory (i.e., memory for unique events that occurred at a particular time and place) in tasks such as recognition and recall of word lists (59). They are also impaired in learning patterned visual material (e.g., faces and patterns) (60), the Brown–Peterson task (53,58), and are prone to proactive interference (i.e., information previously processed interferes with learning of new material) (52).

On the other hand, on certain subtests of the WMS (e.g., mental control, digit span, and paired-associate learning-related pairs), Korsakoff patients perform quite well. These tasks require either highly trained skills (alphabet, counting backward) and well-established semantic associations (related paired associates), or reflect the patient's ability in immediate recall, provided no distraction occurs between stimulus presentation and recall (e.g, digit span; 39). The Korsakoff's syndrome patients are less impaired in their access to semantic memory where highly structured and organized knowledge is stored (56,59).

An interesting exception to the global memory problems of Korsakoff patients is their ability to learn and retain visuoperceptual and motor skills. These patients are able to learn mirror reading of single words (61), bimanual tracking or pursuit rotor tasks (for references, see 61), or a repeated sequence of stimulus positions in a visual reaction time task (62), but they are unable to recall the learning situation or the stimulus material used. Moreover, Korsakoff patients demonstrate a preserved priming effect; for example, in the completion of lists of word fragments, they profit from previous presentation of the words, although they fail if asked to recall the words explicitly (63).

Note that this general pattern of deficits is similar to that induced by benzodiazepines and short-term alcohol intake. Thus, in both cases, digit span and similar measures of short-term memory are normal, whereas recall and recognition memory for longer lists are catastrophically impaired; furthermore, in neither case is there a loss of knowledge memory (3,59). This latter observation distinguishes, on the one hand, organic amnestic syndrome, Korsakoff's syndrome, postencephalitic amnesia, and benzodiazepine- or alcohol-induced amnesias, from Alzheimer's disease and other progressive dementias, which exhibit a loss of both episodic memory (memory for events) and knowledge memory. On the basis of such analogies, some authors (e.g., 64) have argued that benzodiazepine-induced amnesias offer a pharmacologic model for an organic amnestic syndrome.

b. Alcohol Dementia Syndrome. Alcohol dementia syndrome, too, is characterized by dysfunction of short- and long-term memory, but to establish this diagnosis, additional cognitive deficits must be present. Such additional deficits may include aphasia or apraxia, or impairments of abstract thinking, judgment, or personality changes, and a loss of cognitive capacities severe enough to interfere with social and occupational activities (50). The onset of the condition is not distinct, and even Korsakoff patients with an atypical gradual onset may exhibit global cognitive impairments (65). The diagnostic emphasis, therefore, should be on whether there are other intellectual deficits besides the memory impairment (66). Even then, it should not necessarily be assumed that an alcoholic presenting with dementia is suffering from an alcohol amnesia; it may be that, in addition to alcoholism, the patient is also suffering from an underlying amnesia as a result of, for example, Alzheimer's disease, or multi-infarct dementia. These alternative diagnoses are difficult to differentiate clinically.

IV. ANTIDEPRESSANTS AND COGNITIVE FUNCTION

In comparision with benzodiazepines and alcohol, antidepressant use is more circumscribed and generally limited to patient populations. Since depression itself may have markedly debilitating effects on cognitive performance, such as producing pseudodementia (e.g, 67), antidepressants may often improve performance of patients in cognitive tasks. Thus, for instance, Sternberg and Jarvik (68) found improvements on a wide range of memory and learning tests in a group of hospitalized endogenous depressives following 26 days of imipramine treatment, and similar effects have been reported by others for imipramine and amitriptyline (see Ref. 69 for a review).

It should be noted, however, that this is not inevitably the case. Certain tricyclic antidepressants may give rise to delirium or less severe cognitive impairments in depressed patients (70). Clinically, the cognitive impairments associated with antidepressant therapy include overt confusional episodes, sedation, drowsiness, impairment of episodic memory, and speech blockage (71).

In the laboratory setting, using normal volunteers, several antidepressants have been described as having disruptive effects (69). Thus, a single dose of amitriptyline has been reported to worsen performance in DSST (72) and in an information-processing task (73), as well as having consistent effects on immediate (74,75) and delayed recall (76). Other tricyclic antidepressants, including imipramine, 150 mg/day, have been known to impair DSST and time estimation (77). Repeated administration of nortriptyline over 14 days impaired digit span when a backward, but not a forward, recall procedure was used; it also impaired paired associate learning (78). In contrast, 4 weeks of treatment with imipramine in a therapeutic dose range of 200 mg/day led to an improvement of performance on paired-associate learning, but this schedule of treatment led to deficits in the Porteus maze (a measure of foresight and judgment) and a trail-making task (Judd et al., unpublished data cited in Ref. 79). Improvement in paired-associate learning was also seen following 14 days of amitriptyline

(80), although a similar treatment regimen increased the mistakes made in classifying visual and auditory stimuli in a choice–reaction time task, without, however, impairing reaction time (81).

Many of the tricyclic antidepressants, in addition to their ability to inhibit the reuptake of monoamines from the synaptic cleft, also possess marked anticholinergic properties. Branconnier and colleagues (82) suggested that the pattern of cognitive deficits seen with amitriptyline and imipramine resembles that observed under scopolamine administration (e.g., impaired free recall; sparing of iconic and incidental memory), and suggest that the cognitive effects of antidepressants are related to their anticholinergic side effects. In keeping with this hypothesis, a series of antidepressants reported not to possess anticholinergic properties have not impaired cognitive performance (75,83).

On the other hand, Curran et al. (84) point out that several antidepressant drugs are noted for their sedative properties, and that sedatives in general can be expected to impair performance on cognitive tasks demanding psychomotor speed and attention. Consistent with this suggestion, they (84) note that over an 8-day treatment with the tetracyclic, mianserin, tolerance developed at rates similar to its effects on memory processes and indices of sedation (85).

To differentiate between these two hypotheses, Curran and colleagues (84) compared the effects of therapeutically equivalent doses of four antidepressants, two (amitriptyline and protriptyline) with marked anticholinergic effects, and two (viloxazine and trazodone) without. Of these four, protriptyline and viloxazine are classified as being nonsedating, and trazodone and amitriptyline as sedative. Despite the differences in their anticholinergic properties, it was found that the two less-sedating compounds, protriptyline and viloxazine, produced no impairment of memory. In contrast, the two sedating antidepressants produced impairments in symbol copying, symbol substitution, cancellation, choice reaction time, digit span, and visuospatial span. Thus, manual motor speed, attention, recoding skills, and primary memory were all equally affected by the sedating substances.

Nevertheless, amitriptyline and trazodone did differ in tasks involving episodic memory, in which amitriptyline produced the larger impairments, suggesting that the anticholinergic properties do play a part; the ineffectiveness of protriptyline in this test may have come about because at therapeutic doses it is not as potent an anticholinergic as amitryptyline.

This rather elegant demonstration of the importance of sedative effects in the cognition-impairing action of antidepressants is, however, partly contradicted by other comparisons of trazodone and amitriptyline. Thus, Burns et al, (86), using the same dose range as Curran et al. (84), found the two substances to differ in healthy older (more than 60 years old) subjects in measures of response time and vigilance in a computerized version of the Mackworth clock task and of attention in a divided attention task, with amitriptyline showing the larger effects. Consequently, it is not clear whether the larger effects of amitriptyline seen by Curran and her colleagues may not also be attributable to a greater sedative effect.

V. LITHIUM

A number of reports indicate that lithium, in a therapeutic dose range of 1000–1500 mg/day, slows performance, leading to subjective feelings of lack of alertness and efficiency. In objective tests, lithium slowed choice reaction time and performance in the Porteus maze (87). Two-week treatment with lithium led to small decreases in performance in mean IQ scores as well as in the trail-making test (part A) of HRNP, and the DSST (88,89). Weingartner et al. (90,91) have suggested that lithium specifically disrupts memory retrieval, and Judd et al. (92) suggest that the overall effects of lithium, including slowing of performance, are likely to be secondary to a slowing in the rate of central information processing.

VI. NEUROLEPTICS AND COGNITIVE FUNCTION

Given the widespread use of neuroleptics in the treatment of schizophrenia and for the improvement of performance of children with conduct disorders (e.g., 93,94), it is surprising that, in comparison with the benzodiazepines, alcohol, and antidepressants, the data available on the effects of neuroleptics on normal human cognition is sparse. This is the more so, since animal studies have repeatedly suggested negative effects on performance of learning tasks (95). Nevertheless, the limited data available on humans suggest little effect. Thus, Liljequist et al, (78,96) found no effect on digit span, paired-associate learning, or retention, either after a single dose (25 mg) or 2-week administration (first week 30 mg/day, second week 60 mg/day) of low-dose chlorpromazine. Similarly, thioridazine at the same doses affected neither digit span nor paired-associate learning, although, in other studies, single doses of 50 mg thioridazine have been reported both to improve (97) and to impair (98) performance in DSST. In a recent study

(99), haloperidol (4–10 mg) was found to impair performance in DSST, but not in another test, the flexibility of closure test, included to provide a control of nonspecific effects of the neuroleptic on performance.

On the other hand, the administration of small daily doses of sulpiride (150 mg), chlorpromazine (60 mg), or thioridazine (60 mg) did not impair memory or learning in simple tasks that were nevertheless impaired by a benzodiazepine (96). Given the widely accepted effects of neuroleptics on the speed of mental processing, it is rather disturbing that experimental psychopharmacologists have experienced such difficulties in demonstrating these effects in the laboratory. However, this may reflect the doses employed as well as the choice of method employed to investigate cognitive function, more than a lack of effects in a controlled situation.

VII. CONCLUSION

This chapter has attempted to provide an overview of the effects of several commonly used types of psychoactive drugs on cognitive performance in humans. Briefly, it is clear that benzodiazepines, alcohol, and certain antidepressants can all disrupt cognitive activities resulting in mild to severe, but temporary, loss of memory. The extent to which these effects simply reflect the sedative actions of these drug classes cannot be adequately answered, although it is noteworthy that opiates and antihistamines, both of which are known for their sedative properties, do not have a reputation for impairment of cognitive function. The effects of chronic alcohol are different. The severity and permanence of the memory losses of Korsakoff's syndrome reflect organic brain damage that is hardly amenable to treatment.

The effects of benzodiazepines and alcohol, both of which exert at least a part of their pharmacologic effect through actions at receptors sensitive to the brain's major inhibitory transmitter, γ-aminobutyric acid (GABA), are similar. Another group of compounds, also acting in part at this receptor complex, the barbiturates, may possess similar properties (100). Given the ubiquity of GABAergic mechanisms in the brain, it is perhaps surprising how specific these memory effects appear to be, perhaps being limited to effects on encoding of information from working memory into long-term stores. For the experimental psychologist, these properties of benzodiazepines offer a useful tool for the investigation of memory processes; for the patient they represent a more or less considerable nuisance. However, the advent of new types of agents acting at subtypes of benzodiazepine and

GABA receptors is perhaps around the corner, offering anxiolytics that are not amnestic. Similarly, novel antidepressants that are less sedative and with less anticholinergic properties may bring considerable advantages in terms of a lack of cognitive side effects.

To end on a positive note, consider the following: if it is possible that certain types of drugs can slow or disrupt cognitive function, is it also possible that other drugs may accelerate or improve them? This would be an especially worthwhile contribution of psychopharmacology to human existence.

REFERENCES

1. Squire LR. Memory and the brain. New York: Oxford University Press, 1987.
2. Parkin AJ. Memory and amnesia. An introduction. Oxford: Blackwell Scientific, 1987.
3. Roy-Byrne PP, Uhde TW, Holcomb H, Thompson K, King AK, Weingartner H. Effects of diazepam on cognitive processes in normal subjects. Psychopharmacology 1987; 91:30–33.
4. Brown J, Lewis V, Brown M, Horn G, Bowes JB. A comparison between transient amnesias induced by two drugs diazepam or lorazepam and amnesia of organic origin. Neuropsychologia 1982; 20:55–70.
5. Ghonheim MM, Mewaldt SP. Effects of diazepam and scopolamine on storage, retrieval and organisational processes in memory. Psychopharmacology 1975; 44:257–262.
6. Mewaldt SP, Hinrichs JV, Ghonheim MM. Diazepam and memory: support for a duplex model of memory. Mem Cogn 1983; 11:557–564.
7. Lister RG. The amnesic action of benzodiazepines in man. Neurosci Biobehav Rev 1985; 9:87–94.
8. Stephens DN, Duka T, and Andrews JS. Benzodiazepines, β-carbolines and memory. In: Weinman J, Hunter J, eds. Memory, clinical and theoretical aspects. London: Harwood Academic Publishers, 1991:11–42.
9. Brown J, Lewis V, Brown MW, Bones JB. Effects of lorazepam on rate of forgetting on retrieval from semantic memory and on manual dexterity. Neuropsychologia 1983; 21:501–512.
10. Ghonheim MM, Hinrichs JV, Mewaldt SP. Dose response analysis of the behavioral effects of diazepam: I. Learning and memory. Psychopharmacology 1984; 82:291–295.
11. Hinrichs JV, Ghonheim MM, Mewaldt SP. Diazepam and memory: retrograde facilitation produced by interference reduction. Psychopharmacology 1984; 84:158–162
12. Mann RE, Cho-Young J, Vogel-Sprott M. Retrograde enhancement by alco-

hol of delayed free recall performance. Pharmacol Biochem Behav 1984; 20:639–642.
13. Nicaido AM, Ellinwood EH. Comparison of the effects of quazepam and triazolam on cognitive–psychomotor performance. Psychopharmacology 1987; 92:459–464.
14. Tinklenberg J, Taylor J. Assessments of drug effects on human memory functions. In: Squire LR, Butters N, eds. Neuropsychology of memory. New York: Guilford Press, 1984:213–223.
15. Duka T, Goerke D, Dorow R, Höller L, Fichte K. Human studies on the benzodiazepine receptor antagonist β-carboline, ZK 93 426: antagonism of lormetazepam's psychotropic effects. Psychopharmacology 1988; 95:463–471.
16. Lister RG, Weingartner H, Eckardt MJ, Linnoila M. Clinical relevance of effects of benzodiazepines on learning and memory. In: Hindmarch I, Ott H, eds. Benzodiazepine receptor ligands: memory and information processing. Psychopharmacology ser 6. New York: Springer-Verlag, 1988: 117–127.
17. Lader MH, Petursson H. Long-term effects of benzodiazepines. Neuropharmacology 1983; 22:527–533.
18. Sakol MS, Power KG. The effects of long-term benzodiazepine treatment and graded withdrawal on psychometric performance. Psychopharmacology 1988; 95:135–138.
19. Bhatti JZ, Alford CA, Hindmarch I. Lormetazepam, memory and information processing: a review. In: Hindmarch I, Ott H, eds. Benzodiazepine receptor ligands, memory and information processing. Psychopharmacology ser 6. Berlin: Springer-Verlag, 1988:169–179.
20. Goodwin DW, Crane JB, Guze SB. Phenomenological aspects of the alcoholic blackout. Br J Psychiatry 1969; 115:1033–1038.
21. Ryback RS. Alcohol amnesia: observations in seven drinking inpatient alcoholics. Q J Stud Alcohol 1970; 31:616–632.
22. Moskowitz H, Murray JT. Alcohol and backward masking of visual information J Stud Alcohol 1976; 37:40–45
23. Hockey R, MacLean A, Hamilton P. State changes and the temporal patterning of component resources. In: Long J, Baddeley A, eds. Attention and performance. Hillsdale, NJ: Lawrence Erlbaum Associates, 1981:607–621.
24. Jones BM, Jones MK. Alcohol and memory impairment in male and female social drinkers. In: Birnbaum IM, Parker ES, eds. Alcohol and human memory. Hillsdale, NJ: Lawrence Erlbaum Associates, 1977:127–138.
25. Maylor EA, Rabbitt PMA, Kingstone A. Effects of alcohol on word categorization and recognition memory. Br J Psychol 1987; 78:233–239.
26. Weingartner H, Murphy DL. State-dependent storage and retrieval of experience while intoxicated. In: Birnbaum IM, Parker ES, eds. Alcohol and human memory. Hillsdale, NJ: Lawrence Erlbaum Associates, 1977:159–173.
27. Maylor EA, Rabbitt PMA. Effect of alcohol on rate of forgetting. Psychopharmacology 1987; 91:230–235.
28. Wickelgren WA. Alcoholic intoxication and memory storage dynamics. Mem Cogn 1975; 3:385–389.

29. Craik FMI. Similarities between the effects of aging and alcoholic intoxication on memory performance, construed within a "levels of processing" framework. In: Birnbaum IM, Parker ES, eds. Alcohol and human memory Hillsdale, NJ: Lawrence Erlbaum Associates, 1977:9–21.
30. Curran HV, Schiwy W, Eves F, Shine P, Lader M. A levels of processing study of the effect of benzodiazepines on human memory. Hum Psychopharmacol 1988; 3:21–25.
31. Maylor EA, Rabbitt PMA, Kingstone AF. Effects of alcohol on lexical access. Psychopharmacology 1988; 95:119–123.
32. Huntley MS. Effects of alcohol, uncertainty and novelty upon response selection. Psychopharmacologia 1974; 39:259–266.
33. Tharp VK, Rundell OH Jr, Lester K, Williams HL. Alcohol and information processing. Psychopharmacology 1974; 40:33–52.
34. Weingartner H. Models of memory dysfunctions. Ann NY Acad Sci 1985; 444:359–369.
35. Lee K, Moller L, Hardt F, Haubek A, Jensen E. Alcohol induced brain damage and liver damage in young males. Lancet 1979; 2:759–61.
36. Parsons O. Neuropsychological deficits in alcoholics: facts and fancies. Alcoholism 1977; 1:51–56.
37. Matarazzo JD. Wechsler's measurement and appraisal of adult intelligence. Baltimore: Williams & Wilkins, 1972.
38. Oscar-Berman M, Ellis RJ. Cognitive deficits related to memory impairments in alcoholism. Recent Dev Alcohol 1987; 5:59–80.
39. Wilkinson DA, Poulos CX. The chronic effects of alcohol on memory. A contrast between a unitary and dual system approach. Recent Dev Alcohol Res 1987; 5:5–26.
40. Riege WH. Specificity of memory deficits in alcoholism. Recent Dev Alcohol 1987; 5:81–109.
41. Ron MA. The alcoholic brain: CT scan and psychological findings. Psychological medicine. Monogr suppl 3. Cambridge: Cambridge University Press, 1982:1–33.
42. Squire LR. Comparisons between forms of amnesia: some deficits are unique to Korsakoff's syndrome. J Exp Psychol [Learn Mem Cogn] 1982; 8:560–571.
43. Lezak MD. Neuropsychological assessments. New York: Oxford University Press, 1983.
44. Martin PR, Adinoff B, Weingartner H, Mukherjee AB, Eckardt M. Alcoholic organic brain disease: nosology and pathophysiologic mechanisms. Prog Neuropsychopharmacol Biol Psychiatry 1986; 10:147–164.
45. Grant I, Adams KM, Reed R. Aging abstinence, and medical risk factors in the prediction of neuropsychologic deficit among long-term alcoholics. Arch Gen Psychiatry 1984; 41:710–718.
46. Butters N, Cermak LS, Montgomery K. Some comparisons of the memory and visuoperceptive deficits of chronic alcoholics and patients with Korsakoff disease. Alcoholism 1977; 1:73–80.
47. Parsons OA, Prigatano GP. Memory functioning in alcoholics. In: Birnbaum

IM, Parker ES, eds. Alcohol and human memory. Hillsdale, NJ: Lawrence Erlbaum Associates, 1977:185–194.

48. Ryan C, Butters N. Further evidence for a continuum of impairment encompassing male alcoholic Korsakoff patients and chronic alcoholic men. Alcohol Clin Exp Res 1980; 4:190–197.
49. Horvath TB. Clinical spectrum and epidemiologic features of alcoholic dementia. In: Rankin JG, ed. Alcohol, drug and brain damage. Ontario: Addiction Research Foundation of Ontario, 1975:1–16.
50. American Psychiatric Association. Diagnostic and statistical manual of mental disorders, 3rd ed-revised. Washington, DC: American Psychiatric Association, 1987.
51. Leng NRC, Parkin AJ. Aetiological variation in the amnesic syndrome: comparisons using the Brown–Peterson task. Cortex 1989; 25:251–259.
52. Butters N, Martone M, White B, Granholm E, Wolfe J. Clinical validators: comparisons of demented and amnesic patients. In: Poon LW, ed. Handbook for clinical memory assessment of older adults. Washington, DC: American Psychological Association, 1988:337–352.
53. Butters N, Miliotis P. Amnesic disorders. In: Heilmann KM, Valenstein E, eds. Clinical neuropsychology, 2nd ed. New York: Oxford University Press, 1985:403–450.
54. Wilkinson DA, Carlen PL. Relationship of neuropsychological test performance to brain morphology in amnesic and non-amnesic chronic alcoholics. Acta Psychiatrica Scand 1980; 62:89–102.
55. Butters N, Cermak LS. Alcoholic Korsakoff's syndrome: an information processing approach to amnesia. New York: Academic Press, 1980.
56. Salmon DP, Butters N. The etiology and neuropathology of alcoholic Korsakoff's syndrome. Some evidence for the role of the basal forebrain. Recent Dev Alcohol 1987; 5:27–58.
57. Poeck K. Stoerungen von Antrieb und Affektivitaet. In: Poeck K, ed. Klinische Neuropsychologie. Stuttgart: Thieme, 1989:323–329.
58. Longmore BE, Knight RG. The effect of intellectual deterioration on retention deficits in amnesic alcoholics. J Abnorm Psychol 1988; 97:448–454.
59. Weingartner H, Grafman J, Bontelle W, Kaye W, Martin PR. Forms of memory failure. Science 1983; 221:380–382.
60. Moss MB, Albert MS, Butters N, Payne M. Differential patterns of memory loss among patients with Alzheimer's disease, Huntington's disease, and alcoholic Korsakoff's syndrome. Arch Neurol 1986; 43:239–246.
61. Martone M, Butters N, Payne M. Becke JT, Sax DS. Dissociations between skill learning and verbal recognition in amnesia and dementia. Arch Neurol 1984; 41:965–970.
62. Nissen MJ, Willingham D, Hartman M. Explicit and implicit remembering: when is learning preserved in amnesia? Neuropsychologia 1989; 27:341–352.
63. Shimamura AP, Salmon DP, Squire LR, Butters N. Memory dysfunction and word priming in dementia and amnesia. Behav Neurosci 1987; 101:347–351.

64. Wolkowitz OM, Weingartner H, Thopson K, Picker D, Paul SM, Hommer DW. Diazepam-induced amnesia: a neuropharmacological model of an "organic amnesic syndrome." Am J Psychiatry 1987; 144:25–29.
65. Martin PR, Eckardt MJ, Linnoila M. Treatment of chronic organic mental disorders associated with alcoholism. Recent Dev Alcohol 1987; 7:329–350.
66. Eckardt MJ, Martin PR. Clinical assessment of cognition in alcoholism. Alcohol Clin Exp Res 1986; 10:123–127.
67. Grunhaus L, Dilsaver S, Greden JF, Carrol BJ. Depressive pseudodementia: a suggestive diagnostic profile. Biol Psychiatry 1983; 18:215–226.
68. Sternberg DE, Jarvik ME. Memory functions in depression. Improvement with antidepressant medication. Arch Gen Psychiatry 1976; 33:219–224.
69. Thompson PJ, Trimble MR. Non-MAOI antidepressant drugs and cognitive functions: a review Psychol Med 1982; 12:539–548.
70. Meador-Woodruff JH, Akil M, Wisner-Carlson R, Grunhaus L. Behavioral and cognitive toxicity related to elevated plasma tricyclic antidepressant levels. J Clin Psychopharmacol 1988; 8:28–32.
71. Cole JO, Branconnier RJ, Salamon, M, Dessain EC. Tricyclic use in the cognitively impaired elderly. J Clin Psychiatry 1983; 44:14–19.
72. Callaway E. The pharmacology of human information processing. Psychophysiology 1983; 20:359–370.
73. Linnoila M, Johnson J, Dubyoski K, Buchsbaum MS, Schneinin M, Kilts C. Effects of antidepressants on skilled performance. Br J Clin Pharmacol 1984; 18:109S–120S.
74. Peck AW, Hamilton M. Psychopharmacology of bupropion in normal volunteers. J Clin Psychiatry 1983; 44:202–205.
75. Warrington SJ, Ankier SI, Turner P. An evaluation of possible interactions between ethanol and trazodone or amitriptyline. Br J Clin Pharmacol 1984; 18:549–557.
76. Linnoila M. Saariao I, Maki M. Effect of treatment with diazepam or lithium and alcohol on psychomotor skills related to driving. Eur J Clin Pharmacol 1974; 7:337–342.
77. Wittenborn JR, Flaherty CF, McGough WE, Bossange KA, Nash RJ. A comparison of the effect of imipramine, nomifensine, and placebo on the psychomotor performance of normal males. Psychopharmacology 1976; 51:85–90.
78. Liljequist R, Linnoila M, Mattila MJ. Effect of two weeks' treatment with chlorimipramine and nortriptyline, alone or in combination with alcohol on learning and memory. Psychopharmacologia 1974; 39:181–186.
79. Judd LL, Squire LR, Butters N, Salmon DP, Paller KA. Effects of psychotropic drugs on cognition and memory in normal humans and animals. In: Meltzer HY, ed. Psychopharmacology: a third generation of progress. New York: Raven press, 1988:1467–1475.
80. Liljequist R, Seppala T, Mattila MJ. Amitriptyline and mianserin induced changes in acquisition of paired-association learning task. Br J Clin Pharmacol 1978; 5:149–153.

81. Seppälä T. Psychomotor skills during acute and two-week treatment with mianserin (ORG GB 94) and amitriptyline, and their combined effects with alcohol. Ann Clin Res 1977; 9:66–72.
82. Branconnier RJ, de Vitt DR, Cole JO, Spera KF. Amitriptyline selectively disrupts verbal recall from secondary memory of the normal aged. Neurobiol Aging 1982; 3:55–59.
83. Branconnier RJ, Cole JO. Effects of acute administration of trazodone and amitriptyline on cognition, cardiovascular function, and salivation in the normal geriatric subject. J Clin Psychopharmacol 1981; 1:82S–85S.
84. Curran HV, Sakulsriprong M, Lader M. Antidepressants and human memory: an investigation of four drugs with different sedative and anticholinergic profile. Psychopharmacology 1988; 95:520–527.
85. Curran HV, Shine P, Lader M. Effects of repeated doses of fluvoxamine, mianserin and placebo on memory and measures of sedation. Psychopharmacology 1986; 89:360–363.
86. Burns M, Moskowitz H, Jaffe J. A comparison of the effects of trazodone and amitriptyline on skills performance by geriatric subjects. J Clin Psychiatry 1986; 47:252–254.
87. Wetzel CD, Squite LR, Janowsky DS. Methylphenidate impairs learning and memory in normal adults. Behav Neurol Biol 1981; 31:413–424.
88. Judd LL, Hubbard B, Janowsky DS, Huey LY, Attewell PA. The effect of lithium carbonate on affect, mood and personality of normal subjects. Arch Gen Psychiatry 1977; 34:346–351.
89. Judd LL, Hubbard B, Janowsky DS, Huey LY, Takahashi. The effect of lithium carbonate on the cognitive functions of normal subjects. Arch Gen Psychiatry 1977; 34:355–357.
90. Weingartner H, Cohen RM, Bunney WE Jr, Ebert MH, Kaye W. Memory-learning impairments in progressive dementia and depression. Am J Psychiatry 1982; 139:135–136.
91. Weingartner H, Rudorfer MV, Linnoila M. Cognitive effects of lithium treatment in normal volunteers. Psychopharmacology 1985; 86:472–474.
92. Judd LL. Effects of lithium on mood, cognition and personality function in normal subjects. Arch Gen Psychiatry 1979; 36:860–866.
93. Platt JE, Campbell M, Green WH, Grega MD. Effects of lithium carbonate and haloperidol on cognition in aggressive hospitalised school-age children. J Clin Psychopharmacol 1981; 1:8–13.
94. Werry JS, Aman MBV. Methylphenidate and haloperidol in children: effects on attention; memory and activity. Arch Gen Psychiatry 1975; 32:790–795.
95. Oades RD. Impairments of search behaviour in rats after haloperidol treatment, hippocampal or neocortical damage suggest a mesocortical role in cognition. Biol Psychol 1981; 12:77–85.
96. Liljequist R, Linnoila M, Mattila MJ, Saario J, Seppälä T. Effect of two weeks' treatment with thioridazine, chlorpromazine, sulpiride and bromazepam, alone or in combination with alcohol, on learning and memory in man. Psychopharmacologia 1975; 44:205–208.

97. Szabadi E, Bradshaw CM, Gaszner P. The comparison of the effects of DL-308, a potential new neuroleptic agent, and thioridazine on some psychological and physiological functions in healthy volunteers. Psychopharmacology 1980; 68:125–134.
98. Theofilopolous N, Szabadi E, Bradshaw CM. Comparison of the effects of ranitidine, cimetidine and thioridazine on psychomotor functions in healthy volunteers. Br J Clin Pharmacol 1984; 18:135–144.
99. Magliozzi JR, Mungas D, Laubly JN, Blunden D. Effect of haloperidol on a symbol digit substitution task in normal adult males. Neuropsychopharmacology 1989; 2:29–37.
100. Roehrs T, Zorick FJ, Sicklesteel JM, Wittig RM, Hartse KM, Roth T. Effects of hypnotics on memory. J Clin Psychopharmacol 1983; 3:310–313.

7

The Cognitive Effects of Electroconvulsive Therapy

Harold A. Sackeim *College of Physicians and Surgeons, Columbia University, and New York State Psychiatric Institute, New York, New York*

I. INTRODUCTION

Electroconvulsive therapy (ECT) has been in continuous use for more than 50 years, longer than any other form of somatic treatment in psychiatry. It was introduced in the same era in which other dramatic biological treatments, insulin coma and psychosurgery, were first developed (1). In the United States, these other interventions have been virtually abandoned for the treatment of psychiatric conditions. However, the use of ECT remains strong and, in fact, may be increasing. Exact statistics on utilization are uncertain (2), but it can be estimated that up to 100,000 patients per annum receive this treatment in the United States.

The longevity of ECT is due to its efficacy. Among all available treatments for major depressive disorder, ECT is the most effective (3). The antidepressant properties of ECT have been established in a number of ways. A series of double-blind studies have contrasted ECT with the administration of anesthesia alone. With the exception of one study that used what is now known to be an ineffective form of ECT (4), the findings in these comparisons consistently indicated superior therapeutic effects for "real" versus "sham" ECT (3, 5). Other work has suggested that the administration of electrical intensities insufficient to produce a grand mal seizure, that is, subconvulsive treatment, is inferior in efficacy to that of traditional

ECT (6,7). There is also evidence that efficacy is reduced when an anticonvulsant medication (lidocaine), that interferes with and aborts the seizure discharge, is administered with traditional ECT (8). In recent years, it has been demonstrated under double-blind, random assignment conditions that technical factors in ECT administration, involving the interaction between electrode placement and electrical stimulus intensity, have a strong impact on efficacy (9, 10). The combination of bilateral electrode placement and low-stimulus intensity is reliably associated with a response rate of approximately 70%. In contrast, right unilateral electrode placement and very low stimulus intensity is remarkably weak in therapeutic properties with short-term response rates of approximately 20%.

These findings indicate that many of the theories emphasizing psychological factors in accounting for ECTs antidepressant efficacy are untenable (11). Electroconvulsive therapy is a highly ritualized treatment, involving repeated treatment at a schedule of twice or three times a week. The treatment carries high expectancies for clinical recovery, and some have thought that the treatment stimulates and satisfies patient fantasies of being punished. The research demonstrating reduced efficacy when patients are administered anesthesia alone, purely subconvulsive administration, or an anticonvulsant medication concomitant with traditional ECT indicates that the elicitation of a full generalized seizure is a necessary component of the therapeutic process (8,12). The more recent research demonstrating that full seizures can be produced that lack therapeutic properties indicates that the elicitation of a generalized seizure is an insufficient condition for efficacy (13). Rather, the intensity of the ECT stimulus (10,14) and anatomical positioning of electrodes also play a major role (9,13).

Soon after the introduction of antidepressant medications, a series of studies compared the efficacy of these compounds with ECT (e.g., 15,16). In a meta-analysis of this work, Janicak et al. (17) estimated that the percentage of patients responding to ECT exceeded that for tricyclic antidepressant compounds by approximately 20% and that for monoamine oxidase inhibitors by about 45%. Much of this research was methodologically questionable (18), with the dose and duration of medication treatment often below modern standards for what constitutes an adequate medication trial (19–21). Nonetheless, it is generally accepted that the short-term antidepressant properties of ECT are at least equal, if not superior, to those of antidepressant medications. There is also evidence that the quality of clinical response may be superior with ECT. In clinical trials, the criteria used to designate therapeutic response are often sufficiently weak that they produce a considerable range of residual symptomatology in patients classified as responders. The percentage of patients who are asymptomatic following treatment may be higher with ECT than with antidepressant compounds (22).

In part because of these findings, perhaps the most common indication for the use of ECT is failure to respond to other forms of antidepressant treatment (23). In major depression, it has been assumed that response rates to ECT are independent of patient's prior treatment history, with essentially equivalent response rates in medication-naive and medication-resistant patients (24). This assumption has only recently received empirical attention, and the initial findings suggest that patients resistant to adequate trials of antidepressant medication may have both an elevated rate of resistance to ECT (25) and a greater likelihood of early relapse when they do respond to ECT (26). Despite this, it is also evident that a large percentage of depressed patients who fail serial adequate medication trials show marked improvement when administered ECT (21).

The medical risks of antidepressant treatments often exceed those of ECT. In terms of medical morbidity and mortality, ECT has a remarkably high safety profile, with the major risks being cardiovascular and attributable to the administration of general anesthesia (23). Consequently, another major indication for the use of ECT is the presence of medical conditions that contraindicate the use of antidepressant medications or the presence of limiting side effects such that patients cannot tolerate adequate medication trials. Because clinical response may be both more likely and faster with ECT, another indication for its use in major depression is the presence of markedly severe psychiatric symptomatology or associated life-threatening medical conditions. Compared with other treatment modalities, among those who receive ECT, there is an overrepresentation of psychosis and suicidality, as well as debilitation related to severe inanition.

These indications for ECT combine to strongly impinge on the demographics of those who receive the treatment. In recurrent mood disorders, it is believed by some that aging results in greater severity and abruptness of onset of depressive episodes, a shorter period of euthymia between episodes, and greater resistance to conventional antidepressant medications (27–29). Intolerance of antidepressant medications and presentation of medical conditions that contraindicate their use are also particularly likely in the elderly. These factors, combined with an average age of onset of unipolar major depressive disorder between 40 and 50 years of age (29), indicate that a large percentage of patients who receive ECT are elderly. Thus, the cognitive effects of ECT in the elderly is of special concern. Another major demographic factor is gender. The prevalence and incidence of depression is considerably greater among females than males (30,31), resulting in the prototypic ECT patient being a relatively elderly female.

Major depressive illness, either unipolar or bipolar, is by far the most common diagnostic indication for the use of ECT, with survey data indicating that approximately 80% of those who receive ECT in the United States present with this condition (32). However, there is a remarkably broad range of psychiatric and neurological conditions in which the efficacy of ECT is either established or hypothesized. Random assignment, double-blind investigations have shown ECT to be effective in acute mania (33) and schizophrenia (34), and in clinical practice use of ECT in these conditions is usually reserved for medication-resistant patients (23). Less common diagnostic indications include psychotic states secondary to toxic or metabolic abnormalities (35), obsessive–compulsive disorder (36), parkinsonism (37,38), and intractable seizure disorders (39–41). With a few salient exceptions (36,42), virtually all modern research on the cognitive effects of ECT has focused on patients with major depressive disorder. Since the cognitive consequences of ECT are stereotyped and strongly related to technical factors in its administration, it is unlikely that diagnostic factors play an important role in moderating such effects. Nonetheless, this premise has not been investigated empirically.

II. THE COGNITIVE CONSEQUENCES OF ELECTROCONVULSIVE THERAPY: AN OVERVIEW

The clinician will observe drastically different cognitive effects of ECT depending on when patients are examined, and distinctions must be made among acute, subacute, and long-term consequences. Typically, the most profound effects are observed immediately following administration of an ECT treatment. As with spontaneous seizures (43), in the immediate postictal period patients may manifest transient neurological abnormalities (44), profound alterations in consciousness (disorientation, attentional dysfunction) (45,46), sensorimotor abnormalities (47,48) and disturbance in higher cognitive functions, particularly learning and memory (49–52). The severity and persistence of these acute effects show marked sensitivity to technical factors in ECT administration, particularly electrode placement, intensity and type of electrical waveform (e.g., sine wave versus brief pulse, square wave), and the number and spacing of treatments. These factors may determine, for instance, whether patients on average require a few minutes to achieve full reorientation following seizure elicitation or several hours (45,52).

Recovery of cognitive function following a single treatment is rapid. However, with forms of ECT that exert more severe acute cognitive effects (bilateral electrode placement using high intensity sine wave stimulation), recovery may be incomplete by the time of the next treatment. In such cases, repeated acute assessment at the same time points relative to seizure induction demonstrates deterioration over the treatment course (50,53).

For example, at sessions later in the treatment course, patients may take longer to achieve reorientation and may display more severe acute deficits in anterograde and retrograde memory functioning. In extreme cases, patients may develop an organic mental syndrome, with marked disorientation during the ECT course (54–55). Milder forms of ECT have been more recently developed in which cumulative deterioration in cognitive functions does not occur. Indeed, with specific alterations of ECT technique, cumulative improvement in some acute cognitive measures has been demonstrated (52). Depending on how ECT is performed, more than 50% of patients may develop an organic mental syndrome (55), or it may be observed in virtually no patient.

Associations between the magnitude of cognitive effects and ECT treatment parameters rapidly diminish as time from ECT progresses. For example, differences between bilateral ECT (electrodes placed bilaterally over frontotemporal regions) and right unilateral ECT (typically right-sided frontotemporal and parietal placement) in acute cognitive effects are dramatic. Bilateral ECT is associated with a longer period of return to full orientation and greater anterograde and retrograde amnesia, particularly for verbal material (49,51–53,56–57).

After 1 or 2 weeks following the end of the ECT course, differences between electrode placements are more difficult to establish. At this point, in most cognitive domains, depressed patients manifest superior performance relative to their pretreatment baseline. For example, with repeat testing of intelligence, on average, patients will show superior IQ scores shortly following a course of ECT, relative to the untreated depressed state (58). Similarly, before treatment, depressed patients often manifest deficits in the acquisition of information, as revealed by tests of immediate recall or recognition of item lists (59–61). Within several days following the ECT course, patients are typically unchanged or improved in the immediate memory measures, with the change in clinical state being the critical predictor of the magnitude of improvement. In contrast, patients will now often manifest a marked disturbance in their ability to retain information over a delay (62). There is a double dissociation between the effects of depression and ECT on anterograde learning and memory. Depression is associated with an acquisition deficit, most likely related to disturbances in attention and concentration, which frequently recedes following treatment with ECT. In contrast, ECT introduces a new deficit in consolidation or retention, so that information that is newly learned is rapidly forgotten.

A few days after a course of ECT, patients will also display retrograde amnesia. Deficits in the recall or recognition of both personal and public information are usually evident, and there is reason to suspect that these deficits are greatest for events that occurred temporally closest to the treatment (63). Therefore, whereas memory for more remote events is usually intact, patients may have difficulty recalling events that transpired during and several months to years before the ECT course. The retrograde amnesia is rarely dense, and it is more typical for patients to have spottiness in memory for recent events. As time from treatment increases, there is typically improved retrograde functioning, with a return of more distant memories. This temporally graded pattern indicating greatest vulnerability for more recent events is compatible with similar findings of the effects of repeated electroconvulsive shock (ECS) in animals (64).

Usually within a week or so of the end of the ECT course, patients who have shown clinical improvement return to work. Within a few weeks after the end of ECT, objective evidence of persistent cognitive deficit is difficult to obtain (57,65–67). The anterograde amnesia, involving deficits in the retention of information over a delay, typically resolves within a couple of months of ECT termination. The retrograde amnesia will often show a more gradual reduction, with substantial return of memory for events that were seemingly "forgotten" immediately following the treatment course. However, persistent effects of ECT have been identified. Most likely owing to a combination of retrograde and anterograde effects, even when tested at substantial periods after treatment, patients may manifest persistent amnesia for some events that transpired in the interval of several months before and after the ECT course (57).

III. ACUTE AND SUBACUTE COGNITIVE EFFECTS OF ELECTROCONVULSIVE THERAPY

A. Disorientation

After ECT-induced seizures, there is a period of disorientation. The period of disorientation following ECT appears to be exquisitely sensitive to treatment parameters, including electrode placement (bilateral, left unilateral, right unilateral), dose of electrical stimulation or electrical waveform, cumulative treatment number, and the temporal spacing of treatments. The anatomical positioning of ECT-stimulating electrodes has a profound effect on the period of disorientation and some other acute cognitive effects. Of 11 studies that contrasted bilateral and unilateral right electrode placements, 10 studies found substantially quicker orientation recovery with the right unilateral modality (45,52,56,68–75) (Figs. 1–3). All five studies that contrasted left unilateral and right unilateral ECT, found a significant advantage for the right unilateral placement (68,69, 71–73). In contrast, the data contrasting left unilateral and bilateral ECT are equivocal. Three

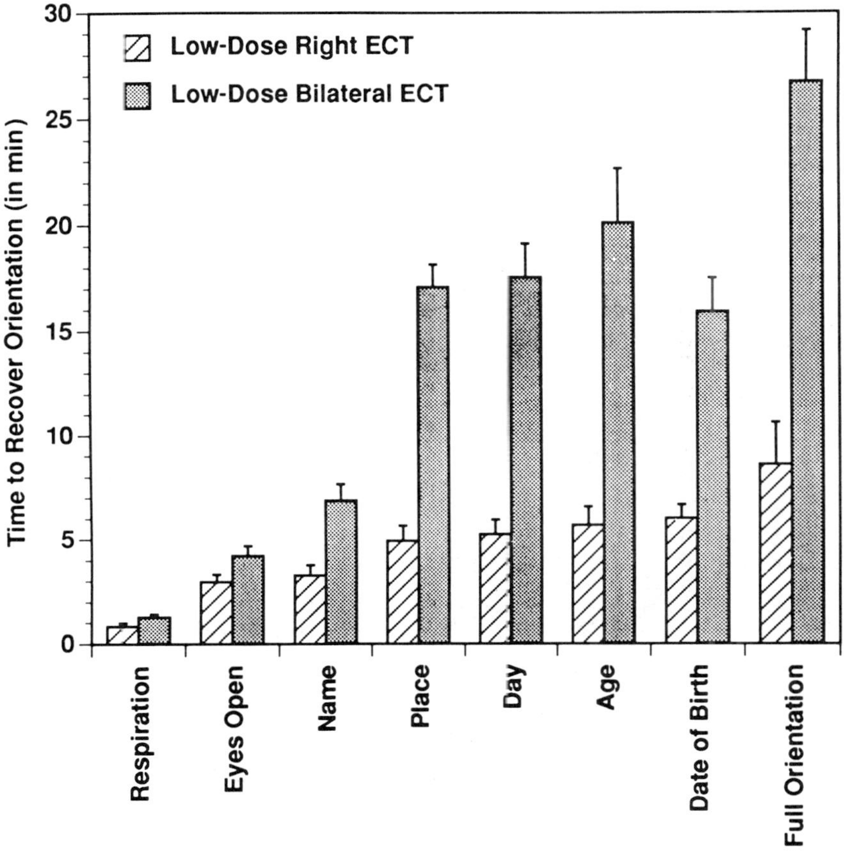

FIGURE 1 Time to recovery of orientation for groups treated with low-dose unilateral right ECT(n=25) and low-dose bilateral ECT (n=24). At each treatment session, time since seizure termination was continuously assessed for return of spontaneous respiration, eyes opening on command, and the orientation components of name, place, day of the week, age, and date of birth. The criterion for full-orientation measure required correct response to four out of five questions, with penalty for not meeting the criterion within 45 min. (Data after Ref. 52.)

studies found that disorientation was longer with bilateral placement (69, 72–73), whereas two studies reported the opposite (68, 71). Site of initial electrical stimulation strongly determines not only the acute neuropsychological effects of the treatment, but acute neurophysiological changes as well. For example, the induction of postictal high-amplitude, slow-wave activity in the electroenchephalogram (EEG) and the reduction in cerebral

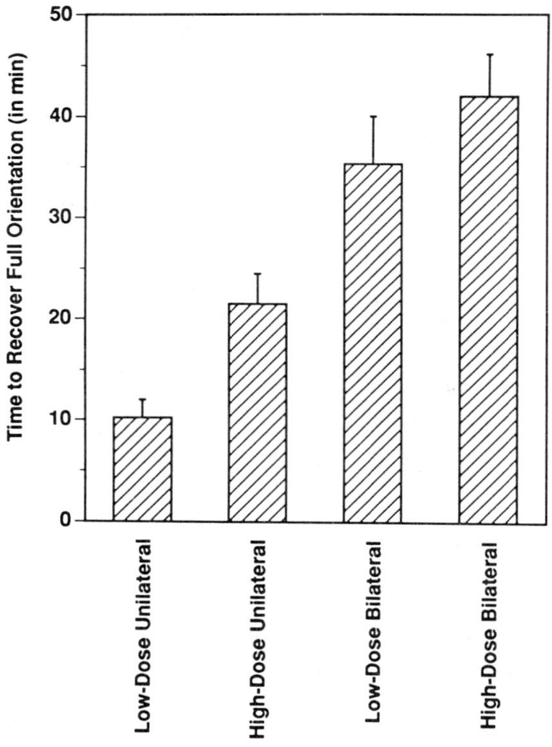

FIGURE 2 Time to recovery of orientation for four groups treated with low- or high-stimulus intensity and unilateral or bilateral ECT (total N=74). Orientation components (name, place, day of the week, age, and date of birth) were assessed continously following seizure termination for 90 min. Orientation recovery required correct response to four of five questions, with penalty for not meeting the criterion by the 90-min cutoff. Main effects of both stimulus intensity (low vs high dose) and electrode placement (unilateral vs bilateral) were obtained.

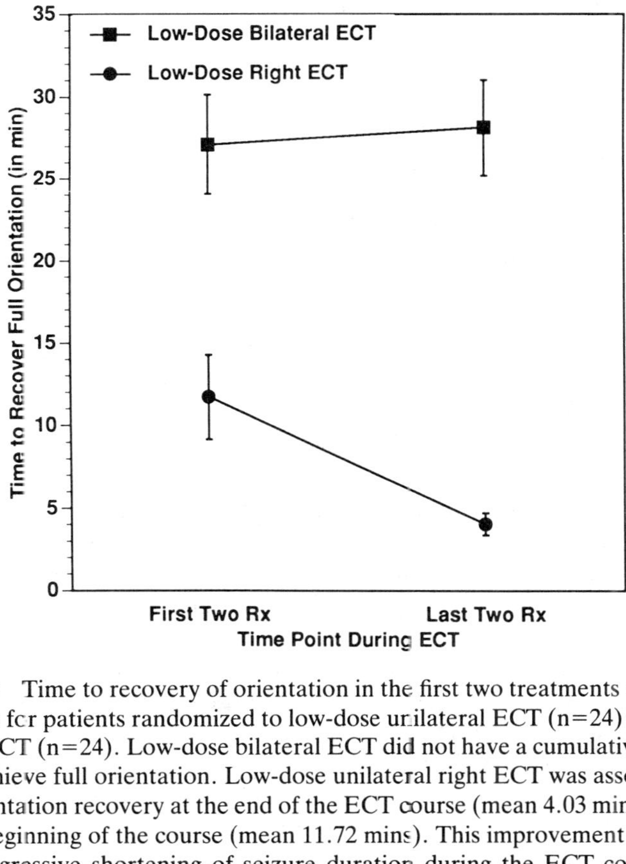

FIGURE 3 Time to recovery of orientation in the first two treatments and last two treatments for patients randomized to low-dose unilateral ECT (n=24) or low-dose bilateral ECT (n=24). Low-dose bilateral ECT did not have a cumulative change in time to achieve full orientation. Low-dose unilateral right ECT was associated with faster orientation recovery at the end of the ECT course (mean 4.03 min) compared with the beginning of the course (mean 11.72 mins). This improvement may be due to the progressive shortening of seizure duration during the ECT course, which covaries with recovery of orientation when using right unilateral ECT. (Data after Ref. 52.)

blood flow is typically most marked in the hemisphere ipsilateral to electrode placement (72, 76, 77).

Various types of electrical waveforms may be used in ECT, with the major alternatives being sine wave (sinusoidal) or square-wave, brief pulse. These waveforms differ in their inherent electrical efficiency in producing seizures. Sine wave stimulation requires about three times the electrical intensity to produce a seizure, compared with brief-pulse stimulation (10, 78). Furthermore, patients vary drastically in their seizure thresholds. With use of a relatively efficient form of brief-pulse stimulation, the minimal electrical intensity needed to produce seizures may vary by a factor of 40 (10, 79). Earlier standard practice had been to administer the same electrical intensity to virtually all patients. Furthermore, until recently almost all information about the effects of ECT stimulus parameters on cognitive functioning came from research that confounded differences in electrical intensity with differences in waveform characteristics. This work usually involved comparisons of a relatively inefficient sine-wave stimulus delivered at high intensity with a brief-pulse stimulus delivered at more moderate intensity.

Valentine et al. (70) contrasted unilateral and bilateral ECT administered with either brief-pulse or sine-wave stimuli, using a factorial design. Electrical dose waveform exerted a large effect, over and above that for electrode placement, with disorientation longest following bilateral, higher-intensity, sine-wave stimulation. Using a similar design, Daniel and Crovitz (45) contrasted the two electrode placements when administered with either brief-pulse (~24 joules) or sine-wave (~62 joules) stimulation. Based on small samples, this work suggested that average time to return to full orientation was about 6 hrs in both the unilateral and bilateral sine wave groups, about 1 hr in the bilateral brief pulse group, and about 15 min in the brief pulse unilateral group. These two studies strongly indicate that electrical intensity or stimulus waveform can have marked effects on time to recover orientation.

More recent research has focused on optimizing administration of the brief-pulse waveform to lessen cognitive effects. In one study, 52 patients were randomized to either right unilateral or bilateral ECT, with the intensity of brief-pulse electrical stimulation titrated to be just above the individual patient's seizure threshold throughout the treatment course (9). Recovery of orientation was assessed continuously following seizure termination at every session. As indicated in Figure 1, recovery of full orientation was relatively rapid in both groups—on average, about 8.5 min following eyes opening upon command for low-dose right unilateral ECT patients and about 27 mins for low-dose bilateral ECT patients (52). Figure 2 presents preliminary findings from a recently completed study in which patients were randomized into four treatment groups, right unilateral ECT and bilateral ECT, administered at lower- or higher-intensity brief-pulse conditions (10). As in the previous study, the low-intensity conditions involved titration of ECT electrical dose to just above patient's seizure threshold. In the higher-intensity conditions, patients were treated with an electrical dose 2.5 times (150% above) the seizure threshold determined in the first treatment. In this study, both electrode placement and electrical dose exerted main effects on time to recovery of orientation. Patients had more prolonged recovery with bilateral and higher-intensity stimulation.

It is commonly believed that the period of postictal disorientation increases with advancing treatment number (53). Five studies have provided data on this issue. Wilson and Gottlieb (80) assessed orientation in each session for the first six treatments in patients receiving either left unilateral, right unilateral, or bilateral ECT. Recovery times deteriorated sequentially in all three groups. Fraser and Glass (74) used a within-patient design, alternating unilateral and bilateral ECT in nine elderly depressed patients (mean age, 72.4 years). In contrasting the first and last treatments with each modality, recovery time deteriorated significantly with bilateral ECT and tended to do so with unilateral ECT. In another study using a between-subjects design with a larger sample, as well as more moderate electrical intensities than in their previous research, Fraser and Glass (75) compared orientation recovery at the first and fifth treatments in patients randomized to bilateral or right unilateral ECT. There was no effect of treatment number in the bilateral group, and patients who received right unilateral ECT had faster recovery at their fifth treatment compared with their first treatment. Daniel and Crovitz (45) contrasted recovery times at the third and eighth treatments in patients randomized to right unilateral or bilateral ECT administered with sine-wave or brief-pulse stimulation. Cumulative deterioration was observed in all groups but the unilateral, low-intensity, brief-pulse condition. Finally, as described earlier, Sackeim et al. (52) tested orientation recovery at all treatments in patients randomized to either bilateral and right unilateral ECT, using minimal brief-pulse stimulus intensity. As seen in Figure 3, with low-dose bilateral ECT, time point during ECT had no effect on recovery time. With right unilateral ECT, there was progressive improvement, dropping from an average of 12 min at the first two treatments to about 4 min at the final two treatments.

These studies suggest that, although progressive lengthening in time to achieve reorientation does occur with an increasing number of treatments, it is an avoidable outcome. Progressive deterioration is particularly likely with the bilateral electrode placement and high-intensity, particularly sine-wave, stimulation. Since sustained disorientation (organic mental syndrome) almost always develops only after several treatments have been administered, it is likely this outcome will most readily occur with this combination of treatment conditions. In contrast, the pairing of the right unilateral electrode placement and low-intensity stimulation may not be associated with progressive deterioration, but indeed, may show progressive improvement. With low-dose unilateral ECT, the duration of seizures is an important predictor of time to recovery of orientation (81). The progressive improvement in orientation times with low-dose right unilateral ECT is likely to be because seizure duration typically decreases over the course of treatment (10, 82).

It is also believed that the spacing of treatments influences orientation recovery (23). To date, only Fraser and Glass (75) provided data on this issue. Within the same patients, a 1-day interval before bilateral treatment resulted in significantly prolonged disorientation, compared with an interval of 2 or more days. Cases of notably prolonged postictal confusion have also been reported with multiple seizure elicitation within the same session (83, 84).

Since there is extraordinary variability in seizure threshold (the minimal electrical intensity necessary to elicit generalized seizures), high absolute electrical doses may be barely suprathreshold for some patients, whereas modest absolute electrical doses may be grossly suprathreshold for other patients. Therefore, it is critical to determine whether the acute cognitive effects of ECT are more tied to the absolute electrical dose administered or to the degree to which that dose exceeds seizure threshold. At stimulus intensity near seizure threshold, for both unilateral and bilateral ECT, there are no relations between absolute electrical dose and cognitive variables (81). Particularly for unilateral ECT, longer seizure durations are associated with greater retrograde amnesia. These findings suggested that when electrical dose is titrated to seizure threshold, the absolute electrical intensity is largely irrelevant in contributing to acute cognitive effects. This raised the possibility that the degree to which electrical dose exceeds seizure threshold is more critical to acute cognitive side effects than the absolute dose administered (82).

Table 1 presents findings from a four-group random assignment study conducted by Sackeim et al. (10). Two alternative measures of time to recover full orientation were examined as dependent measures in simultaneous regressions, with the predictors being assignment to low-dose (threshold) or higher-dose (2.5 times initial threshold) treatment conditions, initial seizure threshold, seizure duration, age, sex, and dose of the anesthetic agent, methohexital. For both right unilateral and bilateral ECT, dose condition was a significant predictor of time to achieve full orientation. In contrast, initial seizure threshold had no predictive power, as in prior research (81). These findings indicate that the degree to which electrical dose

TABLE 1. Predictors of Postictal Time to Recover Full Orientation as a Function of Electrode Placement

Variable	Unilateral ECT n=36				Bilateral ECT n=38			
	Orientation time A		Orientation time B		Orientation time A		Orientation time B	
	t	p	t	p	t	p	t	p
Dosage condition (low vs high)	1.78	0.09	3.71	0.0009	2.46	0.02	2.18	0.04
Age	0.03		0.04		2.84	0.008	2.25	0.03
Sex	−0.14		0.50		0.13		−0.40	
Motor seizure duration	2.22	0.04	2.18	0.04	0.45		−0.19	
Initial seizure threshold	−1.17		−1.16		1.34		0.52	
Methohexital dose	0.08		−0.05		0.24		−0.22	

Orientation time A assessed recovery within a 90-min postictal window; Orientation time B included penalty for failure to orient within the time window. **t** and **p** indicate the values of the t-test and its significance level for the predictor's beta-coefficient in the simultaneous multiple regression on the recovery time dependent measure.

exceeds seizure threshold is probably the critical factor in determining relations between electrical dose and cognitive effects. These findings have important clinical implications. Unless practitioners empirically determine the seizure threshold, they have no certainty that any particular absolute electrical dose is minimally, moderately, or grossly suprathreshold. As we have seen, avoidance of grossly suprathreshold stimulation will likely minimize many of the acute cognitive side effects of ECT. In part, this is why the new clinical standard for the practice of ECT, issued by the American Psychiatric Association, recommends that stimulus parameters be adjusted to the individual patient's needs on a case-by-case basis (23).

Epileptologists have long believed that the duration of spontaneous generalized seizures is associated with the duration of postictal confusion. Table 1 indicates that such a relation holds for right unilateral ECT. It is likely that bilateral ECT results in sufficient lengthening of the time to recover orientation so that relations with seizure duration or other characteristics of the ictal discharge are obscured. In contrast, Table 1 indicates that patient age is a significant predictor of recovery time, with older patients displaying a more prolonged period of disorientation. This provides empirical support for the view that elderly patients may develop more pronounced acute cognitive side effects and that use of right unilateral ECT should be particularly entertained in the elderly (74, 75, 85).

B. Organic Mental Syndrome

It should now be evident that, depending on how ECT is performed, there can be drastic differences in time to recover orientation. For example, Lunn and Tralle (86), using high-intensity bilateral stimulation, without anesthesia or oxygenation, reported that fewer than 40% of patients could report the day of the week 2 hrs postically. In some more modern research with sinusoidal bilateral techniques, the average time to achieve full orientation is several hours. In contrast, low-dose unilateral stimulation may result in average times of a few minutes, even at the end of a full course of treatment.

There has been relatively little research devoted to the development of organic mental syndrome (OMS), which is a state of profound disorientation that does not resolve between treatments. Miller et al. (55) retrospectively examined all clinical cases treated at a New York City facility during 1 year. In 56% of patients, chart notes indicated that the ECT course was interrupted or stopped owing to OMS. This facility used high-intensity, bilateral, sine-wave stimulation, and many elderly patients presented with preexisting medical conditions that may have increased the likelihood of OMS. Summers et al. (54) repeatedly assessed 13 patients who developed OMS during ECT. The average interval to return to baseline functioning was 20.1 days (range 5 to 43). Once OMS develops, it can be frightening to patients and family members and present clinical staff with substantial management problems, owing to the need for close observation. In almost all cases, this is an avoidable outcome. Even with bilateral ECT, in the low-dose study of Sackeim et al. (52), none of the 52 patients developed OMS. Indeed, no patient failed to manifest full orientation when assessed just before each treatment. The use of low electrical intensities titrated to threshold, the avoidance of concomitant treatment with psychotropics, particularly lithium (87, 88), and limiting seizure elicitation to one per treatment (89), and, if necessary, spacing the treatments over wider intervals will mitigate against the development of OMS.

C. Learning and Memory

Virtually all research on post-ECT acute cognitive disturbance has concerned either orientation recovery or learning and memory, with relatively little investigation of perceptual, attentional, or other cognitive processes that are not heavily reliant upon memory (44, 47, 48, 73, 90, 91). Furthermore, the time frame implied by "acute" memory impairment has never been defined. Reviews typically group together studies in which patients were tested from 4 min to 7 days following a treatment (50, 51). This lack of distinction is not trivial, as the processes that are most disrupted acutely and those that display more persistent effects may not be identical. Other methodological points to consider pertain to separating ECT effects on orientation from those on memory, selection bias in the assessment of psychiatric patients, and the nature of sampling of cognitive functions. A number of studies have failed to separate acute orientation effects from effects on memory or other cognitive functions. This issue is particularly consequential in evaluating the claim that bilateral ECT generally results in more pervasive and severe memory disturbance than right unilateral ECT (23, 32, 63, 92). In immediate testing conditions, when orientation is not established before memory assessment (93–96), the relative impairments of the bilaterally treated groups will be magnified.

A significant proportion of psychiatric patients cannot tolerate neuropsychological investigation owing to the severity of their illness. Fortunately, this selection bias is probably inconsequential for determining the cognitive effects of ECT, as there is no evidence that the severity of depressive symptomatology is associated with the nature or extent of ECT-induced impairments. However, a rare group of depressed patients present with pseudodementia (61, 97). Such individuals are typically untestable at pretreatment baseline. When they receive ECT, it is common to observe that a broad range of neuropsychological functions show steady improvement with each treatment, resulting in dissolution of the dementialike profile and clinical recovery (98). The absence of baseline testing in such individuals results in their exclusion from research samples and consequent overestimation of acute deleterious effects of ECT.

The two most common aims in evaluating acute post-ECT cognitive deficits are either to contrast treatment conditions in the nature of the impairments they produce or to specify the profile of ECT-related neuropsychological disturbances by comparing relative impairments for different functions. To accomplish either of these aims, tasks must be internally reliable and possess sufficient discriminating power such that floor and ceiling effects are avoided (99, 100). Particularly for the second aim, tasks should be matched on psychometric properties, so that findings of relative deficits are not simply due to differences in task discriminating power. A number of the negative or conflicting findings in this area are likely due to the use of tasks with inadequate psychometric properties. For example, there have been comparisons of treatment conditions using a retrograde memory task that comprised a single item (101). Not surprisingly, no effects were found.

1. *Effects of Electrode Placement*

Despite these limitations, there is a consensus on some central points. Both anterograde and retrograde verbal memory disturbances are greater following unilateral left and bilateral ECT than following unilateral right ECT (49, 52, 70, 71, 102–107). Studies of retrograde amnesia typically have involved deliberate learning of a stimuli list before a treatment, with delayed testing following the treatment. The bulk of these studies have focused on performance within an hour following seizure termination. Studies of anterograde memory functioning have also involved deliberate list learning followed by immediate and delayed testing, but the bulk of these investigations have examined patients several hours or days after ECT. Only a small group of studies have contrasted left unilateral and bilateral ECT. For retrograde verbal memory, despite the widespread view that bilateral ECT results in more profound deficits than unilateral ECT, the opposite was found in two studies (68, 80), and no significant difference was obtained with five tasks used in four studies (71, 72, 103, 108). For anterograde verbal memory, deficits were greater following left unilateral ECT than bilateral ECT in two studies with long ECT test intervals (69, 103), and not significantly different in two other studies (69, 102). These findings indicate that the extent of amnesia for verbal material, retrograde or anterograde, is greatest for treatments that involve the greatest direct stimulation of the left hemisphere (left unilateral and bilateral ECT) and that there may be no advantage to left unilateral ECT compared with bilateral ECT. In general, the magnitude of verbal memory deficits, as well as the specificity to modality, appear to decrease with greater intervals between ECT and cognitive assessment.

Characterization of the literature on anterograde and retrograde memory for nonverbal material is more difficult. First, only three studies have examined acute retrograde effects on nonverbal material (52, 109, 110). Second, across the anterograde–retrograde dimension, the majority of studies have used tasks that are likely to be inappropriate. The aim, presumably, in assessing nonverbal memory is to determine the impact of ECT on cognitive functions subserved to a greater extent by the right than left hemisphere. The tasks used in the bulk of studies have been recognition of common objects or recognition of geometric designs (e.g., 49, 72). Such tasks do not preferentially call upon right hemisphere processing, as a picture of a chair may be encoded and stored as the word *chair* perhaps more readily than as a visual image (111–113).

When this distinction is applied to ECT studies, greater anterograde nonverbal memory deficits were obtained for right unilateral relative to left unilateral ECT, when tasks sampled material difficult to encode verbally (unfamiliar face recognition, recognition of nonsense shapes) (69, 102, 104,

105). On the other hand, without exception, studies that obtained no difference between the unilateral modes used "nonverbal" tasks that sampled material easily subject to verbal encoding (e.g., 105, 114). With this type of task, bilateral ECT has consistently shown greater anterograde nonverbal memory deficits than right unilateral ECT (49, 52, 109, 115, 116). Often, no difference between bilateral and right unilateral ECT has been observed with purer nonverbal tasks (52, 57, 62, 69, 110, 114, 116–118). Therefore, in terms of acute effects for deliberately learned material, it is likely that bilateral ECT results in a broader range of anterograde and retrograde deficits than does right unilateral ECT. However, the two modalities may be more equivalent than had been suspected in the magnitude of deficits for purer nonverbal material.

Figure 4 summarizes findings from the study by Sackeim et al. (52) in which patients were randomized to low-dose unilateral right or bilateral ECT. Several minutes prior to each treatment, patients were asked to commit to memory a list of words, geometric shapes, and nonsense shapes. Retrograde word recall and recognition and shape recognition were tested as part of a larger neuropsychological battery, once patients meet criteria for full orientation during the postictal period. In addition, at randomly selected treatments, patients were also asked to memorize a set of unfamiliar faces with postictal retrograde recognition testing. At the sessions in which retrograde face recognition testing was omitted, the same task was administered with an anterograde format during the postictal period.

Regardless of electrode placement, there was virtually complete amnesia when retrograde memory for the word lists was tested with a recall format. With recognition testing, right unilateral ECT group resulted in superior performance for the retrograde word, geometric shape, and nonsense shape tasks. The two groups were equivalent in retrograde and anterograde recognition memory for unfamiliar, emotionally neutral faces. In line with the concerns about the verbal encodability of geometric shapes, recognition accuracy on this task strongly covaried with the performance on the retrograde word recognition task, whereas performance on the nonsense task was independent of both the word and geometric shape tasks. Nonetheless, the finding of greater impairment with bilateral ECT for nonsense shape recognition supports the claim that this modality produces greater retrograde memory disturbance for information processing principally mediated by either the left or right hemisphere (32, 49). However, there is substantial evidence that neutral face recognition is particularly dependent on the integrity of right hemisphere processes (112, 119). The equivalence of the treatment groups on the retrograde and anterograde versions of these tasks raises the possibility that there may be specificity in the types of right hemisphere cognitive functions that are differentially affected by bilateral and right

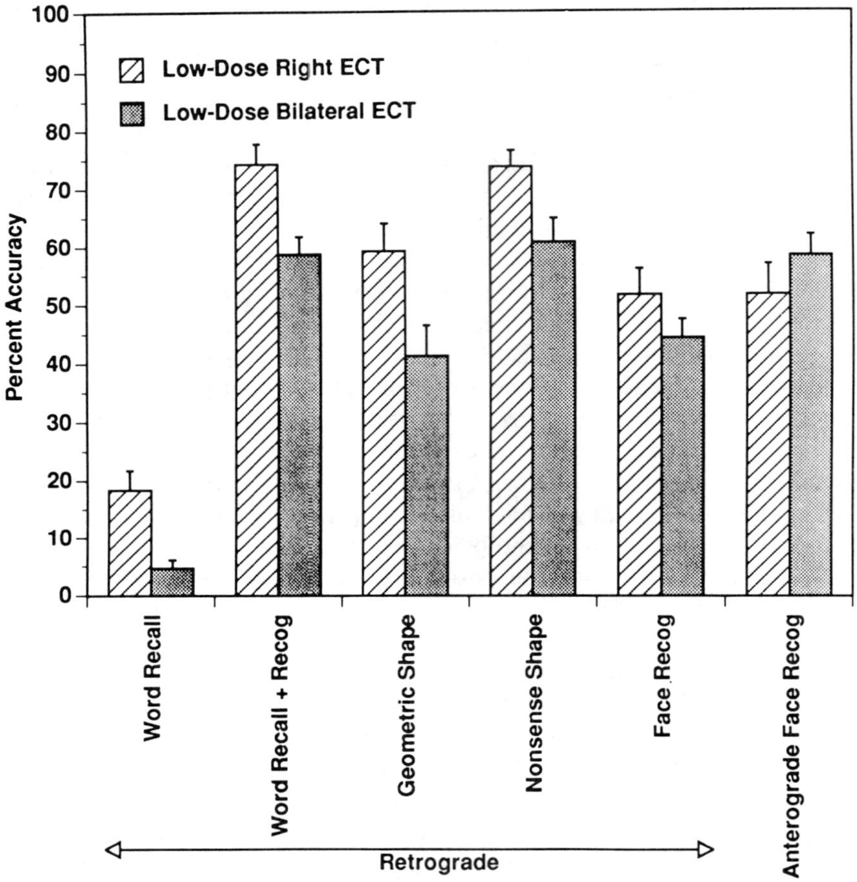

FIGURE 4 Neuropsychological performance during the acute postictal period. Prior to each treatment, patients randomized to low-dose right unilateral ECT (n=25) or low-dose bilateral ECT (n=22) committed to memory a set of six words, two geometric shapes, two nonsense shapes, and eight neutral faces. After recovery of orientation, retrograde recall (words) and recognition (words, shapes, faces) was tested, followed by anterograde immediate memory for neutral faces. Values represent accuracy of performance at postictal assessment. Unilateral right ECT was associated with superior performance for all but the neutral face recognition tasks. (Data after Ref. 52.)

unilateral ECT (52). These two modalities differ not only in the lateralization of current distributions in the brain, but also in the regional distributions within the right hemisphere (120, 121).

For methodological reasons, the emphasis on the study of retrograde and anterograde amnesia for deliberately learned material is understandable. However, from an ecological viewpoint, such procedures sample only a small portion of memory functions. Much of what we have available in memory was never subject to deliberate learning and, regardless of the strategies used in learning, was first subject to encoding over variable time frames, often extending to much earlier in the past. Furthermore, it would not be unexpected for patients to be more concerned about memory loss for personally significant information than for difficulties in retaining relatively meaningless lists of items (122, 123). In this context, it may be useful to make distinctions among incidental and deliberate learning, semantic and episodic memory, and episodic memory for personal and impersonal or public information.

The distinction between incidental and deliberate learning and memory is related to the distinction between effortful or controlled processing and automatic processing (124). Generally speaking, before treatment, patients with major depression evidence learning deficits on tasks that require effortful, complex processing or independent structuring of information relative to preexisting knowledge (62, 125–127). Depressed patients often do not show impairment on tasks tapping automatic and shallow processing. This specificity may reflect diminished capacity, inflexibility, or variability in the allocation of attention (61, 66, 128, 129). Therefore, it would be expected that depressed patients do not evidence pretreatment performance deficits on incidental learning tasks, although this has yet to receive significant empirical investigation. Surprisingly, it is also unknown whether incidental learning and memory are affected by ECT.

Squire and Chase (130) reported the most ambitious attempt to evaluate incidental memory in ECT patients. They contrasted bilateral, right unilateral, and a non-ECT patient control group 6–9 months after hospitalization. Assignment was not random, and pretreatment baseline testing was not available. Subjects were questioned on the type and order of psychological tests and the appearance of the examiner at a visit 2 weeks earlier. No differences among the groups were obtained in incidental memory performance. However, one should note that the time point of testing was certainly out of the acute–subacute period and at this time point no differences were obtained on a series of other tasks that assessed immediate and delayed memory performance for deliberately learned verbal and nonverbal material. Daniel et al. (131), in a very small sample of patients, reported that bilateral ECT and sine-wave administration both had main effects in producing greater "autobiographical" memory deficit than right unilateral ECT and brief-pulse stimulation. Although patients in this study were assessed during the ECT course and, therefore, were more likely to manifest amnestic disturbance, only one of the four items used in the memory test sampled incidental learning and memory. Therefore, the question of whether ECT results in impairment of incidental learning and memory is essentially unexplored. This issue is both of practical and theoretical significance. In the general neuropsychological literature, it is unknown whether amnestic deficits for incidental and deliberate learning covary.

Tasks that assess incidental or deliberate learning and memory typically require that subjects be exposed to new sets of information. Such episodic learning and memory has been distinguished from semantic memory, with the suggestion that the two types form separate memory systems (e.g., 126, 132). *Semantic memory* refers to "the representation of structured and organized information, or knowledge in memory, which serves as a basis for appreciating, interpreting, and encoding ongoing experience" (126, p. 381). For the most part, if ECT has any impact on semantic memory, it is detectable only shortly after a treatment. Pratt and Warrington (94, 133, 134) used left and right unilateral ECT in within-patient designs to establish lateralization of language functions. At very short postictal intervals, disturbance in naming based on verbal description was a sensitive discriminator of the treatment modalities. With these procedures, Geffen and Caudrey (135) found that in 31 of 32 cases there was agreement in identification of language dominance between acute postictal testing and pre-ECT evaluation with a dichotic monitoring procedure. However, much of this work may have confounded assessment of dysnomia with postictal confusion. In contrast, we have used similar testing procedures during the postictal period once patients have met the criteria for return of full orientation. With repeated assessment following each treatment, we have observed no impairments in patients receiving either bilateral ECT or right unilateral ECT, with performance equivalent to pre-ECT baseline. Similarly, it is common to observe that scores on the Wechsler's Adult Intelligence Scale (WAIS) vocabulary and information subtests are unchanged or improved following a course of ECT (58). The sparing of semantic memory may pertain to other instances of nonepisodic knowledge. Skill retention also does not seem to be influenced by this treatment (136).

A major focus of investigation has been retrograde memory for impersonal (public) or personal events, in part because of indications that if long-term impairments accrue with ECT, they pertain to this domain (137). Retrograde amnesia following some types of brain trauma displays a temporal gradient, with events closest to the trauma most susceptible to loss, and recovery of functioning over time occurring first for the more remote events

(138, 139). Squire demonstrated similar phenomena in ECT patients (140–142). One hour after the fifth treatment, memory for the names of television programs was disturbed for those programs aired 1–3 years before treatment, but not those that aired earlier (141). In contrast, a right unilateral ECT group showed no acute deficit and at 6–9 months post-ECT, bilateral and right unilateral patients were equivalent to controls. Squire et al. (142) found that the ability to make judgments about the temporal order of television programs was impaired in a temporally graded fashion 1–2 weeks after bilateral ECT. Weiner et al. (57) used tasks assessing retrograde memory for famous public events and for the faces of famous people. They found that the performance of patients randomly assigned to bilateral ECT significantly deteriorated with testing 2–3 days following ECT termination, both in relation to themselves at pre-ECT baseline and in relation to a depressed comparison group that did not receive ECT. The deficits on both tasks were greater with bilateral than right unilateral ECT, and the right unilateral ECT group did not differ from the non-ECT comparison patients.

It was originally suggested by Janis (143–145) that memory for personal events is more disturbed following ECT than memory for impersonal, public events. In two studies in schizophrenic patients, amnesia for recent personal events was found 1 month after treatment, particularly for events that were emotionally disturbing. Stieper et al. (146) reported similar findings for recent personal memory functioning. However, methodological problems with these studies preclude putting much weight on the findings. Squire et al. (147) had a small group of bilateral ECT patients and non-ECT comparison patients report details about their personal history, with the time frame of questions extending from the very recent day of hospitalization to elementary school. There was a marked deficit in the number of autobiographical details that could be recalled shortly after bilateral ECT. At 7-month follow-up, overall there was no difference between the groups in remote memory performance. However, when the data was examined discretely for the items inquiring about the most recent events, a persistent deficit was noted in the ECT sample. Strain et al. (117) observed that 10 days following ECT, testing of personal memories showed the largest deficit in an extensive neuropsychological battery, although there was recovery by 1 year (148, 149). Weeks et al. (65) did not observe a long-term deficit in personal memory performance with 4 and 7 months post-ECT testing. The importance of this negative result was compromised by the failure of their custom-designed task to manifest a deficit at an acute testing interval, raising the issue of task sensitivity. In contrast, Weiner et al. (57), using an extensive interview schedule to elicit a large corpus of details of personal history at pretreatment, with confirmation by interviewing family informants, found that deficits in personal memory were the most sensitive of a variety of memory-testing procedures in distinguishing among different forms of ECT and in discriminating patients who received ECT from a non-ECT-treated comparison group. Two or three days after ECT, patients who received bilateral ECT or sine-wave stimulation had the greatest deficits. Patients who had received right unilateral ECT administered with brief-pulse stimulation did not differ from the non-ECT comparison group. Of particular concern, at retesting 6 months after the ECT course, patients who received bilateral ECT evidenced significantly greater amnesia than controls, and patients who received sine-wave stimulation tended to manifest persistent retrograde deficits. Although sample sizes were small, this report provides some of the first objective evidence for persistent amnesia 6 months after termination of ECT. Furthermore, within a large neuropsychological battery involving assessment of both anterograde learning and memory and retrograde personal and impersonal memory functioning, deficits at 6 months post-ECT were only observed for the personal memory task. This may well have been because this task sampled memory for events that occurred in relatively close proximity to the ECT course.

2. *Effects of Stimulus Intensity and Electrical Waveform*

As in the effects on orientation recovery, acute and subacute memory functioning following ECT is sensitive to the electrical dose or waveform administered. Only the classic study by Ottosson (8) and ongoing research by the Columbia University group (10) have examined the effects of electrical intensity on memory functioning, without confounding electrical dose with electrical waveform characteristics. Ottosson (8) found that markedly suprathreshold bilateral ECT resulted in greater anterograde amnesia after the first treatment compared with moderate electrical stimulation. He concluded that electrical stimulus dose has a powerful effect on memory performance and was of greater consequence than seizure duration.

Figure 5 illustrates preliminary findings from the Columbia University study (10). Patients were randomized under double-blind conditions to four treatment conditions, right unilateral or bilateral ECT administered with low electrical dose (just above the seizure threshold) or at higher dose (2.5 times the seizure threshold). A neuropsychological battery was administered at each treatment session. In acute testing of retrograde amnesia for word and shape stimuli, there were main effects of both electrode placement and stimulus intensity. Generally, retrograde amnesia was greater with bilateral than unilateral stimulation and with higher relative to lower electrical intensity. In this study, this pattern was maintained across a host of measures of acute and subacute memory functioning, with the magnitude of the objective amnestic effects attributable to electrode placement typically greater than that attributable to stimulus intensity.

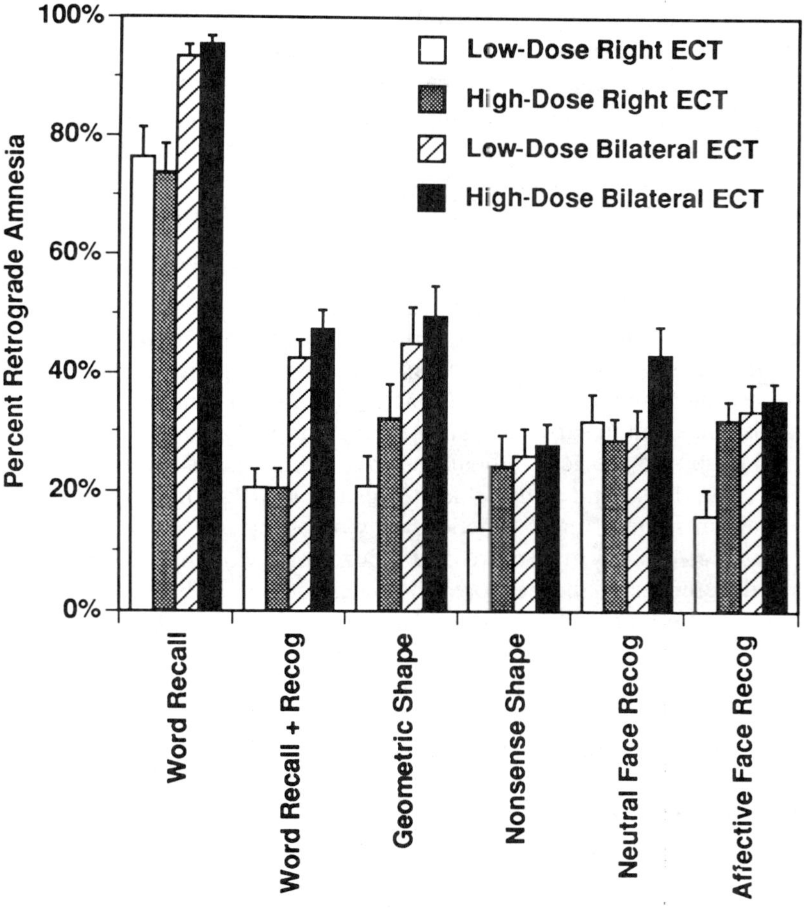

FIGURE 5 Acute retrograde amnesia in patients randomized to low- or high-stimulus intensity and unilateral right or bilateral ECT (total N=87). Patients committed to memory a set of words, geometric shapes, nonsense shapes, and neutral or affectively expressive faces before each treatment session, with immediate recall or recognition testing following presentation of each type of stimulus material. After recovery of orientation, retrograde memory was assessed with repeat recall and/or recognition testing. Values represent the percentage of material reported before the treatment that was not reported at postictal assessment (percentage forgetting). Across the tasks, both dosage condition and electrode placement exerted main effects, with the effects of electrode placement generally being more consequential than electrical dose.

Therefore, it appears that both anterograde and retrograde memory are sensitive to the dose of electrical stimulation. This view is consonant with a large set of studies that have contrasted the effects on acute cognitive functioning of electrical waveforms that differed in intensity. The early workers in this area claimed that brief-pulse or other low-intensity stimuli had less amnestic properties than higher-intensity sine-wave stimulation (e.g., 150). For the most part, from the earliest to contemporary studies, this claim has been supported (57, 70, 93, 150–156).

A small group of studies have failed to find waveform effects on cognition (96, 101, 157, 158). In much of this work, the tasks used are known to be insensitive to ECT-induced impairments. For instance, Goldstein et al. (157) administered the Halstead–Reitan battery to patients treated with brief-pulse and sine-wave stimulation. A number of studies have shown that Halstead–Reitan subscales, such as finger tapping, finger agnosia, and grooved pegboard are generally insensitive to differences among ECT modalities (159, 160), and with subacute testing shortly following ECT improvement in some of these functions may be observed (58). Of particular note is a recent study by Squire and Zouzounis (96), that reported only limited differences in the neuropsychological effects of brief-pulse versus sine-wave stimulation. The authors noted that brief-pulse patients had been treated at what was essentially the maximum output of the ECT device, averaging approximately 52 joules. They suggested that the advantages with respect to side effects of brief-pulse stimulation may be compromised when this form of treatment is used with high-intensity stimulation.

3. *Effects of Cumulative Treatment Number*

Acute and subacute cognitive deficits are sensitive to the number of treatments administered, with the magnitude of acute deficits increasing as treatment progresses. Daniel and Crovitz's (53) review identified 16 studies that made comparisons of deficits following treatments earlier and later in the ECT course. In 13 of these studies, evidence of significant deterioration was obtained. Of the 3 studies that failed to observe a cumulative effect with advancing treatment number, 1 study (109) found no change and 2 studies (161, 162) found a decrease in deficits. Various methodological problems characterized these studies, including administration of the same form of tasks, thereby maximizing practice effects (162), use of a short number of intervening treatments between testing occasions (109, 161), and ceiling effects in performance which limited capacity to observe change (109).

That 13 of 16 studies found significant cumulative deterioration effects underscores the robustness of the phenomenon. In many of these studies, relatively few treatments intervened between "early" and "late" testing. Frequently, only single-testing occasions entered into the comparisons, with a consequent lack of reliability owing to limited sampling, and often tasks were used that were relatively insensitive in revealing amnestic deficits (80, 106, 108, 140, 163–165).

The Columbia University group reexamined the issue of cumulative deterioration, using ECT techniques involving an efficient waveform and adjustment of stimulus intensity relative to each patient's seizure threshold. In one study, involving only low-dose right unilateral and low-dose bilateral ECT, no evidence was obtained for cumulative deterioration over the treatment course (52). To maximize the probability of identifying such effects, patients were tested at each treatment session with a battery examining a variety of neuropsychological functions, including anterograde and retrograde memory. A number of the tasks used showed strong sensitivity in differentiating right unilateral from bilateral ECT, and acute ECT-induced impairment was established for both groups relative to pretreatment baseline testing. Nonetheless, the magnitude of amnestic and other cognitive deficits at the final two treatments was essentially equivalent to that observed at the first two treatments for almost all measures, in both the right unilateral ECT and bilateral ECT conditions. In ongoing work (10), the absence of cumulative deterioration with low-intensity stimulation has been replicated. Whether or not the traditional pattern of increased magnitude of deficit emerges in patients treated at higher-stimulus intensity is currently under investigation in this work.

These findings suggest that technical factors in ECT administration, particularly stimulus intensity, may strongly affect whether or not acute cognitive deficits show a cumulative pattern. This is of particular importance clinically, since one would expect that the magnitude of subacute deficits and their persistence would be related to the slope of cognitive functioning during the ECT course. For other technical parameters, the literature is inconsistent. Cumulative deterioration has been observed repeatedly with both right unilateral and bilateral ECT, but there is uncertainty whether the slope of this function differs for the two modalities (68, 80, 117, 148). When differences have been obtained, bilateral ECT resulted in more rapid deterioration in cognitive measures (117, 148).

IV. LONG-TERM COGNITIVE CONSEQUENCES OF ELECTROCONVULSIVE THERAPY

Subacute deficits several days following the end of the ECT course have been identified and pertain mainly to aspects of anterograde and retrograde memory. One of the most critical issues in this field concerns the relative persistence of these deficits. Are these deficits transient or are patients left with permanent disabilities?

There is a large literature that addresses this question, and several reviews are available (1, 23, 32, 63, 84, 166–168). The reader is referred particularly to Weiner (137) for a critical discussion of the evidence. Here, emphasis will be given only to the most general conclusions that can be drawn from this literature, as well as consideration of some of the methodological difficulties that limit interpretation. Following conventions in this literature, *persistent deficits* are defined as those documented 10 or more days following the ECT course.

Publications bearing on the persistence of ECT-induced cognitive effects comprise case reports, retrospective studies (with and without control or comparison groups), prospective studies involving no control or comparison groups, prospective studies with comparison of different ECT modalities, and prospective studies with comparison to non-ECT patient or normal control groups.

A. Retrospective Studies

Much of the evidence from retrospective studies has concentrated on patients with chronic schizophrenia, many of whom have received numerous ECT treatments in the distant past, often unmodified by anesthesia and oxygenation (164, 169, 170). Although, in some of this work, there were indications that former ECT samples had greater cognitive impairment than comparison groups, characteristically there was either evidence that the ECT sample was more chronically or severely ill or the possibility of such intergroup differences was not addressed (164, 169, 171). More recent retrospective comparisons, focusing primarily on depressed patients, have failed to identify persistent effects (130, 172).

A particularly important retrospective study was conducted by Freeman et al. (173). Through newspaper advertisements, they recruited 26 individuals who had received ECT in the past and believed that they had sustained memory loss. This group was contrasted with 13 former ECT patients without memory complaints and 56 demographically matched normal controls. Blind neuropsychological testing indicated that the combined patients groups differed from normal controls on 8 of 19 cognitive measures. However, the patient samples differed from normal controls in current psychiatric status and recent medication history. Furthermore, the group of patients with memory complaints evidenced greater current psychopathology and were receiving greater intensity of pharmacologic treatment than the noncomplaining ECT sample. After attempting to control statistically for the influence of current psychopathology and medication levels, the group of ECT complainers showed significantly inferior performance on 2 of the 19 tests (a face–name association task and a verbal learning task).

This study represents the only attempt to date to examine with objective neuropsychological measures a group of patients who believe that ECT has resulted in persistent impairment. In large part, the findings were indeterminate. At a technical level it is questionable whether large differences with comparison groups in levels of psychopathology and medication effects can or should be controlled through covariance techniques (174). Substantively, the presence of group differences may suggest that ECT had some persistent deleterious effects, particularly in those with complaints. On the other hand, at times individuals who attribute cognitive difficulties and other disabilities to ECT may be particularly motivated to document impairments. There are no acceptable techniques by which to estimate the influence of such a factor on neuropsychological test scores. In addition, in much of the research on patient perceptions of memory functioning, the most critical predictor of memory complaints is the level of current pyschopathology. However, viewing persisting memory complaints as only a reflection of psychopathology, from the perspective of the patient and others, may be tantamount to "blaming the victim." Nonetheless, it is a common observation that various forms of psychopathology are associated with cognitive impairments. Therefore, it should be expected that patient groups selected for ECT complaints have neuropsychological deficits that may be independent of their psychiatric treatment history. This circumstance illustrates the need for more creative approaches to the selection of comparison groups, and certainly this is an area of research that requires more attention.

B. Uncontrolled, Prospective Studies

A variety of uncontrolled prospective studies have contrasted long-term neuropsychological performance in patients to their own pre-ECT baselines (e.g., 142, 175, 176). These comparisons have indicated no change or improvement at follow-up testing. Such findings are not particularly enlightening. Lingering cognitive deficits may be masked by the improvements associated with clinical recovery or by practice efforts.

More helpful are studies that contrast prospectively patient groups randomly assigned to different forms of ECT. Because such groups should be comparable in all major respects at baseline, differences between them at long-term follow-up is more telling that at least some forms of ECT may be associated with persistent impairment. A large number of such comparative trials have been conducted. With only two exceptions (69, 162), there has been a remarkable absence of documentation that forms of ECT that differ in technical features (electrode placement or electrical waveform) also differ in cognitive sequelae 2 weeks or later after the ECT course (75,

85, 117, 148). This outcome is particularly surprising given the robustness of the acute and subacute effects on cognition that have been attributed to variations in ECT method. Consequently, this large group of negative findings also certify that recovery of function is typically rapid following termination of the ECT course. The two exceptional studies had positive findings of treatment group differences that were of uncertain significance. Halliday et al. (69) at a 3-month follow-up found 3 significant effects out of 18 comparisons, with the important qualification that many patients had received additional ECT during the follow-up period. Cronin et al. (162) examining patients 4–6 weeks post-ECT, found 1 significant effect out of 24 comparisons of treatment conditions. However, without a non-ECT comparison group, these studies are not informative on whether persistent deficits characterized the total patient sample.

C. Controlled Prospective Studies

Prospective studies that contrast the performance of ECT patients with comparison groups that do not receive ECT are the most critical source of information. In such studies, comparison samples have involved demographically matched normal controls (62), poorly or unmatched patient comparison groups (146, 177–179), and well-matched patient comparison groups (57, 65–66, 114, 180, 181). Particularly because baseline and follow-up cognitive performance is expected to vary with the presence and severity of psychopathology (29, 61, 99), we will focus on studies that have used well-matched patient control groups.

Jackson (114) randomly assigned 34 patients to one of three forms of ECT (left unilateral, right unilateral, bilateral ECT) or a non-ECT comparison category. Immediate testing demonstrated that the neuropsychological battery was sensitive to ECT effects, both in comparison to baseline performance and the non-ECT group. With follow-up testing 10 days following ECT, there was no difference between the ECT patients and the non-ECT group, with return to at least baseline in all memory measures.

During the 1970s, a series of double-blind trials comparing real ECT (electrical stimulation and seizure induction) to "sham ECT" (induction of anesthesia without electrical stimulation) were conducted in the United Kingdom. Although such trials offered a remarkable opportunity for controlled investigation of long-term cognitive effects, this was rarely done. Frith et al. (66, 182) randomly assigned 70 depressed patients to real or sham ECT and compared these groups with a nondepressed, non-ECT psychiatric outpatient sample matched for age and sex. An extensive neuropsychological battery was administered at time points corresponding to pretreatment, subacutely following eight treatments, and at 6-month follow-up. Before treatment the depressed patients in the real and sham ECT groups performed poorer than controls on a variety of measures. At subacute testing, relative to the sham ECT group, the real ECT group was impaired on measures of vigilance, word list recognition, and rapidity of learning. At 6-month follow-up, the real and sham groups were equivalent in all measures (including assessments of clinical state), and with but one exception (word list recall), no longer differed from the non-ECT controls.

A particularly comprehensive investigation was conducted by Weeks et al. (65). Fifty-one depressed patients who received ECT (right unilateral ECT n=15; bilateral ECT n=36) were matched on demographic variables and severity of depression to 51 patients who were not treated with ECT. A second comparison group of 51 normal controls was also used, matched to the patients groups on the same demographic variables. The neuropsychological battery, blindly administered, contained 17 tests, with a high concentration that sampled components of memory. The groups were tested at comparable intervals, corresponding to pretreatment baseline, 3-month, and 6-month follow-ups in the ECT sample. Despite matching on observer and self-ratings of severity of depressive illness, patients who received ECT had poorer baseline performance on a number of measures relative to the patient comparison group who, in turn, were significantly more impaired than the normal controls. This pattern illustrates that in the absence of random assignment to ECT and comparison conditions, the nature of the patient populations referred for ECT may result in differences in neuropsychological profiles, even when groups are matched on general clinical indices of illness severity. Indeed, Weeks et al. (65) noted that the ECT group had a greater representation of endogenous features.

At the 3-month follow-up, there was scant evidence that ECT was associated with persistent cognitive deficits. At this point, the ECT group performed worse than the non-ECT patient controls on memory for famous personalities of the 1970s, but significantly better than patient controls on a test of capacity to shift mental sets. At 6-month follow-up, there was one difference between the patient groups. The ECT sample had superior performance on a logical memory (paragraph recall) task. The importance of these null results was reinforced by the observation that the two patient groups were equivalent in depression severity measures at both follow-up intervals. Weeks et al. (65) concluded that their study supported the view that "ECT when used in everyday clinical circumstances to treat depressed patients does not cause lasting cognitive impairment" (p. 33).

Similar negative findings regarding long-term cognitive impairment were reported by Gangadhar et al. (181). In this study, 32 depressed patients were randomized to either bilateral ECT or sham ECT plus imipramine. Although 3-month and 6-month follow-up data indicated no differences in impairment indices, relatively insensitive neuropsychological testing was used, and the spacing of ECT treatments was nontraditional.

It is evident that this series of controlled prospective comparisons has yielded largely negative findings on long-term cognitive deficits induced by ECT. However, although some of these studies included acceptable measures of anterograde learning and memory, with the exception of Weeks et al. (65), retrograde memory, particularly for autobiographical material, was poorly sampled in this work. Another set of investigations has indicated that this domain may be the most likely to show persistence of memory impairment.

The work of Janis (143–145, 180) in the early 1950s was the first to suggest that this domain may be especially vulnerable to persistent ECT effects. In studies of schizophrenic patients who received unmodified treatment (no anesthesia, oxygenation, or muscle relaxation), Janis described an amnesia for events of personal significance that persisted for at least 1-month after ECT. These studies, and similar early work (146), were characterized by a variety of methodological problems, including poor matching of comparison samples and non-blind evaluation of personal memory using open-ended questioning. Subsequently, the possibility of persistent deficits in this domain was reasserted by Squire et al. (147). Small and poorly matched patient samples were asked to provide details about personal (e.g., day of hospitalization) and impersonal events (e.g., Watergate scandal), with the time frame of events ranging from elementary school to the very recent past. A bilateral ECT and comparison non-ECT patient group were tested at intervals corresponding to baseline, during or shortly after the ECT course, and at 7 months following ECT. At the later two testing intervals, recognition cues were given when patients failed to report specific details spontaneously.

In terms of overall performance, the groups were equivalent both at baseline and at 7-month follow-up, but the ECT patients evidenced a deficit at the immediate and intermediate testing intervals. When items were dichotomized for remote or recent (within 3 years) retrograde memory, a persistent memory deficit was identified for the ECT patients for two of the three items in the recent memory grouping. Furthermore, the cue-reminding procedure was 100% effective in the non-ECT group in prompting recognition of nonrecalled details, but only 71% effective in the ECT patients. Therefore, this study provided some evidence that ECT may result in persistent impairment in retrograde memory for recent events.

Unfortunately, there has been only one comprehensive and methodologically rigorous investigation of this issue. Weiner et al. (57) randomized 53 depressed patients to four types of ECT, crossing the factors of electrode placement (unilateral right versus bilateral) with waveform morphology (brief pulse versus sine wave). An additional 21 non-ECT patients were matched to the total ECT sample for demographic and clinical features, including global estimates of illness severity. Patients were evaluated at baseline, 2–3 days after ECT termination and at 6-month follow-up. At last follow-up the total ECT sample was reduced to 39 patients with 13 non-ECT controls. The neuropsychological battery was particularly comprehensive in assessment of anterograde and retrograde memory. In particular, a detailed personal memory questionnaire was utilized, inquiring about both recent and remote events.

At intermediate testing Weiner et al. (57) found that sine-wave stimulation and bilateral electrode placement produced more severe disturbances of personal memory. Relative to controls, patients that had received brief-pulse unilateral ECT did not evidence any deficit at the intermediate interval. The remaining three ECT groups showed substantial deficits, with recall failures most marked with the combination of bilateral electrode placement and sine wave stimulation. Most critically, at the 6-month testing interval, patients who received bilateral ECT displayed deficits relative to the right unilateral ECT groups and relative to non-ECT patient controls. At this point, patients who received right unilateral ECT (either brief pulse or sine wave) were equivalent to controls, and there was an indication that, among patients who had received bilateral ECT, sine wave stimulation was associated with the most marked persistent deficits. Upon completion of the 6-month recall testing, patients were given a series of recognition trials on the items for which there was a discrepancy in content between responses at baseline and at long-term follow-up. Patients assessed whether the baseline report was correct, the follow-up report was correct, or whether they were uncertain about which response was correct. Using this self-corroboration method, and deleting equivocal items (e.g., initial information at baseline judged by the patient to be incorrect), the differences among the groups were further magnified. For example, the percentage of baseline items consistently not recalled at the intermediate and long-term testing intervals was approximately 10% in the non-ECT controls and both right unilateral groups. It was approximately 20% with brief-pulse bilateral ECT and approximately 30% with sine-wave bilateral ECT. Preliminary internal analyses of recall failures have suggested that events in the most recent past were most vulnerable to persistent amnesia. The significance of these findings was enhanced by the fact that assessment of retrograde personal memory was the only domain in an extensive memory battery to show persistent deficit.

D. Comments

This summary of the evidence concerning long-term cognitive consequences indicates that findings of persistent deficit in anterograde learning and memory 10 or more days following the ECT course are scarce. The same applies to remote retrograde memory. For persistent deficits, it appears that information acquired in time frames proximal to the administration of ECT is the most likely area of persistent deficit. It is presently unclear whether this persistent retrograde amnesia for recent events is particularly pronounced for autobiographical information or extends equally to memory for recent public events. Of note, Squire and Slater (123) asked 31 patients who had received bilateral ECT 3 years earlier to indicate the portions of time for which they presently had difficulties remembering. On average, these patients indicated spottiness in memory for a period extending 6 months before ECT and 2 months after the treatment. Of course, in such naturalistic work it is difficult to tease out the contribution of acquisition deficits during the period of depression to later recall deficits for events that occurred prior to ECT. Indeed, these same patients when assessed 3 years earlier, before ECT, reported difficulties in remembering events in the 5-month period before the treatment. Nonetheless, it is noteworthy that patients' reports of the boundaries of persistent amnesia tend to correspond to the limited evidence from objective testing.

The research on the long-term cognitive consequences of ECT leaves many unanswered questions. Among them is the concern that, given the nature of the scientific method, virtually all the objective evidence we have about persisting cognitive effects comes from group comparisons. The nature of such comparisons involves pooling of data across individuals, so that outliers who may have suffered more extensive or persistent deficits may be missed. Based on very limited data, it is estimated that approximately 1:200 former ECT patients will report that the treatment had a profound and persistent impact on their cognitive functioning, such that they may no longer be able to engage in former occupations or have dense amnesia reaching far back into the past for events of personal significance (23). The validity of these claims is extremely difficult to determine. If the suggested base rates are accurate, within any single research program such individuals would be too rare for meaningful analysis. Furthermore, it must be recognized that not only may persistent psychopathology exert a strong influence on a variety of measures of cognitive function, but that marked deterioration in neuropsychological function may well be part of the natural progression of some chronic mental disorders, irrespective of treatment history (29, 183). Studies that specifically recruit patients who believe they have suffered persistent cognitive deficits need to be conducted in a sophisticated fashion (e.g., 173).

Another difficulty in this area concerns the breadth of cognitive functions examined. As in our review of the acute and subacute effects of ECT, it is evident that the focus of research on long-term consequences has used highly structured tasks, typically involving deliberate list learning. In contrast, the one area where there is evidence of persistent deficit concerns mainly retrograde memory for autobiographical information. Rarely does one deliberately memorize (with forewarning of later testing) the details of personal events. The aberrant process that contribute to the persistent retrograde amnesia needs to be identified and, more generally, a wider range of ecologically valid assessments of cognitive function needs to be employed.

Finally, in our review of acute and subacute effects, the degree to which technical factors in ECT administration (electrical dose, electrode placement, waveform morphology, spacing of treatments) affects cognitive functioning was striking. Electroconvulsive therapy is far from a single form of treatment and its cognitive consequences can be strongly modified, depending on how it is performed. Likewise, although the research by Weiner et al. (57) provided the strongest evidence for persistent cognitive deficits with ECT, it also suggested that with attention to treatment parameters such persistent effects may be avoided.

V. PATIENT PERCEPTIONS OF ELECTROCONVULSIVE THERAPY EFFECTS ON MEMORY

In addition to objective evaluation of cognitive function, there has been concerted investigation of the perceptions of former patients about ECT effects on memory. Space limitations prevent a detailed review of this area, and only the central conclusions will be highlighted. With use of a variety of instruments to elicit self-reports and to assess memory, no investigator has observed significant relations between changes in subjective and objective measures of memory functioning at either subacute or long-term testing intervals (e.g., 57, 66, 123, 154, 184). With noted consistency, the symptomalogical state of patients has been a critical predictor of the patient evaluations of their memory functioning (57, 66, 123, 130, 146, 185). Early studies by Squire (122, 123, 130) suggested that shortly after right unilateral ECT, there was no change in the level of memory complaints, but that with bilateral ECT, there was an increase in memory complaints and a redistribution in the nature of perceived deficits. With testing several months after ECT, patients who had received bilateral stimulation showed a reduction of memory complaints, reaching the global level that was observed in unilateral ECT patients, but nonetheless showing a persistent redistribution in the nature of complaints. As with the findings for objective memory deficits, technical factors in how ECT is performed may affect alterations in subjective complaints. The work by Squire typically involved high-intensity electrical stimulation in patients who were not randomly assigned to unilateral or bilateral electrode placements. Since then, Pettinati and Rosenberg (185) found that shortly after treatment, patients randomly assigned to brief-pulse unilateral right or bilateral ECT showed pronounced improvement in self-evaluations of memory functioning. There was no evidence that the treatment groups differed in the global level or distribution of perceived memory difficulties. Likewise, Weiner et al. (57) observed that within 2–3 days after ECT termination there was a marked improvement in global self-ratings of memory function compared with pre-ECT baseline, with no differences between ECT patients and non-ECT-matched controls. Similarly, in three separate, large samples the Columbia University group has repeatedly observed that patients report fewer memory difficulties within a week of the ECT course than they had before the course.

In general, it would appear that, in group data, ECT has little, if any, persistent negative effects on patient evaluations of their memory functioning. It may be surprising that most current research indicates that memory complaints decrease during the course of ECT. However, it should be recalled that a large group of cognitive functions show improvement shortly after the ECT course, particularly with tests that were heavily influenced by the adequacy of attention and concentration. It is unlikely that, within their own subjective experience, patients can readily tease out deficits related to the retention of information over delays or the recall of recent events from improvements in capacity to acquire new information or to attend to their surroundings. Furthermore, there is evidence that even among normal samples, level of depressed mood has a strong impact on self-ratings of memory functioning (186). With the marked change in clinical state that typically occurs with ECT, there is often improvement self-evaluations of cognitive capacities.

VI. SUMMARY AND IMPLICATIONS

It is evident that after 50 years of use, much has been learned about the cognitive effects of ECT, but also that much remains unresolved. For the clinicians or patients considering this modality, some facts are central. The most profound cognitive side effects are experienced during and shortly following the treatment course. These relatively acute deficits show rapid resolution. However, within a few weeks of ECT, patients may continue to have impairments in their ability to retain new information over delays and in their ability to recall events from the recent past. Even at acute testing many other aspects of cognition that had been impaired by the psychiatric illness will be improved relative to pretreatment baseline. The anterograde memory deficit should resolve within a couple of months of the termination of ECT. However, deficits in the recall of recent events may persist and may be permanent. Patients may be left with a spottiness in memory for events that transpired during the period extending from several months before ECT until a couple of months following treatment.

The magnitude of the acute and subacute side effects are strongly determined by how ECT is performed. It should be recognized that the nature and quality of ECT practice varies considerably among institutions. Factors such as electrode placement, electrical intensity, and waveform morphology display lawful relations to side effect profiles. Indeed, initial evidence suggests that "softer" forms of ECT may not only moderate considerably the acute and subacute side effects, but may also fail to produce the persistent retrograde amnesia.

At the same time, it should be recognized that we have relatively little information on the patient characteristics that may be predictive of variation in the severity of cognitive side effects. Patients who receive the same form of ECT do vary considerably in the magnitude of acute and subacute deficits. Although clinically we suspect that some of this variability may be related to age, preexisting neurological impairment, and adverse interactive effects with specific concomitant medications, such relations have yet to be established empirically. At the concrete level, we can not say with certainty that the depressed patient with a history of cerebrovascular disease or other neurological impairment is more at risk for severe side effects than the patient with a negative neurological history.

Furthermore, in informing patients about ECT, it is important to relate that a few individuals report profound and long-lasting cognitive impairment that they attribute to this treatment modality. Clearly, this phenomenon has not been established with objective testing, and the reasons for this discrepancy are not clear. Complicating this issue are the effects of current psychopathology on cognitive functions, the natural progression of some forms of psychiatric illness, and the effects of current and past treatments other than ECT. In addition, because of the public and scientific attention that has been given to the cognitive side effects of ECT, patients who receive this modality are likely to be more primed to attribute perceived changes in cognitive functioning to this treatment relative to other modalities or to the aging process (63).

From a basic science viewpoint it is critical that the most significant amnestic effects of ECT are stereotyped, are well modeled by animal studies with ECS, and largely pertain to discrete aspects of the retention of new information and the recall or recognition of recent events. As noted by others (63, 187), this suggests that ECT has particularly important effects of medial temporal structures long implicated as subserving amnestic functions. A large number of theories have been offered to account for the selective amnestic effects of ECT (13). Among the most attractive is the view that the anterograde and retrograde memory disturbances reflect dysfunctions of consolidation. Months to years after encoding, information may be vulnerable to loss, since the process of consolidation is not complete. Memories that are more remote in time may be least vulnerable, whereas interference with consolidation may result in permanent loss of recently acquired information. Drugs that reversibly inhibit protein synthesis interfere with long-term, but not short-term memory (188). In both animals and humans, seizure elicitation results in a reversible inhibition of protein synthesis (e.g., 189). It is possible, therefore, that ECT transiently disrupts the plasticity mechanisms needed for consolidation or maintenance of long-term memories. Although such a mechanism fits well with what has been learned about ECT amnestic effects, there has been no attempt to directly link the cognitive consequence of ECT with assessment of disruption of protein synthesis.

At a clinical level, it is evident that modifications in ECT technique have transformed this treatment modality. Further advances are possible. In animals ECS is a standard screening procedure for pharmacologic compounds that may have beneficial effects on memory. A large variety of agents have been shown to diminish or block ECS amnestic effects. Typically, when the efficacy of such agents has been evaluated in humans, it has been in the context of clinical trials targeted at various forms of dementia, often with disappointing results. Surprisingly, there have been few attempts to moderate pharmacologically the cognitive side effects of ECT in the human (190–192), despite the wealth of candidate agents and the close similarities in the effects of ECS and ECT. This approach holds considerable promise for further improving this form of treatment.

ACKNOWLEDGMENT

The work presented herein was supported in part by grant MH35636 from the National Institute of Mental Health. I thank D. P. Devanand and Richard D. Weiner for their comments. Many individuals contributed to the findings presented here. These include Kathlene Briscoe, Richard P. Brown, Eliza Coleman, Paolo Decina, D.P. Devanand, Linda Fitzsimons, Judith Kiersky, Martin McElhiney, Bobba Moody, Stephanie Portnoy, Joan Prudic, and Francis R. Ross.

REFERENCES

1. Fink M. Convulsive therapy: theory and practice. New York: Raven Press, 1979.
2. Thompson JW, Blaine JD. Use of ECT in the United States in 1975 and 1980. Am J Psychiatry 1987; 144:557–562.

3. Devanand DP, Sackeim HA. Electroconvulsive therapy. In: Pohl R, Gershon S, eds. The biological basis of psychiatric treatment. Basel: S Krager, 1990:170–210.
4. Lambourn J, Gill D. A controlled comparison of simulated and real ECT. Br J Psychiatry 1978; 133:514–519.
5. Crow TJ, Johnstone EC. Controlled trials of electroconvulsive therapy. Ann NY Acad Sci 1986; 462:12–29.
6. Ulett GA, Smith K, Gleser GC. Evaluation of convulsive and subconvulsive shock therapies utilizing a control group. Am J Psychiatry 1956; 112:795–802.
7. Fink M, Kahn RL, Green MA. Experimental studies of the electroshock process. Dis Nerv Syst 1958; 19:113–18.
8. Ottosson J-O. Experimental studies of the mode of action of electroconvulsive therapy. Acta Psychiatr Scand [Suppl] 1960; 145:1–141.
9. Sackeim HA, Decina P, Kanzler M, Kerr B, Malitz S. Effects of electrode placement on the efficacy of titrated, low-dose ECT. Am J Psychiatry 1987; 144:1449–1455.
10. Sackeim HA, Devanand DP, Prudic J. Stimulus intensity, seizure threshold, and seizure duration: impact on the efficacy and safety of electroconvulsive therapy. Psychiatr Clin North Am (in press).
11. Miller E. Psychological theories of E.C.T.: a review. Br J Psychiatry 1967; 113:301–311.
12. Ottosson J-O. Use and misuse of electroconvulsive treatment. Biøl Psychiatry 1985; 20:933–46.
13. Sackeim HA. Mechanisms of action of electroconvulsive therapy. In: Hales RE, Frances J, eds. Annu Rev Psychiatry 1988; 7:436–457.
14. Robin A, De Tissera S. A double-blind controlled comparison of the therapeutic effects of low and high energy electroconvulsive therapies. Br J Psychiatry 1982; 141:357–366.
15. Greenblatt M, Grooser GH, Wechsler HA. Differential response of hospitalized depressed patients in somantic therapy. Am J Psychiatry 1964; 120:935–943.
16. Shepherd M. Clinical trial of the treatment of depressive illness. Br Med J 1965; 1:881–6.
17. Janicak PG, Davis JM, Gibbons RD, Ericksen S, Chang S, Gallagher P. Efficacy of ECT: a meta-analysis. Am J Psychiatry 1985; 142:297–302.
18. Rifkin A. ECT versus tricyclic antidepressants in depression: a review of the evidence. J Clin Psychiatry 1988; 49:3–7.
19. Quitkin FM, Rabkin JG, Ross D, McGrath PJ. Duration of antidepressant drug treatment: what is an adequate trial? Arch Gen Psychiatry 1984; 41:238–245.
20. Quitkin FM. The importance of dosage in prescribing antidepressants. Br J Psychiatry 1985; 147:593–597.
21. Sackeim H, Prudic J, Devanand D. Treatment of medication-resistant depression with electroconvulsive therapy. In: Tasman A, Goldfinger S, Kaufmann C, eds. Annu Rev Psychiatry 1990; 9:91–115.
22. Hamilton M. The effect of treatment on the melancholias (depressions). Br J Psychiatry 1982; 140:223–230.

23. American Psychiatric Association (Weiner R, Fink M, Hammersley D, Moench L, Sackeim HA, Small I). The practice of ECT: recommendations for treatment, training and privileging—report of the APA Task Force on ECT. Washington, DC: American Psychiatric Press, 1990.
24. Fink M. How does ECT work? Neuropsychopharmacology 1990; 3:77–82.
25. Prudic J, Sackeim H, Devanand D. Medication resistance and clinical response to electroconvulsive therapy. Psychiatry Res 1990; 31:287–296.
26. Sackeim H, Prudic J, Devanand D, Decina P, Kerr B, Malitz S. The impact of medication resistance and continuation pharmacotherapy on relapse following response to electroconvulsive therapy in major depression. J Clin Psychopharmacol 1990; 10:96–104.
27. Krauthammer C, Klerman GL. The epidemiology of mania. In: Shopsin B, ed. Manic illness. New York: Raven Press, 1979:11–28.
28. Roy-Byrne PP, Post RM, Uhde TW, Porcu T, Davis D. The longitudinal course of recurrent affective illness: life chart data from research patients at the NIMH. Acta Psychiatr Scand [Suppl] 1985; 317:1–34.
29. Goodwin FK, Jamison KR. Manic-depressive illness. New York: Oxford University Press, 1990.
30. Weissman MM, Kleramn GL. Sex differences and the epidemiology of depression. Arch Gen Psychiatry 1977; 34:98–111.
31. Weissman MM, Leaf PJ, Tischler GL, Blazer DG, Karno M, Bruce ML, Florio LP. Affective disorders in five United States communities. Psychol Med 1988; 18:141–153.
32. American Psychiatric Association (Frankel FH, Bidder TG, Fink M, Mandel MR, Small IF, Wayne GJ, Squire LR, Dutton EN, Gurel L). Electroconvulsive therapy, task force report no. 14. Washington DC: American Psychiatric Association, 1978.
33. Small JG, Klapper MH, Kellams JJ, Miller MJ, Milstein V, Sharpley PH, Small IF. Electroconvulsive treatment compared with lithium in the management of manic states. Arch Gen Psychiatry 1988; 45:727–732.
34. Brandon S, Cowley P, McDonald C, Neville P, Palmer R, Wellstood-Eason S. Leicester ECT trial: results in schizophrenia. Br J Psychiatry 1985; 146:177–83.
35. Rosen AM, Mukherjee S, Shinbach K. The efficacy of ECT in phencyclidine-induced psychosis. J Clin Psychiatry 1984; 45:220–222.
36. Khanna S, Gangadhar BN, Sinha V, Rajendra PN, Channabasavanna SM. Electroconvulsive therapy in obsessive-compulsive disorder. Convulsive Ther 1988; 4:314–320.
37. Balldin J, Edën S, Granërus AK, Modigh K, Svanborg A, Walinder J, Wallin L. Electroconvulsive therapy in Parkinson's syndrome with "on-off" phenomenon. J Neural Transm 1980; 47:11–21.
38. Douyon R, Serby M, Klutchko B, Rotrosen J. ECT and Parkinson's disease revisited: a "naturalistic" study. Am J Psychiatry 1989; 146:1451–1455.
39. Caplan G. Electrical convulsion therapy in treatment of epilepsy. J Ment Sci 1946; 92:784–793.

40. Sackeim HA, Decina P, Prohovnik I, Malitz S, Resor SR. Anticonvulsant and antidepressant properties of electroconvulsive therapy: a proposed mechanism of action. Biol Psychiatry 1983; 18:1301–1310.
41. Schnur DB, Mukherjee S, Silver J, Degreef G, Lee C. Electroconvulsive therapy in the treatment of episodic aggressive dyscontrol in psychotic patients. Convulsive Ther 1989; 5:353–361.
42. Milstein V, Small JG, Miller MJ, Sharpley PH, Small IF. Mechanisms of action of ECT: schizophrenia and schizoaffective disorder. Biol Psychiatry 1990; 27:1282–1292.
43. Trimble MR, Thompson PJ. Neuropsychological and behavioral sequelae of spontaneous seizures. Ann NY Acad Sci 1986; 462:284–292.
44. Kriss A, Blumhardt LD, Halliday AM, Pratt RT. Neurological asymmetries immediately after unilateral ECT. J Neurol Neurosurg Psychiatry 1978; 41:1135–1144.
45. Daniel WF, Crovitz HF. Disorientation during electroconvulsive therapy: technical, theoretical, and neuropsychological issues. Ann NY Acad Sci 1986; 462:293–306.
46. Sackeim HA. Acute cognitive side effects of ECT. Psychopharm Bull 1986; 22:482–484.
47. Altman JA, Balonov LJ, Deglin VL. Effects of unilateral disorder of the brain hemisphere function in man on directional hearing. Neuropsychologia 1979; 17:295–301.
48. Ringo JL, Guttmacher LB. Amnesia for the McCollough effect following unilateral electroconvulsive therapy: implications for laterality. Biol Psychiatry 1988; 24:384–390.
49. Squire LR, Slater P. Bilateral and unilateral ECT: effects on verbal and nonverbal memory. Am J Psychiatry 1978; 135:1316–1320.
50. Daniel WF, Crovitz HF. Acute memory impairment following electroconvulsive therapy. 1. Effects of electrical stimulus waveform and number of treatments. Acta Psychiatr Scand 1983; 67:1–7.
51. Daniel WF, Crovitz HF. Acute memory impairment following electroconvulsive therapy. 2. Effects of electrode placement. Acta Psychiatr Scand 1983; 67:57–68.
52. Sackeim HA, Portnoy S, Neeley P, Steif BL, Decina P, Malitz S. Cognitive consequences of low-dosage electroconvulsive therapy. Ann NY Acad Sci 1986; 462:326–340.
53. Daniel WF, Crovitz HF. Recovery of orientation after electroconvulsive therapy. Acta Psychiatr Scand 1982; 66:421–428.
54. Summers WK, Robins E, Reich T. The natural history of acute organic mental syndrome after bilateral electroconvulsive therapy. Biol Psychiatry 1979; 14:905–912.
55. Miller ME, Siris SG, Gabriel AN. Treatment delays in the course of electroconvulsive therapy. Hosp Community Psychiatry 1986; 37:825–7.
56. Lancaster N, Steinert R, Frost I. Unilateral electroconvulsive therapy. J Ment Sci 1958; 104:221–227.

57. Weiner RD, Rogers HJ, Davidson JR, Squire LR. Effects of stimulus parameters on cognitive side effects. Ann NY Acad Sci 1986; 462:315–325.
58. Malloy FW, Small IF, Miller MJ, Milstein V. Changes in neuropsychological test performance after electroconvulsive therapy. Biol Psychiatry 1982; 17:61–67.
59. Cronholm B, Ottosson J-O. Memory functions in endogenous depression. Before and after electroconvulsive therapy. Arch Gen Psychiatry 1961; 5:193–199.
60. Sternberg DE, Jarvik ME. Memory function in depression: improvement with antidepressant medication. Arch Gen Psychiatry 1976; 33:219–224.
61. Sackeim HA, Steif BL. The neuropsychology of depression and mania. In: Georgotas A, Cancro R, eds. Depression and mania. New York: Elsevier, 1988:265–289.
62. Steif BL, Sackeim HA, Portnoy S, Decina P, Malitz S. Effects of depression and ECT on anterograde memory. Biol Psychiatry 1986; 21:921–930.
63. Squire LR. Memory functions as affected by electroconvulsive therapy. Ann NY Acad Sci 1986; 462:307–314.
64. McGaugh JL, Herz MM. Memory consolidation. San Francisco: Albion Publishing, 1972.
65. Weeks D, Freeman CP, Kendell RE. ECT: III: enduring cognitive deficits? Br J Psychiatry 1980; 137:26–37.
66. Frith CD, Stevens M, Johnstone EC, Deakin JF, Lawler P, Crow TJ. Effects of ECT and depression on various aspects of memory. Br J Psychiatry 1983; 142:610–617.
67. Abrams R, Taylor MA. A prospective follow-up study of cognitive functions after electroconvulsive therapy. Convulsive Ther 1985; 1:4–9.
68. Gottlieb G, Wilson I. Cerebral dominance: temporary disruption of verbal memory by unilateral electroconvulsive shock treatment. J Comp Physiol Psychol 1965; 60:368–372.
69. Halliday A, Davison K, Browne M, Kreeger L. A comparison of the effects on depression and memory of bilateral ECT and unilateral ECT to the dominant and non-dominant hemispheres. Br J Psychiatry 1968; 114:997–1012.
70. Valentine M, Keddie K, Dunne D. A comparison of techniques in electroconvulsive therapy. Br J Psychiatry 1968; 114:989–996.
71. Sutherland EM, Oliver JE, Knight DR. E.E.G., memory and confusion in dominant, non-dominant and bi-temporal E.C.T. Br J Psychiatry 1969; 115:1059–1064.
72. d'Elia G. Unilateral electroconvulsive therapy. Acta Psychiatr Scand [Suppl] 1970; 215:1–98.
73. Deglin VL. A clinico-experimental study of unilateral electroconvulsive seizures. Zh Nevropatol Psikhiatr 1973; 73:1609–1621.
74. Fraser RM, Glass IB. Recovery from ECT in elderly patients. Br J Psychiatry 1978; 133:524–528.
75. Fraser RM, Glass IB. Unilateral and bilateral ECT in elderly patients. A comparative study. Acta Psychiatr Scand 1980; 62:13–31.
76. Prohovnik I, Sackeim HA, Decina P, Malitz S. Acute reductions of regional

cerebral blood flow following electroconvulsive therapy: interactions with modality and time. Ann NY Acad Sci 1986; 462:249–262.
77. Silfverskiöld P, Gustafson L, Risberg J, Rosën I. Acute and late effects of electroconvulsive therapy: clinical outcome, regional cerebral blood flow, and electroencephalogram. Ann NY Acad Sci 1986; 462:236–248.
78. Weiner RD. ECT and seizure threshold: effects of stimulus wave form and electrode placement. Biol Psychiatry 1980; 15:225–241.
79. Sackeim HA, Decina P, Prohovnik I, Malitz S. Seizure threshold in electroconvulsive therapy. Effects of sex, age, electrode placement, and number of treatments. Arch Gen Psychiatry 1987; 44:355–360.
80. Wilson IC, Gottlieb G. Unilateral electroconvulsive shock therapy. Dis Nerv Syst 1967; 28:541–545.
81. Sackeim HA, Decina P, Portnoy S, Neeley P, Malitz S. Studies of dosage, seizure threshold, and seizure duration in ECT. Biol Psychiatry 1987; 22: 249–268.
82. Sackeim HA, Decina P, Prohovnik I, Portnoy S, Kanzler M, Malitz S. Dosage, seizure threshold, and the antidepressant efficacy of electroconvulsive therapy. Ann NY Acad Sci 1986; 462:398–410.
83. Strain JJ, Bidder TG. Transient cerebral complication associated with multiple monitored electroconvulsive therapy. Dis Nerv Syst 1971; 32:95–100.
84. Abrams R. Electroconvulsive therapy. New York: Oxford University Press, 1988.
85. Heshe J, Roeder F, Theilgaard A. Unilateral and bilateral ECT: a psychiatric and psychological study of therapeutic effect and side effects. Acta Psychiatr Scand [Suppl] 1978; 275:1–180.
86. Lunn V, Trolle E. On the initial impairment of consciousness following electric convulsive therapy: a preliminary communication. Acta Psychiatr Neurol Scand 1949; 24:33–57.
87. Small JG, Kellams JJ, Milstein V, Small IF. Complications with electroconvulsive treatment combined with lithium. Biol Psychiatry 1980; 15:103–112.
88. Weiner RD, Whanger AD, Erwin CW, Wilson WP. Prolonged confusional state and EEG seizure activity following concurrent ECT and lithium use. Am J Psychiatry 1980; 137:1452–1453.
89. Roemer RA, Dubin WR, Jaffe R, Lipschultz L, Sharon D. An efficacy study of single versus double ECT induction in major affective disorder. J Clin Psychiatry 1990; 51:473–478.
90. Price TR. Short- and long-term cognitive effects of ECT. Part II—effects on nonmemory associated cognitive functions. Psychopharmacol Bull 1982; 18:91–101.
91. Sackeim HA, Portnoy S, Decina P, Malitz S, Warmflash V, Vingiano WA, Yudofsky SC. Left-side visual neglect in ECT patients. Psychopharmacol Bull 1983; 19:83–85.
92. Squire LR. ECT and memory loss. Am J Psychiatry 1977; 134:997–1001.
93. Medlicott RW. Brief stimuli electroconvulsive therapy. NZ Med J 1948; 47:29–37.

94. Pratt RT, Warrington EK, Halliday AM. Unilateral ECT as a test for cerebral dominance, with a strategy for treating left-handers. Br J Psychiatry 1971; 119:79–83.
95. Williams M. Errors in picture recognition after E.C.T. Neuropsychologia 1973; 11:429–436.
96. Squire LR, Zouzounis JA. ECT and memory: brief pulse versus sine wave. Am J Psychiatry 1986; 143:596–601.
97. Caine E. The neuropsychology of depression: the pseudodementia syndrome. In: Grant I, Adams KM, eds. Neuropsychological assessment of neuropsychiatric disorders. New York: Oxford University Press, 1986:221–243.
98. Price TR, McAllister TW. Safety and efficacy of ECT in depressed patients with dementia: a review of clinical experience. Convulsive Ther 1989; 5:61–74.
99. Chapman LJ, Chapman JP. Disordered thought in schizophrenia. Englewood Cliffs, NJ: Prentice-Hall, 1973.
100. Calev A, Erwin P. Recall and recognition in depressives: use of matched tasks. Br J Clin Psychol 1985; 24:127–128.
101. Daniel WF, Crovitz HF, Weiner RD, Rogers HJ. The effects of ECT modifications on autobiographical and verbal memory. Biol Psychiatry 1982; 17:919–924.
102. Cohen BD, Noblin CD, Silverman AJ, Penick SB. Functional asymmetry of the human brain. Science 1968; 162:475–477.
103. Fleminger JJ, de Horne DJ, Nair NP, Nott PN. Differential effect of unilateral and bilateral ECT. Am J Psychiatry 1970; 127:430–436.
104. Berent S, Cohen BD, Silverman A. Changes in verbal and nonverbal learning following a single left or right unilateral electroconvulsive treatment. Biol Psychiatry 1975; 10:95–100.
105. d'Elia G, Lorentzson S, Raotma H, Widepalm K. Comparison of unilateral dominant and non-dominant ECT on verbal and non-verbal memory. Acta Psychiatr Scand 1976; 53:85–94.
106. Squire LR, Miller PL. Diminution of anterograde amnesia following electroconvulsive therapy. Br J Psychiatry 1974; 125:490–495.
107. Squire LR, Nadel L, Slater PC. Anterograde amnesia and memory for temporal order. Neuropsychologia 1981; 19:141–145.
108. Costello CG, Belton GP, Abra JC, Dunn BE. The amnesic and therapeutic effects of bilateral and unilateral ECT. Br J Psychiatry 1970; 116:69–78.
109. Zinkin S, Birtchnell J. Unilateral electroconvulsive therapy: its effects on memory and its therapeutic efficacy. Br J Psychiatry 1968; 114:973–988.
110. Ashton R, Hess N. Amnesia for random shapes following unilateral and bilateral electroconvulsive shock therapy. Percept Mot Skills 1976; 42:669–670.
111. Kimura D. Dual functional asymmetry of the brain in visual perception. Neuropsychologia 1966; 4:275–278.
112. Milner B. Visual recognition and recall after right temporal-lobe excision in man. Neuropsychologia 1968; 6:191–209.
113. Hecaen H, Albert ML. Human neuropsychology. New York: John Wiley & Sons, 1978.

114. Jackson B. The effects of unilateral and bilateral ECT on verbal and visual spatial memory. J Clin Psychol 1978; 34:4–13.
115. Dornbush R, Abrams R, Fink M. Memory changes after unilateral and bilateral convulsive therapy (ECT). Br J Psychiatry 1971; 119:75–78.
116. Robertson AD, Inglis J. Memory deficits after electroconvulsive therapy: cerebral asymmetry and dual-encoding. Neuropsychologia 1978; 16:179–187.
117. Strain JJ, Brunschwig L, Duffy JP, Agle DP, Rosenbaum AL, Bidder TG. Comparison of therapeutic effects and memory changes with bilateral and unilateral ECT. Am J Psychiatry 1968; 125:50–60.
118. Fromholt P, Christensen AL, Strömgren LS. The effects of unilateral and bilateral electroconvulsive therapy on memory. Acta Psychiatr Scand 1973; 49:466–478.
119. Benton AL. The neuropsychology of face recognition. Am Psychologist 1980; 35:176–186.
120. Weaver L, Williams R, Rush S. Current density in bilateral and unilateral ECT. Biol Psychiatry 1976; 11:303–312.
121. Sackeim HA, Mukherjee S. Neurophysiological variability in the effects of the ECT stimulus. Convulsive Ther 1986; 2:267–276.
122. Squire LR, Wetzel CD, Slater PC. Memory complaint after electroconvulsive therapy: assessment with a new self-rating instrument. Biol Psychiatry 1979; 14:791–801.
123. Squire LR, Slater PC. Electroconvulsive therapy and complaints of memory dysfunction: a prospective three-year follow-up study. Br J Psychiatry 1983; 142:1–8.
124. Hasher L, Zacks R. Automatic and effortful processes in memory. J Exp Psychol [Gen] 1979; 108:356–388.
125. Cohen R, Weingartner H, Smallberg S, Pickar D, Murphy D. Effort and cognition in depression. Arch Gen Psychiatry 1982; 39:593–597.
126. Weingartner H, Grafman J, Boutelle W, Kaye W, Martin PR. Forms of memory failure. Science 1983; 221:380–382.
127. Roy-Bryne PP, Weingartner H, Bierer LM, Thompson K, Post RM. Effortful and automatic cognitive processes in depression. Arch Gen Psychiatry 1986; 43:265–267.
128. Byrne D. Affect and vigilance performance in depressive illness. J Psychiatr Res 1977; 13:185–191.
129. Caudrey D, Kirk K, Thomas P, Ng K. Perceptual deficit in schizophrenia: a defect in redundancy utilization, filtering or scanning? Br J Psychiatry 1980; 137:352–360.
130. Squire LR, Chace PM. Memory functions six to nine months after electroconvulsive therapy. Arch Gen Psychiatry 1975; 32:1557–1564.
131. Daniel WF, Weiner RD, Crovitz HF. Autobiographical amnesia with ECT: an analysis of the roles of stimulus wave form, electrode placement, stimulus energy, and seizure length. Biol Psychiatry 1983; 18:121–126.
132. Corkin S. Acquisition of motor skill after bilateral medial temporal-lobe excision. Neuropsychologia 1968; 6:255–265.

133. Pratt RT, Warrington EK. The assessment of cerebral dominance with unilateral ECT. Br J Psychiatry 1972; 121:327–328.
134. Warrington EK, Pratt RT. Language laterality in left-handers assessed by unilateral E.C.T. Neuropsychologia 1973; 11:423–428.
135. Geffen G, Caudrey D. Reliability and validity of the dichotic monitoring test for language laterality. Neuropsychologia 1981; 19:413–423.
136. Squire LR, Cohen NJ, Zouzounis JA. Preserved memory in retrograde amnesia: sparing of a recently acquired skill. Neuropsychologia 1984; 22:145–152.
137. Weiner RD. Does ECT cause brain damage? Behav Brain Sci 1984; 7:1–53.
138. Russell WR, Nathan PW. Traumatic amnesia. Brain 1946; 69:280–300.
139. Talland GA. Deranged memory. New York: Academic Press, 1965.
140. Squire LR. Amnesia for remote events following electroconvulsive therapy. Behav Biol 1974; 12:119–125.
141. Squire LR, Slater PC, Chace PM. Retrograde amnesia: temporal gradient in very long term memory following electroconvulsive therapy. Science 1975; 187:77–79.
142. Squire LR, Chace PM, Slater PC. Retrograde amnesia following electroconvulsive therapy. Nature 1976; 260:775–777.
143. Janis IL. Psychologic effects of electric convulsive treatments. (I. Posttreatment amnesias). J Nerv Ment Dis 1950; 111:359–382.
144. Janis IL. Psychologic effects of electric convulsive treatments. (II. Changes in word association reactions). J Nerv Ment Dis 1950; 111:383–397.
145. Jans IL. Psychologic effects of electric convulsive treatments. (III. Changes in affective disturbances). J Nerv Ment Dis 1950; 111:469–489.
146. Stieper DR, Williams M, Duncan CP. Changes in impersonal and personal memory following electroconvulsive therapy. J Clin Psychol 1951; 7:361–366.
147. Squire LR, Slater PC, Miller PL. Retrograde amnesia and bilateral electroconvulsive therapy. Long-term follow-up. Arch Gen Psychiatry 1981; 38:89–95.
148. Bidder TG, Strain JJ, Brunschwig L. Bilateral and unilateral ECT: follow-up study and critique. Am J Psychiatry 1970; 127:737–745.
149. Brunschwig L, Strain JJ, Bidder TG. Issues in the assessment of post-ECT memory changes. Br J Psychiatry 1971; 119:73–74.
150. Liberson WT, Wilcox PH. Electric convulsive therapy: comparison of "brief stimuli technique" with Friedman–Wilcox–Reiter technique. Dig Neurol Psychiatr 1945; 13:291–302.
151. Liberson WT. Brief stimulus therapy: Physiological and clinical observations. Am J Psychiatry 1948; 105:28–39.
152. Epstein J, Wender L. Alternating current vs. unidirectional current for electroconvulsive therapy—comparative studies. Confin Neurol 1956; 16: 137–46.
153. Kendall BS, Mills WB, Thale T. Comparison of two methods of electroshock in their effect on cognitive functions. J Consult Psychol 1956; 20:423–19.
154. Cronholm B, Ottosson J-O. Ultrabrief stimulus technique in electroconvulsive therapy. I. Influence on retrograde amnesia of treatments with the Elther ES electroshock apparatus, Siemens Konvulsator III and of lidocane-modified treatment. J Nerv Ment Dis 1963; 137:117–123.

155. Weiner RD. The role of stimulus waveform in therapeutic and adverse effects of ECT. Psychopharmacol Bull 1982; 18:71–72.
156. Daniel WF, Crovitz HF, Weiner RD, Swartzwelder HS, Kahn EM. ECT-induced amnesia and postictal EEG suppression. Biol Psychiatry 1985; 20:344–348.
157. Goldstein SG, Filskov SB, Weaver LA, Ives JO. Neuropsychological effects of electroconvulsive therapy. J Clin Psychol 1977; 33:789–806.
158. Warren EW, Groome DH. Memory test performance under three different waveforms of ECT for depression. Br J Psychiatry 1984; 144:370–375.
159. McAndrew J, Berkey B, Matthews C. The effects of dominant and non-dominant unilateral ECT as compared to bilateral ECT. Am J Psychiatry 1967; 124:483–490.
160. Small IF, Small JG, Milstein V, Sharpley P. Interhemispheric relationships with somatic therapy. Dis Nerv Syst 1973; 34:170–177.
161. Cronholm B, Lagergren A. Memory disturbances after electroconvulsive therapy. Acta Psychiatr Neurol Scand 1959; 34:283–310.
162. Cronin D, Bodley P, Potts L, Mather MD, Gardner RK, Tobin JC. Unilateral and bilateral ECT: a study of memory disturbance and relief from depression. J Neurol Neurosurg Psychiatry 1970; 33:705–713.
163. Miller E. The effect of ECT on memory and learning. Br J Med Psychol 1970; 43:57–62.
164. Goldman H, Gomer FE, Templer DI. Long-term effects of electroconvulsive therapy upon memory and perceptual–motor performance. J Clin Psychol 1972; 28:32–34.
165. Reichert H, Benjamin J, Neufeldt AH, Marjerrison G. Bilateral and non-dominant unilateral ECT. Part II—development of prograde effects. Can Psychiatr Assoc J 1976; 21:79–86.
166. Harper RG, Wiens AN. Electroconvulsive therapy and memory. J Nerv Ment Dis 1975; 161:245–254.
167. Price TR. Short- and long-term cognitive effects of ECT: Part I—effects on memory. Psychopharmacol Bull 1982; 18:81–91.
168. Taylor JR, Tompkins R, Demers R, Anderson D. Electroconvulsive therapy and memory dysfunction: is there evidence for prolonged defects? Biol Psychiatry 1982; 17:1169–93.
169. Templer DI, Penick SB, Buonpane N. Memory change following EST and drug treated depression. J Med Soc NJ 1973; 70:453–454.
170. Exner JE Jr, Murillo LG. A long term follow-up of schizophrenics treated with regressive ECT. Dis Nerv Syst 1977; 38:162–168.
171. Teuber HL, Corkin S, Twitchell TE. A study of cingulotomy in man. Final report. MIT contract NO1-HU-6-211.
172. Shellenberger W, Miller MJ, Small IF, Milstein V, Stout JR. Follow-up study of memory deficits after ECT. Can J Psychiatry 1982; 27:325–329.
173. Freeman CP, Weeks D, Kendell RE. ECT: II: patients who complain. Br J Psychiatry 1980; 137:17–25.
174. Lord FM. A paradox in the interpretation of group comparisons. Psychol Bull 1967; 68:304–305.

175. Luborsky LB. Psychometric changes during electric shock. J Nerv Ment Dis 1948; 107:531–536.
176. Cronholm B, Molander L. Memory disturbances after electroconvulsive therapy. Acta Psychiatr Scand 1964; 40:212–216.
177. Huston PE, Strother CR. The effect of electric shock on mental efficiency. Am J Psychiatry 1947; 104:707–712.
178. Korin H, Fink M, Kwalwasser S. Relation of changes in memory and learning to improvement in electroshock. Confin Neurol 1956; 16:83–96.
179. Hemsi LK, Whitehead A, Post F. Cogntiive functioning and cerebral arousal in elderly depressives and dements. J Psychosom Res 1968; 12:145–156.
180. Janis IL, Astrachan M. The effects of electroconvulsive treatments on memory efficiency. J Abnorm Soc Psychol 1951; 46:501–511.
181. Gangadhar BN, Kapur RL, Kalyanasundaram S. Comparison of electroconvulsive therapy with imipramine in endogenous depression: a double blind study. Br J Psychiatry 1982; 141:367–371.
182. Johnstone EC, Deakin JFW, Lawler P, Frith CD, Stevens M, McPherson K, Crow TJ. The Northwick Park electroconvulsive therapy trial. Lancet 1980; 2:1317–1320.
183. Waddington JL, Youssef HA. Tardive dyskinesia in bipolar affective disorder: aging, cognitive dysfunction, course of illness, and exposure to neuroleptics and lithium. Am J Psychiatry 1988; 145:613–616.
184. Squire LR, Zouzounis JA. Self-ratings of memory dysfunction: different findings in depression and amnesia. J Clin Exp Neuropsychol 1988; 10:727–738.
185. Pettinati HM, Rosenberg J. Memory self-ratings before and after electroconvulsive therapy: depression- versus ECT-induced. Biol Psychiatry 1984; 19:539–548.
186. Larrabee GJ, Levin HS. Memory self-ratings and objective test performance in a normal elderly sample. J Clin Exp Neuropsychol 1986; 8:275–284.
187. Inglis J. Shock, surgery and cerebral asymmetry. Br J Psychiatry 1970; 117:143–148.
188. Davis H, Squire L. Protein synthesis and memory. Psychol Bull 1984; 96:518–559.
189. Siesjô BK, Ingvar M, Wieloch T. Cellular and molecular events underlying epileptic brain damage. Ann NY Acad Sci 1986; 462:207–223.
190. Lerer B, Zabow T, Egnal N, Belmaker RH. Effect of vasopressin on memory following electroconvulsive therapy. Biol Psychiatry 1983; 18:821–824.
191. Ezzat DH, Ibraheem MN, Makhawy B. The effect of piracetam on ECT-induced memory disturbances. Br J Psychiatry 1985; 146:720–721.
192. Nasrallah HA, Varney N, Coffman JA, Bayless J, Chapman S. Opiate antagonism fails to reverse post-ECT cognitive deficits. J Clin Psychiatry 1986; 47:555–556.

III

COGNITIVE DISORDERS OF LATE YEARS

8

Alzheimer's Disease

Douglas Galasko and Leon J. Thal *University of California at San Diego and San Diego Veterans Affairs Medical Center, San Diego, California*

I. INTRODUCTION

Dementia refers to the loss of intellectual abilities, resulting in impairment of social or occupational function at an early stage, and inability to communicate or care for basic needs at an advanced stage. Alzheimer's disease (AD) is the most common cause of dementia in the elderly and, in recent years, it has been the focus of an intensive research effort. In this review we cover clinical aspects of AD as well as the underlying neuropathology and changes in neurotransmitter systems that are involved in the production of symptoms in AD. Treatment of dementia is evolving, and we shall focus on the rationale for current and future therapeutic strategies.

II. POSSIBLE ETIOLOGY

A. Epidemiology

The prevalence of AD depends on the longevity and age distribution of the population surveyed. Because most samples include relatively few subjects over age 85 or 90, the greatest uncertainty concerning age-specific prevalence exists in this group of the "old old." An issue crucial to the epidemiology of AD is choosing accurate diagnostic clinical criteria. Prevalence studies have adopted varying approaches, ranging from including only moderate or severe AD to using somewhat arbitrary cutoff points on psychometric tests. This lack of uniformity accounts for some of the variation in reported rates.

In the United States, about 4–5% of persons over 65 have severe dementia, leading to the inability to function independently; a further 10% have mild or moderate dementia(1). These figures translate to 1.3 million people with severe, and 2.8 million with mild to moderate, dementia. Of these, at least 60% have AD, and an additional 15–20% have a combination of AD and vascular dementia(1). Recent community surveys of AD in persons over 65, using a variety of diagnostic criteria, have reported prevalence figures ranging from 5.8%(2) to 10%(3) or 11%(4). Thus, AD is a major health problem in the elderly and will increase in importance as average life expectancy rises. Alzheimer's disease is strongly associated with aging: data from a recent report suggested that 3% of persons aged 65–74, 18.7% aged 75–84, and 47.2% of those over 85 met clinical criteria for AD(3). International comparisons of AD have been limited. In developed countries the prevalence of AD has not been shown to vary dramatically(2). Additional studies of dementia in developing countries are currently under way.

Analytical epidemiology has examined potential factors that may influence the risk of developing AD (Table 1), using primarily case–control methodology. Age is the strongest risk factor for AD in every study, and the incidence appears to increase with advancing age. There are no clinical or epidemiological criteria that distinguish between presenile and senile

TABLE 1 Potential Risk Factors for Alzheimer's Disease

Definite
Age
Heredity
Possible
Gender: women > men
Low educational level
Head injury
Aluminum
Nonsteroidal anti-inflammatory drugs (?protective)
Myocardial infarction
Unlikely
Viral infection
Smoking

dementia. Gender may contribute to the risk of dementia, since even after their increased life expectancy is taken into account, women develop AD at a higher rate than men (5,6). A contentious issue is whether education is a protective factor against AD(7). The hypothesis that low levels of education may lower the threshold for developing symptoms of AD is being pursued. A major bias that must be carefully controlled in these studies is that persons with relatively few years of formal education may perform suboptimally on many tasks in standard neuropsychological tests, although they are not impaired on activities of daily living.

A number of environmental factors have been examined in AD. Patients with AD had a history of head injury more commonly than controls in two reports (8,9); however, recent studies failed to confirm these findings (10,11). Surveys concerning occupational or other exposure to toxic agents have not yielded any positive associations in patients with AD(2). Exposure to aluminum, thought by some to play a part in neuropathological changes in AD, is difficult to assess reliably because of the diverse routes and sources of aluminum intake. Cigarette smoking does not appear to promote AD(10). An excessive rate of other illnesses, such as cancer, thyroid disease, and autoimmune conditions, has not been found in AD. A recent report(12) suggested that patients with rheumatoid arthritis who took nonsteroidal anti-inflammatory drugs over many years had a lower-than-expected prevalence of AD, possibly because of a protective effect of the medication. Unless convincing associations between defined environmental factors and AD are found, the role of the environment remains tentative. Age still remains the strongest predictor of AD.

B. Genetics

Over 20 families have been reported with clearcut autosomal dominant AD(13,14). Apart from a strikingly younger age of onset in most familial AD (FAD) pedigrees, there are no clinical or neuropathological differences between subjects with FAD and sporadic AD. A provocative issue is whether a late-onset gene with a high frequency in the general population may contribute to sporadic cases. An equally compelling question is whether genetic factors are sufficient to produce AD or require an interaction with environmental factors.

A traditional genetic approach is to measure concordance rates for a trait in twins. Currently, 14 of 32 monozygotic twin pairs and 3 of 7 dizygotic twins have been reported as concordant for AD(15). In concordant pairs, the age of onset of AD varied by as much as 10 years(16). This suggests either that genetic predisposition is insufficient to cause AD or that environmental factors may affect the expression of AD genes.

Numerous case–control studies have assessed the genetic contribution to sporadic AD by comparing the prevalence of probable AD in first-degree relatives of subjects with AD and nondemented elderly controls. Since many first-degree relatives of subjects with AD may have died of "competing" illnesses before manifesting AD, life-table adjustments, such as the Kaplan–Meier method, have been used. In general, these studies have included a few very elderly subjects, resulting in a great deal of variance in estimates of the risk of developing dementia after the age of 80. Some results suggest that the risk of developing AD approaches 50% for first-degree relatives of AD patients if they survive to age 90(17–19). This is consistent with an autosomal dominant gene with varying penetrance. However, the community prevalence studies cited earlier indicate that longevity alone may be associated with a similarly high risk of AD by the age of 85–90(3), and some case–control studies have failed to show an excess risk of AD in relatives of AD probands compared with controls(20,21). Again, the contribution of heredity to apparently sporadic AD awaits clarification; a biological marker of AD would greatly improve further studies.

Molecular genetic investigation of FAD with use of restriction fragment length polymorphism (RFLP) probes represents the most direct and powerful study of AD genetics. The finding that persons with Down syndrome inevitably develop neuropathological changes characteristic of AD by their fourth decade(22) has prompted an intensive search for a gene locus on chromosome 21. In 1987, statistically significant linkage between FAD and a site on the proximal part of chromosome 21 was reported(14). Subsequent studies have produced positive(23) and negative results(24,25) in additional families. Other candidate loci for FAD have not yet been supported by linkage studies. When additional well-defined FAD pedigrees are identified, the gene for FAD may be located and its product determined, permitting the interaction between genetics and environment in AD to be explained.

C. Environmental Factors: Viral Infections and Aluminum Neurotoxicity

Unconventional or slow virus infections include Creutzfeld–Jakob disease (CJD), an uncommon dementing illness that is usually more rapidly progressive than AD. The transmissable nature of this disease was shown by the inoculation of brain extracts from CJD patients into the brains of primates, which produced a spongiform encephalopathy. Similar attempts using brains from FAD and sporadic AD have failed to transmit AD(26). Recently, vacuolar changes were induced in the brains of hamsters inoculated with leukocyte preparations from living AD patients or their relatives(27). Although this result is provocative, it did not adequately reproduce AD pathology. Molecular studies have identified the prion protein, which is encoded by mammalian cells, as playing an important role in the formation of amyloid plagues in CJD and the Gerstman–Straussler syndrome of late onset ataxia and dementia(28). However, the neuropathological hallmarks of AD do not contain prions.

Several findings have implicated aluminum in AD. In the 1970s, dialysis dementia emerged as a major cause of mortality in renal patients and was associated with vastly increased levels of aluminum in the brain(29). With strict control of aluminum in dialysis water, the problem has all but disappeared. Intracerebral inoculation of aluminum into rabbits produced neurofibrillary degeneration resembling the tangles of AD(30). Elevated levels of aluminum have been detected in senile plaque cores(31) and in tangle-bearing neurons in AD(32). Aluminum is difficult to assay in the brain, and a recent report using neutron activation found no increase in aluminum in AD(33). An epidemiological study that tried to correlate geographic variation in the prevalence of AD with levels of aluminum in drinking water tentatively suggested a weak relationship(34). In a case–control study, the use of antiperspirants or deodorants containing aluminum was not significantly greater in the AD group(35). Overall, the weight of evidence for aluminum as a primary factor in AD is not compelling.

III. NEUROPATHOLOGY

Both the gross and microscopic features of AD occur, to some extent, in brains of nondemented elderly individuals. The age of the subject at death and the severity of pathological findings must, therefore, be taken into account in diagnosing AD. Grossly, the "typical" AD brain has marked atrophy of gyri and sulci, primarily in the association areas of the frontal, temporal, and parietal lobes, accompanied by enlargement of the lateral and third ventricles. Brain weight is reduced by about 10% compared with age-matched controls(36), with considerable overlap.

At a microscopic level, large-diameter neocortical neurons are especially depleted(37), glial cells are increased, and dendritic branching of surviving neurons is reduced(38). The hippocampus, particularly the CA1 region and subiculum, is among the most severely affected areas of the neocortex(39). Certain subcortical areas, notably the amygdala, locus coeruleus, and cholinergic neurons of the nucleus basalis of Meynert(40) also show extensive neuronal depletion.

The neuropathological hallmarks of AD are senile plaques (SPs) and neurofibrillary tangles (NFTs), which also occur in the brains of nondemented elderly individuals, but are more abundant in AD. Since NFTs occur in other conditions such as parkinsonism–dementia of Guam, Hallevorden–Spatz disease, and dementia pugilistica, the finding of SP is essential for the diagnosis of AD. The seminal studies of Blessed et al.(41,42) showed that the density of SPs in the neocortex correlated with scores on a mental state test and a scale measuring activities of daily living in demented and nondemented elderly individuals.

The SPs are spherical structures, with a central amorphous core containing extracellular deposits of amyloid protein, surrounded by abnormal-appearing neurites and glial cells. The varying morphology of SPs has led to suggestions of progressive stages of plaque evolution in aging and AD(43). Amyloid fibrils composed of a 4-kd peptide called β-protein or A4 are found in plaque cores, in the walls of cerebral blood vessels, and as deposits in the neuropil in AD(44,45). The origin of the β-protein deposits is controversial, and a major focus of research concerns the metabolism of the much larger precursor protein that gives rise to β-protein(46,47). Interest has been sparked by the localization of the gene for this precursor to chromosome 21, and the identification of several forms of the precursor, some of which contain protease-inhibiting sequences(48–50). Deposition of the precursor in the brain in Down syndrome precedes the development of senile plaques or abnormal neurites(51). Normally, the precursor proteins are secreted from cells, a process that involves cleavage of the precursor in the middle of the β-region, which would prevent amyloid formation(52,53). A major focus of research concerns the mechanisms allowing intact β-protein to reach extracellular sites(54). In addition, the physiological role of β-protein requires clarification, since both toxic(55) and trophic(56,57) functions have been postulated.

Many other proteins have been identified in SPs, although their presence may not reflect primary or early events in SP formation. Abnormal-appearing neurites surround mature plaques. These neurites contain a mixture of neurofilaments and are readily visualized with silver stains. They arise from several different neurotransmitter systems and may be part of an aberrant sprouting response in AD(58).

Several structural abnormalities of neurons in AD are related to the cytoskeleton, notably NFTs, granular–vacuolar degeneration (GVD), and Hirano bodies. The NFTs are composed of paired helical filaments (PHF) and may also contain straight filaments. Several constituents of NFTs have been identified, notably the microtubule-associated proteins tau and MAP 2(59,60), and A68(61,62), a protein enriched in AD brain. A biochemical assay, using antibodies to A68 and related proteins, showed that these proteins were increased in brain homogenates from AD, compared with those of controls and other neurological diseases(63), indicating that this test will be helpful in supporting the pathological diagnosis of AD. Ubiquitin, a member of the heat-shock protein family that binds to proteins destined for degradation, is also associated with NFTs(64). Neurons bearing NFTs may eventually disintegrate, leaving extracellular PHFs as "ghost" neurons. The sequence of events leading to NFT formation is under intensive study at a molecular level.

The primary or inciting event in the neuropathological changes of AD remains to be determined and separated from the chain of secondary processes.

IV. NEUROTRANSMITTER SYSTEMS

Deficiencies of several neurotransmitter systems occur in AD (Table 2) and can be correlated with the neuropathologic changes of AD and with cognitive measures obtained during life. In animals, lesions that selectively reduce the levels of certain neurotransmitters can impair learning. Subcortical nuclei projecting to the neocortex produce many neurotransmitters found in the cortex, and reduced levels of acetylcholine (ACh), norepinephrine (noradrenaline; NA), and serotonin reflect loss of nerve terminals from neurons originating in the brain stem.

The first neurotransmitter deficit reported in AD was a 50–90% decrease of choline acetyltransferase (ChAT), the biosynthetic enzyme for acetylcholine (ACh), in the hippocampus and neocortex(65–67). A later study, using temporal lobe biopsies from patients with early AD, found that the cholinergic deficiency was the most prominent transmitter abnormality at this early stage(68). The basal forebrain, notably the nucleus basalis of Meynert and septal nuclei, contains cholinergic neurons ascending to the cortex, and extensive neuronal loss and NFT formation occurs in these regions(40). The relative preservation of cholinergic muscarinic receptors in the cortex(65,69) supported the concept that degeneration of subcortical neurons was responsible for the cholinergic deficit. Strengthened by animal data showing that selective depletion or pharmacologic blockade of ACh impaired learning, the cholinergic theory of memory dysfunction in AD was proposed(70) and has influenced attempts to treat AD by enhancing cholinergic function.

Brain stem monoaminergic nuclei also show extensive pathological changes in AD. In the locus coeruleus, neuronal depletion and abundant NFTs result in a reduction in norepinephrine in the neocortex(71); similarly, involvement of the raphe nuclei results in decreased serotonin(71). Dopamine is only slightly depleted in AD brain(72). Monoamine oxidase (MAO) B, which breaks down dopamine and exogenous amines, is increased in AD brain, primarily at nonneuronal sites(73).

The excitatory amino acids glutamate and aspartate are widely distributed throughout the cortex, and neurons that normally use these neurotransmitters may be especially vulnerable in AD(74). Overactivity of these

TABLE 2 Neurotransmitters, Peptides, and Receptors in the Brain in Alzheimer's Disease

Transmitter	Level	Ref.	Receptor	Level	Ref.
Acetylcholine	↓	65–67	M_1	Nl	65
			M_2	↓	88
			N	↓	89
Dopamine	sl ↓	71,72	D_1	↓	90
			D_2	↓	90
Norepinephrine	Nl	71			
Epinephrine	↓	71			
Serotonin	↓	71	S_1	↓	91
			S_2	↓	91
Glutamate	↓	74	NMDA	↓	92
			Quis	↓	92
GABA	↓	75	A	↓	93,94
			B	↓	93
Neuropeptides					
Somatostatin	↓	77,78	S_1	↓	78
			S_2	↓	78
Neuropeptide Y	Nl	79,80			
Vasopressin	Nl	81			
CRF	↓	82		↑	82
Oxytocin	↓	83			
Cholecystokinin	Nl	84			
VIP	Nl	85			
TRH	Nl	86			
Neurotensin	Nl	87			
Substance P	Nl	87			
Galanin	Nl	76			

Abbreviations: sl, slightly; Nl, normal; CRF, corticotropin-releasing factor; VIP, vasoactive intestinal peptide; TRH, thyrotropin-releasing hormone. Receptors: M_1, postsynaptic muscarinic; M_2, presynaptic muscarinic; N, nicotinic; D_1, presynaptic dopaminergic; D_2, postsynaptic dopaminergic; NMDA, *N*-methyl-D-aspartate receptor; Quis, quisqualate receptor; for serotonin, somatostatin and GABA, 1 and 2 or A and B refer to receptor subtypes defined by ligand binding.

excitatory transmitters may cause neuronal damage under circumstances such as ischemia, and it is possible that they contribute to pathological changes in AD. The most abundant inhibitory transmitter, γ-aminobutyric acid (GABA), is not altered in AD(75); its receptors are decreased by over 40%(93).

Neuropeptides localize to many populations of neurons, and they may be selectively involved in AD. The concentrations of many peptides, including cholecystokinin (CCK), vasoactive intestinal polypeptide (VIP), thyrotropin-releasing hormone (TRH), neurotensin, and galanin probably do not change in AD(76). The most consistent neuropeptide change is a decrease in somatostatin in the cortex(77), accompanied by a reduction of postsynaptic somatostatin receptors(78). Neuropeptide Y, corticotropin-releasing factor (CRF), and vasopressin are also decreased in AD.

Receptors for neurotransmitters have also been examined in AD (see Table 2). The data are difficult to interpret, because altered levels may be secondary to up- or down-regulation in response to neurotransmitter decreases. For the cholinergic system, reports indicate that presynaptic (M_2) muscarinic receptors are decreased in the cortex, whereas postsynaptic (M_1) receptors are unchanged(88). Nicotinic receptors are reduced. Decreases in receptors for dopamine (D_2), serotonin (S_1 and S_2), somatostatin, and GABA have been reported, whereas CRF receptors are increased.

Neurotrophic factors, which in low concentration can support the survival or growth of select populations of neurons, have been intensively studied and are covered in detail in Chapter 13. Cholinergic neurons of the basal forebrain respond to nerve growth factor (NGF), the best characterized of these. In AD brain, the levels of NGF and its mRNA are unchanged (95), as is the message for its receptor(96).

V. CLINICAL ASPECTS

A. The Diagnostic Approach

The syndrome of dementia can result from numerous conditions, of which AD is the most common, and a structured clinical approach helps to reduce diagnostic errors. In several recent series, the accuracy rate of clinical diagnosis of AD was over 80%(97–99). The initial question to be answered is whether or not the patient is demented. The *DSM-III-R* criteria stipulate that the patient should have an insidious onset of cognitive symptoms severe enough to interfere with social or occupational function. In addition, the symptoms should be present for at least 3 months, in the absence of clouding of consciousness, which distinguishes dementia from delirium. On mental status examination, findings must include impairment of memory and at least one other cognitive capacity such as abstraction, judgment, language, praxis, or visuospatial function. Several brief screening tests of mental function have been widely used in dementia and AD, notably the Mini-Mental State Examination(100) and the Blessed Information–Memory–Concentration (BIMC) test(41). Inquiry about performance of tasks of daily living is a useful adjunct to mental status examination.

An expert panel convened by the National Institute of Neurological and Communicative Disorders and Stroke (NINCDS), and the Alzheimer's Disease and Related Disorders Association (ADRDA) established clinical criteria for diagnosing AD(101) (Table 3). These have an accuracy rate of over 80% in studies for which neuropathological confirmation of AD was obtained(98). The criteria include a screening mental status test, augmented by formal neuropsychological assessment, neurological examination to exclude other disease processes such as stroke, and screening blood tests to rule out metabolic abnormalities and thyroid disease. A neuro-

TABLE 3 Criteria for the Clinical Diagnosis of Alzheimer's Disease

I. *Criteria for the clinical diagnosis of **probable AD***
- Dementia documented by mental status testing (e.g., the Mini-Mental Test or Blessed Dementia Scale)
- Progressive deficits in memory and at least one other area of cognition
- No disturbance of consciousness
- Absence of systemic or brain disorders capable of producing progressive deficits in memory and cognition.

II. *Supportive evidence*
- Progressive deterioration of language (aphasia), motor skills (apraxia), or perception (agnosia)
- Impaired activities of daily living and altered behavior
- Compatible laboratory results (e.g., normal lumbar puncture; normal or non-specifically abnormal EEG; cerebral atrophy on CT)

III. *Clinical features that may be part of probable AD*
- Plateaus in the course
- Symptoms of depression, insomnia, incontinence, delusions, illusions, hallucinations, catastrophic outbursts, sexual disorders, and weight loss
- Neurological abnormalities in advanced AD (e.g., increased muscle tone, myoclonus, gait disorder, or seizures)
- CT normal for age

IV. *Features making probable AD unlikely*
- Sudden onset
- Early focal neurological findings, abnormal gait or seizures

V. *Criteria for the clinical diagnosis of **possible AD***

Same features as probable AD, but with
- Atypical onset, presentation or clinical course; *or*
- A second illness capable of causing dementia, which is not thought to be the major cause

VI. *Criteria for **definite AD***
- Clinical criteria for probable AD with histopathological evidence from brain biopsy or autopsy

Source: Modified from Ref. 101.

imaging test is desirable to document the absence of lesions that might cause dementia.

Occasionally, the evaluation and laboratory workup of dementia will detect conditions amenable to treatment, the so-called reversible dementias. Great enthusiasm for the notion of treatable dementia was sparked by reports suggesting that as many as 20% of patients with dementia fall into this category. A recent review of studies in which dementia was thought to be reversible and had improved with treatment of the underlying disorder, provides a more cautious viewpoint(102): about 10% of demented patients had potentially treatable conditions, but only 3% were documented to have improved.

B. Clinical Features and Course

The usual symptoms of AD reflect dysfunction of widespread regions of the cerebral cortex. Memory loss is the cardinal and, frequently, the presenting complaint. Initially, the patient has difficulty learning new information, such as names or details of conversation, whereas remote memories are relatively preserved. A feature of the amnesia of AD is the failure to recall recently presented information, even when given cues(103). With progression, the memory loss worsens to include remote memory.

Language is frequently normal early in AD. A subtle early finding at this stage is impairment of verbal fluency for categories, for instance names of animals or words beginning with a particular letter. As dementia progresses, many patients become dysphasic(104). Initially, there may be dysnomia, mild loss of fluency, paraphasic errors, and relative preservation of repetition, a pattern resembling transcortical sensory aphasia(105). At a later stage, language is obviously nonfluent and repetition impaired; terminally, the patient may be reduced to a state of near-mutism.

Visuospatial impairment results in symptoms such as misplacing objects or getting lost, and difficulty with tasks such as drawing complex figures. Difficulty with calculation, including skills such as handling money, apraxia, and agnosia are further problems that develop in AD. Early in AD, judgment and abstraction are often impaired, suggesting involvement of the frontal lobes.

Behavioral or psychiatric symptoms may compound intellectual deficits in AD. Over and above a general decline of activity and interest in virtually all AD patients, depressive symptoms occur in about 25%(106), although severe depression is uncommon. Delusions, usually simple persecutory, are common, although they are rarely systematized, as in schizophrenia. The spectrum of behavioral abnormalities includes wandering, agitation, insomnia, and disinhibition.

Many AD patients have abnormal neurological findings, which are more noticeable in advanced stages(107). Primitive reflexes and extrapyramidal features of muscle rigidity and bradykinesia are frequent, and myoclonus and seizures occur in up to 10% of AD patients.

As neuronal degeneration progresses, all of the foregoing symptoms worsen, and eventually patients become uncommunicative, unable to care for themselves, to walk, and to maintain continence. In end-stage AD, death usually results from the complications of being bedbound, such as aspiration pneumonia, urinary tract infections, sepsis, or pulmonary embolism(108).

The course of AD and the combination of symptoms that manifest in each patient are markedly heterogeneous, which makes prognostication difficult. On average, life expectancy following the initial symptoms of AD is reduced, compared with age-matched controls(109,110). Mean survival after diagnosis is about 6 years(111), but may range from 2 to 20 years. Certain factors may predict more rapid deterioration in AD, in particular the early development of aphasia, psychosis, extrapyramidal signs, or myoclonus(112–114). Predictors of the need for institutional placement of AD are less clear(115), because factors such as community and caregiver resources interact with the severity of cognitive impairment and associated behavioral symptoms to influence this decision.

C. Neuroimaging and Quantitative Techniques

Imaging of the brain or measuring its metabolism has the potential of supporting the early clinical diagnosis of AD, as well as providing a biological marker of the disease. Studies of several of these techniques have revealed limitations, including a substantial overlap with controls and a difficulty in quantifying radiographic images.

The electroencephalogram (EEG) may be normal or show mild diffuse slowing early in AD. Brain electrical activity mapping (BEAM) converts EEG recordings into spectral frequency maps, and may show different patterns in AD(116). Late components of evoked potentials, in particular the P_{300} wave, show increased latency in AD, compared with controls, but do not clearly separate early AD from normal aging(117).

Anatomical imaging of the brain with computerized tomography (CT) is of value in ruling out strokes or mass lesions. The cortical atrophy and ventricular enlargement usually seen in AD also occur in normal aging, although these changes progress more rapidly in AD than in controls(118). Magnetic resonance imaging (MRI) provides even more precise detail of brain structure, allowing imaging and volumetric measurement of the hippocampus(119). Atrophy of this area in AD has been visualized in a few patients, but confirmatory studies are needed.

Advances in metabolic imaging of the brain have permitted cerebral blood flow, glucose utilization, and ligand binding to neurotransmitter receptors to be imaged. In AD, positron emission tomography (PET) has shown decreased glucose metabolism in the parietal and temporal cortex in AD, even in early stages(120). Similar claims have been made for measures of regional cerebral blood flow(121). The simpler technique of single-photon emission computerized tomography (SPECT) has demonstrated similar findings in the temporoparietal cortex(122). Further validation of these radiological methods, particularly in patients with early AD and other dementias, is needed.

VI. THERAPEUTIC APPROACHES

There are several strategies or levels for treating AD, and useful analogies may be drawn from the approach to Parkinson's disease (PD). First, therapy may be directed at controlling or relieving symptoms of AD. This can be approached without understanding the processes responsible for neuronal degeneration. Secondary symptoms, particularly depression and agitation, which often impair the day-to-day function of patients with AD, can be treated with a variety of drugs, most commonly antidepressants or neuroleptics. Clinical trials of these medications have suffered from too few subjects and other methodological flaws, and elderly patients have an increased risk of developing side effects. Consequently, further studies are needed to establish which drugs provide safe and effective control of secondary symptoms. Guidelines for treating secondary symptoms in AD are discussed in a companion volume in this series(123).

Memory impairment is a primary symptom of AD, and this is the major target of many treatment trials. Treatment of memory in AD is likely to be most effective early in the course of the disease, with a declining response as neuronal degeneration worsens. One attractive rationale is the enhancement of neurotransmitter function, particularly the cholinergic system (reviewed in Ref. 124). Clinical trials of four pharmacologic approaches for improving cholinergic function have been conducted: increasing acetylcholine synthesis by administering precursors; enhancing the synaptic release of acetylcholine; inhibiting the enzymatic breakdown of acetylcholine; and using agonists to directly stimulate postsynaptic receptors. Lecithin and choline, precursors of acetylcholine, and 4-aminopyridine, which enhances release, have failed to improve memory in patients with AD. Inhibitors of acetylcholinesterase such as physostigmine and tacrine (tetrahydroaminoacridine) augment cholinergic function by preventing the hydrolysis of ACh. In many small investigator-sponsored trials, these agents have been reported to augment verbal memory, and several large-scale clinical trials are under way. In two recent multicenter studies of tacrine, a clinically significant improvement of memory was not achieved (125,126). However, both studies had relatively few subjects, and used crossover designs, which resulted in carryover effects in one study. Attempts to enhance cholinergic transmission by intraventricular infusion of bethanechol, which acts directly at postsynaptic receptor sites, have not improved memory in AD (127). In general, cholinomimetic agents have been limited by side effects, poor crossing of the blood–brain barrier, and short duration of action. It is possible that improvements in drug design may yield better results.

Another group of drugs that may improve memory has a less well-understood mode of action and may be referred to as "cognitive enhancers." This category includes vasodilators and nootropics. The vasodilator most frequently used for AD is dihydroergotoxine, a mixture of ergoloid mesylates, which is reported to improve orientation, depression, mental alertness, and self-care, but has not been shown to affect memory(128). As a result, although this drug is often given to patients with AD, its value is uncertain. Nootropics, such as piracetam, can be shown to improve memory in laboratory animals. Their mode of action in the brain is unknown, and at best, they are claimed to improve attention in AD, but have not been shown to benefit memory(129).

An appealing strategy involves slowing the rate of progression of AD. The recent report that deprenyl, which attenuates the toxicity of 1-methyl-4-phenyl-1,2,3,6-tetrahydropyridine (MPTP) in an animal model of PD, significantly retarded the rate of progression of PD(130) illustrates the potential of this approach. There are several candidate drugs that may be similarly applied to AD: a brief list includes membrane-stabilizing agents such as acetyl-L-carnitine, calcium channel blockers, inhibitors of excitatory neurotransmitters, and trophic factors such as nerve growth factor.

A more basic level of treatment would require an understanding of the earliest events in AD at a molecular level, coupled with the ability to diagnose AD at an extremely early stage, perhaps even before the onset of symptoms. Treatment would then aim to delay the development of symptoms. For example, if a critical amount of amyloid deposition in the brain is a necessary precursor of overt AD, treatment could be aimed at retarding the rate of amyloid formation. Alternatively, if environmental factors are important in the pathogenesis of AD, their modification may prove useful. The therapeutic challenge of preventing AD from developing awaits novel approaches at the basic science as well as clinical levels.

Note added in proof: Goate et al. (Nature 1991;349:704–706) recently reported a mutation in the APP gene in members of 2 familial AD pedigrees, but excluded this mutation in 15 other families with early-onset AD.

ACKNOWLEDGMENT

Supported by Department of Veterans Affairs and NIH grant AG05131.

REFERENCES

1. Katzman R. The prevalence and malignancy of Alzheimer's disease: a major killer. Arch Neurol 1976; 33:217–218.
2. Rocca WA, Amaducci LA, Schoenberg BS. Epidemiology of clinically diagnosed Alzheimer's disease. Ann Neurol 1986; 19:415–424.
3. Evans DA, Funkenstein HH, Albert MS, Scherr PA, Cook NR, Chown MJ, Hebert LE, Hennekens CH, Taylor JO. Prevalence of Alzheimer's disease in a community population of older persons. JAMA 1989; 262:2551–2556.
4. Pfeffer RI, Afifi AA, Chance JM. Prevalence of Alzheimer's disease in a retirement community. Am J Epidemiol 1987; 125:420–435.
5. Molsa PK, Marttila RJ, Rinne UK. Epidemiology of dementia in a Finnish population. Acta Neurol Scand 1982; 65:541–552.
6. Schoenberg BS, Anderson DW, Haerer AF. Severe dementia: prevalence and clinical features in a biracial US population. Arch Neurol 1985; 42:740–743.
7. Filley CM, Brownell HH, Albert ML. Education provides no protection against Alzheimer's disease. Neurology 1985; 35:1781–1784.
8. Heyman A, Wilkinson WE, Stafford JA, Helms MJ, Sigmon AH, Weinberg T. Alzheimer's disease: a study of epidemiological aspects. Ann Neurol 1984; 15:335–341.
9. Mortimer JA, French LR, Hutton JT, Schuman LM. Head injury as a risk factor for Alzheimer's disease. Neurology 1985; 35:264–267.
10. Amaducci LA, Fratiglioni L, Rocca WA, Fieschi S, Livrea P, Pedone D, Bracco L, Lippi A, Gandolfo C, Bino G, Prencipe M, Bonatti ML, Girotti F, Carella F, Tavolato B, Ferla S, Lenzi GL, Carolei A, Gambi A, Grigoletto F, Schoenberg BS. Risk factors for clinically diagnosed Alzheimer's disease: a case–control study in an Italian population. Neurology 1986; 36:922–931.
11. Chandra V, Kokmen E, Schoenberg BS, Beard CM. Head trauma with loss of consciousness as a risk factor for Alzheimer's disease. Neurology 1989; 39:1576–1578.
12. McGeer PL, McGeer E, Rogers R, Sibley J. Anti-inflammatory drugs and Alzheimer's disease. Lancet 1990;335:1037.
13. Nee LE, Polinsky RJ, Eldridge R, Weingartner H, Smallberg S, Ebert M. A family with histologically confirmed Alzheimer's disease. Arch Neurol 1983; 40:203–208.
14. St George-Hysloph, Tanzi R, Polinsky RJ, Haines JL, Nee L, Watkins PC, Myers RH, Feldman RG, Pollen D, Drachman D, Growdon J, Bruni A, Foncin J-F, Salmon D, Frommelt P, Amaducci L, Sorbi S, Piacentini S, Stewart GD, Hobbs WJ, Conneally PM, Gusella JF. The genetic defect causing familial Alzheimer disease maps on chromosome 21. Science 1987; 235:885–890.

15. Creasey H, Jorm A, Longley W, Broe GA, Henderson AS. Monozyzgotic twins discordant for Alzheimer's disease. Neurology 1989; 39:1474–1476.
16. Nee LE, Eldridge R, Sunderland T, Thomas CB, Katz D, Thompson KE, Weingartner H, Weiss H, Julian C, Cohen R. Dementia of the Alzheimer type: clinical and family study of 22 twin pairs. Neurology 1987; 37:359–363.
17. Breitner JCS, Silverman JS, Mohs RC, David KL. Familial aggregation in Alzheimer's disease: comparison of risk among early- and late-onset cases and among male and female relatives in successive generations. Neurology 1988; 38:207–212.
18. Heston LL, Mastri AR, Anderson E, White J. Dementia of the Alzheimer type. Clinical genetics, natural history and associated conditions. Arch Gen Psychiatry 1981; 31:1085–1090.
19. Heyman A, Wilkinson WE, Hurwitz BJ, Schmechel G, Sigmon AH, Weinberg T, Helms MJ, Swoft M. Alzheimer's disease: genetic aspects and associated clinical disorders. Ann Neurol 1983; 14:507–515.
20. Chandra V, Philipose V, Bell PA, Schoenberg BS. Case-control study of late-onset "probable Alzheimer's disease." Neurology 1987; 37:1295–1300.
21. Farrer LA, O'Sullivan DM, Cupples LA, Growdon JH, Myers RH. Assessment of genetic risk for Alzheimer's disease among first-degree relatives. Ann Neurol 1989; 25:485–493.
22. Wisniewski KE, Wisniewski HM, Wen GY. Occurrence of neuropathological changes and dementia of Alzheimer's disease in Down's syndrome. Ann Neurol 1985; 17:278–282.
23. Goate AM, Haynes AR, Owen MJ, Farrall M, James LA, Lai LYC, Mullan MJ, Roques P, Rossor MN, Williamson R, Hardy JA. Predisposing locus for AD on chromosome 21. Lancet 1989; 1:352–355.
24. Pericak-Vance MA, Yamaoka LH, Haynes CS, Speer MC, Haines JL, Gaskell PC, Hung W-Y, Clark CM, Heyman ALO, Trofatter JA, Eisenmenger JP, Gilbert JR, Lee JE, Alberts MJ, Dawson DV, Bartlett RJ, Earl NL, Siddique T, Vance JM, Conneally PM, Roses AD. Genetic linkage studies in Alzheimer's disease families. Exp Neurol 1988; 102:271–279.
25. Schellenberg GD, Bird TD, Wijsman EM, Moore DK, Boehnke M, Bryant EM, Lampe TH, Nochlin T, Sumi SM, Deeb SS, Beyreuther K, Martin GM. Absence of linkage of chromosome 21q21 markers to familial Alzheimer's disease. Science 1988; 241:1507–1510.
26. Goudsmit J, Morrow CH, Asher DM, Yanagihara RT, Masters CL, Gibbs CH, Gajdusek DC. Evidence for and against the transmissability of Alzheimer's disease. Neurology 1980; 30:945–950.
27. Manuelides EE, de Figueiredo JM, Kim JH, Fritch WW, Manuelides L. Transmission studies of blood from Alzheimer's disease patients and healthy relatives. Proc Natl Acad Sci USA 1988; 85:4898–4901.
28. Prusiner SP. Prions and neurodegenerative disease. N Engl J Med 1987; 317:1571–1581.
29. Alfrey AC, Le Gendre GR, Kaehny WD. The dialysis encephalopathy syndrome: possible aluminum intoxication. N Engl J Med 1976; 294:184–188.

30. Klatzo I, Wisniewski H, Steicher E. Experimental production of neurofibrillary degeneration. J Neuropathol Exp Neurol 1965; 24:187–199.
31. Candy JM, Klinowski J, Perry RH, Perry EK, Fairbairn A, Oakley AE, Carpenter TA, Atack JR, Blessed G, Edwardson JA. Aluminosilicates and senile plaque formation in Alzheimer's disease. Lancet 1986; 1:354–356.
32. Perl DP, Brody AR. Alzheimer's disease: x-ray spectrometric evidence of aluminum accumulation in neurofibrillary tangle-bearing neurons. Science 1980; 208:297–299.
33. Markesbery WR, Ehmann WD, Hussain TIM, Allaudin M, Goodin T. Instrumental neutron activation analysis of brain aluminum in Alzheimer disease and aging. Ann Neurol 1981; 10:511–516.
34. Martyn CN, Barker DJP, Osmond C, Harris EC, Edwardson JA, Lacey RF. Geographical relationship between Alzheimer's disease and aluminum in drinking water. Lancet 1989; 1:59–62.
35. Graves AB, White E, Koepsell TD, Reifler BV, Van Belle G, Larson EB. The association between aluminum-containing products and Alzheimer's disease. J Clin Epidemiol 1990; 43:35–44.
36. Terry RD, Peck A, De Teresa R, Schechter R, Horoupian D. Some morphometric aspects of the brain in senile dementia of the Alzheimer type. Ann Neurol 1981; 10:122–126.
37. Hansen LA, De Teresa R, Davies P, Terry RD. Neocortical morphometry, lesion counts, and choline acetyltransferase levels in the age spectrum of Alzheimer's disease. Neurology 1988; 38:48–54.
38. Scheibel AB. Structural aspects of the aging brain: spine systems and the dendritic arbor. In: Katzman R, Terry RD, Bick KL, eds. Aging, vol. 7. Alzheimer's disease: senile dementia and related disorders. New York: Raven Press, 1978:353–373.
39. Hyman BT, Van Hoesen GW, Damasio AR, Barnes CL. Alzheimer's disease; cell-specific pathology isolates the hippocampal formation. Science 1984; 225:1168–1170.
40. Whitehouse PJ, Price DL, Struble RG, Clark AW, Coyle JT, DeLong MR. Alzheimer's disease and senile dementia: loss of neurons in the basal forebrain. Science 1982; 215;1237–1239.
41. Blessed G, Tomlinson BE, Roth M. The association between quantitative measures of dementia and of senile change in the cerebral grey matter of elderly subjects. Br J Psychiatry 1968; 114:797–811.
42. Tomlinson BE, Blessed G, Roth M. Observations on the brains of demented old people. J Neurol Sci 1970; 11:205–242.
43. Wisniewski HM, Terry RD. Reexamination of the pathogenesis of the senile plaque. Prog Neuropathol 1973; 2:1–26.
44. Glenner GG, Wong CW. Alzheimer's disease. Initial report of the purification and characterization of a novel cerebrovascular amyloid protein. Biochem Biophys Res Commun 1984; 120:885–890.
45. Masters CL, Simms G, Weinmann NA, Multhaup G, McDonald BL, Beyreu-

ther K. Amyloid plaque core protein in Alzheimer's disease and Down's syndrome. Proc Natl Acad Sci USA 1985; 82:4245–4249.
46. Dyrks T, Weidemann A, Multhaup G, Salbaum JM, Lemaire HG, Kang J, Muller-Hill B, Masters CL, Beyreuther K. Identification, transmembrane orientation and biogenesis of the amyloid A4 precursor of Alzheimer's disease. EMBO J 1988; 7:949–957.
47. Weidemann A, Konig G, Bunke D, et al. Identification, biogenesis, and localization of precursors of Alzheimer's disease A4 amyloid protein. Cell 1989; 57:115–126.
48. Kitaguchi N, Takahashi Y, Tokushima Y, Shiojiri S, Ito H. Novel precursor of Alzheimer's disease amyloid protein shows protease inhibitory activity. Nature 1988; 331:530–532.
49. Ponte P, Gonzalez-De Whitt P, Shilling J, Miller J, Hsu G, Greenberg B, Davis K, Wallace W, Lieberberg I, Fuller F, Cordell B. A new A4 amyloid mRNA contains a domain homologous to serine protease inhibitors. Nature 1988; 331:525–527.
50. Tanzi RE, McClatchey AI, Lamperti ED, Villa-Komaroff L, Gusella JF, Neve RL. Protease inhibitor domain encoded by an amyloid protein precursor mRNA associated with Alzheimer's disease. Nature 1988; 311:528–530.
51. Giacone G, Tagliavini F, Linoli G, Bouras C, Frigerio L, Frangione B, Bugiani O. Down patients: extracellular preamyloid deposits precede neuritic degeneration and senile plaques. Neurosci Lett 1989; 97:232–238.
52. Sisodia S, Koo EH, Beyreuther K, Unterbeck A, Price DL. Evidence that beta-amyloid protein in Alzheimer's disease is not derived by normal processing. Science 1990; 248:492–495.
53. Esch FS, Keim PS, Beattie EC, Blacher RW, Culwell AR, Oltersdorf T, McClure D, Ward P. Cleavage of amyloid beta peptide during constitutive processing of its precursor. Science 1990;248:1122–1124.
54. Selkoe D. Deciphering Alzheimer's disease: the amyloid precursor protein yields new clues. Science 1990; 248:1058–1060.
55. Yankner BA, Dawes LR, Fisher S, Villa-Komaroff L, Oster-Granite ML, Neve RL. Neurotoxicity of a fragment of the amyloid precursor associated with Alzheimer's disease. Science 1989; 245:417–420.
56. Whitson JS, Selkoe DJ, Cotman CW. Amyloid beta protein enhances the survival of hippocampal neurons in vitro. Science 1989; 243:1488–1490.
57. Saitoh T, Sundsmo M, Roch J-M, Kimura N, Cole G, Schubert D, Oltersdorf T, Schenk DB. Secreted form of amyloid beta protein precursor is involved in the growth regulation of fibroblasts. Cell 1989; 58:615–622.
58. Terry RD, Katzman R. Senile dementia of the Alzheimer type. Ann Neurol 1983; 14:497–506.
59. Kosik KS, Joachim CL, Selkoe DJ. Microtubule-associated protein tau is a major antigenic component of paired helical filaments in Alzheimer's disease. Proc Natl Acad Sci USA 1986; 85:4884–4888.
60. Wischik CM, Novak M, Edwards PC, Klug A, Tichelaar W, Crowther RA. Structural characterization of the core of the paired helical filament of Alzheimer's disease. Proc Natl Acad Sci USA 1988; 85:4884–4888.

61. Nukina N, Kosik K, Selkoe D. The monoclonal antibody Alz50 recognizes tau proteins in Alzheimer's disease brain. Neurosci Lett 1987; 87:240–246.
62. Wolozin B, Davies P. Alzheimer-related neuronal protein A68: specificity and distribution. Ann Neurol 1987; 22:521–526.
63. Ghanbari HA, Miler BE, Haigler HJ, Arato M, Bissette G, Davies P, Nemeroff CB, Perry EK, Perry R, Ravid R, Swaab DF, Whetsell WO, Zemlan FP. Biochemical assay of Alzheimer's disease-associated protein(s) in human brain tissue. JAMA 1990; 263:2907–2910.
64. Mori H, Kondo J, Ihara Y. Ubiquitin is a component of paired helical filaments in Alzheimer's disease. Science 1987; 235:1641–1644.
65. Bowen DM, Smith CB, White P, Davison AN. Neurotransmitter-related enzymes and indices of hypoxia in senile dementia and other abiotrophies. Brain 1976; 99:459–496.
66. Davies P, Verth AH. Selective loss of central cholinergic neurons in Alzheimer's disease. Lancet 1977; 1:668–670.
67. White P, Goodhardt MJ, Keet JP, Hiley CR, Carrasco LH, Williams TEI, Bowen DM. Neocortical cholinergic neurons in elderly people. Lancet 1977; 1:668–670.
68. Francis PT, Palmer AM, Sims NR, Bowen DM, Davison AN, Esiri MM, Nearey D, Snowden JS, Wilcock GK. Neurochemical studies of early-onset Alzheimer's disease. Possible influence on treatment. N Engl J Med 1985; 313:7–11.
70. Bartus RD, Dean RL, Beer B, Lippa AS, The cholinergic hypothesis of geriatric memory dysfunction. Science 1982; 217:408–417.
71. Adolfsson R, Gottfries CG, Roos BE, Winblad B. Changes in brain catecholamines in patients with dementia of Alzheimer type. Br J Psychiatry 1979; 135:216–223.
72. Yates CM, Allison Y, Simpson J, Maloney AFJ, Gordon A. Dopamine in Alzheimer's disease and senile dementia. Lancet 1979; 2:851–852.
73. Oreland L, Gottfries C-G. Platelet and brain monoamine oxidase in aging and in dementia of Alzheimer's type. Prog Neuropsychopharmacol Biol Psychiatry 1986; 10:533–540.
74. Hyman BT, Van Hoesen GW, Damasio AR. Alzheimer's disease: glutamate depletion in the hippocampal perforant pathway zone. Ann Neurol 1987; 22:37–40.
75. Rossor MN, Garret NJ, Johnson AJ, Mountjoy CQ, Roth M, Iversen LL. A post-mortem study of cholinergic and GABA systems in senile dementia. Brain 1982; 105:313–330.
76. Katzman R, Thal LJ. Neurochemistry of Alzheimer's disease. In: Siegel G, Agranoff B, Albers RW, Molinoff P, eds. Basic neurochemistry: molecular, cellular and medical aspects, 4th ed. New York: Raven Press, 1989:827–838.
77. Davies P, Katzman R, Terry R. Reduced somatostatin-like immunoreactivity in cerebral cortex from cases of Alzheimer's disease and Alzheimer senile dementia. Nature 1980; 288:279–280.
78. Beal MF, Mazurek MF, Tran VT, Chatta G, Bird ED, Martin JB. Reduced numbers of somatostatin receptors in the cerebral cortex in Alzheimer's disease. Science 1985; 229:289–291.

79. Allen JM, Ferrier IN, Roberts GW, Cross AJ, Adrian TE, Crow TJ, Bloom SR. Elevation of neuropeptide Y (NPY) in substantia innominata in Alzheimer's type dementia. J Neurol Sci 1984; 64:321–325.
80. Beal MF, Mazurek MF, Chattha GK, Svendsen CN, Bird ED, Martin JB. Neuropeptide Y immunoreactivity is reduced in cerebral cortex in Alzheimer's disease. Ann Neurol 1986; 20:282–288.
81. Mazurek MF, Beal MF, Bird ED, Martin JB. Vasopressin in Alzheimer's disease: a study of postmortem brain concentrations. Ann Neurol 1986; 20;665–670.
82. De Souza EB, Whitehouse PJ, Kuhar MJ, Price D, Vale WW. Reciprocal changes in corticotropin-releasing factor (CRF)-like immunoreactivity and CRF receptors in cerebral cortex of Alzheimer's disease. Nature 1986; 319:593–595.
83. Mazurek MF, Beal MF, Bird ED, Martin JB. Oxytocin in Alzheimer's disease: postmortem brain levels. Neurology 1987; 37:1001–1003.
84. Perry RH, Dockray GJ, Dimaline R, Perry EK, Blessed G, Tomlinson BE. Neuropeptides in Alzheimer's disease, depression and schizophrenia: a postmortem analysis of vasoactive intestinal peptide and cholecystokinin in cerebral cortex. J Neurol Sci 1981; 51:465–472.
85. Rossor MN, Fahrenkrug J, Emson PC, Mountjoy CQ, Iversen LL, Roth M. Reduced choline acetyltransferase activity in senile dementia of Alzheimer type is not accompanied by changes in vasoactive intestinal peptide. Brain Res 1980; 201:249–253.
86. Yates CM, Harmar AG, Rosie R, Sheward J, Sanchez De Levy G, Simpson J, Maloney AFJ, Gordon A, Fink G. Thyrotropin releasing hormone, luteinizing hormone-releasing hormone and substance P immunoreactivity in postmortem brain from cases of Alzheimer type dementia and Down's syndrome. Brain Res 1983; 258:445–452.
87. Ferrier IN, Cross AJ, Johnson JA, Roberts GW, Crow TJ, Corsellis JA, Lee YC, O' Shaughnessy D, Adrian TE, McGregor GP. Neuropeptides in Alzheimer type dementia. J Neurol Sci 1983; 62:159–170.
88. Mash DC, Flynn DD, Potter LT. Loss of M_2 muscarinic receptors in the cerebral cortex in Alzheimer's disease and experimental cholinergic denervation. Science 1985; 228:1115–1117.
89. Whitehouse PJ, Martino AM, Price DL, Kellar KJ. Reductions in nicotinic but not muscarinic cholinergic receptors in Alzheimer's disease measured using ^{3}H acetylcholine. Ann Neurol 1985; 18:145.
90. Cross AJ, Crow TJ, Ferrier IN, Johnson JA, Markakis D. Striatal dopamine receptors in Alzheimer type dementia. Neurosci Lett 1984; 52:1–6.
91. Cross AJ, Crow TJ, Ferrier IN, Johnson JA, Bloom SR, Corsellis JAN. Serotonin receptor changes in dementia of the Alzheimer type. J Neurochem 1984; 43:1574–1581.
92. Greenamyre JT, Penney JT, Young AB, D'Amato CJ, Hicks SP, Shoulson I. Alterations in L-glutamate binding in Alzheimer's and Huntington's disease. Science 1985; 227:1496–1499.

93. Chu DCM, Penney JB, Young AB. Cortical $GABA_A$ and $GABA_B$ receptors in Alzheimer disease. Neurology 1987; 37:1454–1459.
94. Reisine TD, Yamamura HI, Bird ED, Spokes E, Enna SJ. Pre- and postsynaptic alterations in Alzheimer's disease. Brain Res 1978; 159:477–481.
95. Goedert M, Fine A, Hunt SP, Ullrich A. Nerve growth factor mRNA in peripheral and central rat tissues and in the human central nervous system: lesion effects in the rat brain and levels in Alzheimer's disease. Mol Brain Res 1986; 1:85–92.
96. Goedert M, Fine A, Dawbarn D, Wilcock GK, Chao MN. Nerve growth factor receptor mRNA distribution in human brain: normal levels in basal forebrain in Alzheimer's disease. Mol Brain Res 1989; 5:1–7.
97. Molsa PK, Paljavi L, Rinne JO, Rinne UK, Sako E. Validity of clinical diagnoses in dementia: a prospective clinicopathological study. J Neurol Neurosurg Psychiatry 1985; 48:1085–1090.
98. Tierney MC, Fisher RH, Lewis AJ, Zorzitto ML, Snow WG, Reid DW, Nieuwstraten P. The NINCDS–ADRDA Work Group criteria for the clinical diagnosis of probable Alzheimer's disease: a clinicopathologic study of 57 cases. Neurology 1988; 38:359–364.
99. Wade JPH, Mirsen TR, Hachinski VC, Fisman M, Lau C, Merskey H. The clinical diagnosis of Alzheimer's disease. Arch Neurol 1987; 44:24–29.
100. Folstein MF, Folstein SE, McHugh PR: Mini-Mental State: a practical method for grading the cognitive state of patients for the clinician. J Psychiatr Res 1975;12:189–198.
101. McKhann G, Drachman D, Folstein MF, Katzman R, Price D, Stadlan EM. Clinical diagnosis of Alzheimer's disease: report of the NINCDS–ADRDA work group. Neurology 1984; 34:939–944.
102. Clarfield AM. The reversible dementias: do they reverse? Ann Intern Med 1988; 109:476–486.
103. Shimamura AP, Salmon DP, Squire LR, Butters N. Memory dysfunction and word priming in dementia and amnesia. Behav Neurosci 1987; 101:347–351.
104. Faber-Langendoen K, Morris JC, Knesevich JW, LaBarge E, Miller JP, Berg L. Aphasia in senile dementia of the Alzheimer type. Ann Neurol 1988;23:365–370.
105. Cummings JL, Benson DF, Hill MA, Read S. Aphasia in dementia of the Alzheimer type. Neurology 1985; 35:394–397.
106. Cummings JL, Miller B, Hill MA, Neshkes R. Neuropsychiatric aspects of multi-infarct dementia and dementia of the Alzheimer type. Arch Neurol 1987; 44:389–393.
107. Huff FJ, Boller F, Luchelli F, Querrirera R, Beyer J, Belle S. The neurologic examination in patients with probable Alzheimer's disease. Arch Neurol 1987; 44:929–932.
108. Molsa PK, Marttila RJ, Rinne UK. Survival and cause of death in Alzheimer's disease and multi-infarct dementia. Acta Neurol Scand 1986; 74:103–107.
109. Martin DC, Miller JK, Kapoor W, Arena VC, Boller F. A controlled study of survival with dementia. Arch Neurol 1987; 44:1122–1126.

110. Wang HS. Prognosis in dementia and related disorders in the aged. In: Katzman R, Terry RD, Bick KL, eds. Aging, vol 7: Alzheimer's disease: senile dementia and related disorders. New York: Raven Press, 1978:309–313.
111. Barclay LL, Zemcov A, Blass JP, Sansone J. Survival in Alzheimer's disease and vascular dementias. Neurology 1985; 35:834–840.
112. Chui HC, Teng ET, Henderson VW, Moy AC. Clinical subtypes of dementia of the Alzheimer type. Neurology 1985; 35:1544–1550.
113. Mayeux RT, Stern Y, Spanton S. Heterogeneity in dementia of the Alzheimer type: evidence of subgroups. Neurology 1985; 35:453–461.
114. Stern Y, Mayeux R, Sano M, Hauser WA, Bush T. Predictors of disease course in patients with probable Alzheimer's disease. Neurology 1987; 37:1649–1653.
115. Hutton JT, Dippel RL, Loewenson RB, Mortimer JA, Christians BL. Predictors of nursing home placement of patients with Alzheimer's disease. Tex Med 1985; 81:40–43.
116. Duffy FH, Albert MS, McAnulty J. Brain electrical activity in patients with presenile and senile dementia of the Alzheimer type. Ann Neurol 1984; 16:439–448.
117. Gordon E, Kriuhin C, Harris A, Meares R, Howson A. The differential diagnosis of dementia using P_{300} latency. Biol Psychiatry 1986; 21:1123–1132.
118. Creasey H, Schwartz M, Frederickson H, Jaxby JV, Rapoport SI. Quantitative computerized tomography in dementia of the Alzheimer type. Neurology 1986; 36:1563–1568.
119. Press GA, Amaral DG, Squire LR. Hippocampal abnormalities in amnesic patients revealed by high-resolution magnetic resonance imaging. Nature 1989; 341:54–57.
120. Haxby JV, Grady CL, Duara R, Schlageter N, Berg G, Rapoport SI. Neocortical metabolic abnormalities precede nonmemory cognitive deficits in early Alzheimer's-type dementia. Arch Neurol 1986; 43:882–885.
121. Prohovnik I, Mayeux RT, Sackeim HA, Smith G, Stern Y, Alderson PO. Cerebral perfusion as a diagnostic marker of early Alzheimer's disease. Neurology 1988; 38:931–937.
122. Johnson KA, Holman BL, Mueller SP, Rosen TJ, English R, Nagel JS, Growdon JH. Single photon emission computed tomography in Alzheimer's disease. Arch Neurol 1988; 45:392–396.
123. Cummings JL, Miller BL. Alzheimer's disease: treatment and long-term management. New York, Marcel Dekker, 1990.
124. Thal LJ. Pharmacological treatment of memory disorders. In: Boller F, Grafman J, eds. Handbook of neuropsychology, vol. 3. Amsterdam: Elsevier Science Publishers, 1989:247–267.
125. Chatellier G, Lacomblez L. Tacrine (tetrahydroaminoacridine; THA) and lecithin in senile dementia of the Alzheimer type: a multicentre trial. Br Med J 1990; 300:395–399.
126. Gauthier S, Bouchard R, Lamontagne A, Bailey P, Bergman H, Ratner J, Tesfaye Y, Saint-Martin M, Bacher Y, Carrier L, Charbonneau R, Clarfield

AM, Collier B, Dastoor D, Gauthier L, Germain M, Kissel C, Krieger M, Kushnir S, Masson H, Morin J, Nair V, Neirinck L, Suissa S. Tetrahydroaminoacridine–lecithin combination treatment in patients with intermediate-stage Alzheimer's disease. N Engl J Med 1990; 322:1272–1276.

127. Penn RD, Martin EM, Wilson RS, Fox JH, Savoy SM. Intraventricular bethanechol infusion for Alzheimer's disease: results of double-blind and escalating dose trials. Neurology 1988; 38:219–222.
128. Hollister LE, Yesavage J. Ergoloid mesylates for senile dementia: unanswered questions. Ann Intern Med 1984; 100:894–898.
129. Waters CH. Nootropics. In: Cummings JL, Miller BL, eds. Alzheimer's disease: treatment and long-term management. New York: Marcel Dekker, 1990:53–68.
130. The Parkinson Study Group. Effect of deprenyl on the progression of disability in early Parkinson's disease. N Engl J Med 1989; 321:1364–1371.

9

Cognitive Dysfunction in Parkinson's Disease and Related Disorders

Christopher F. O'Brien and Ira Shoulson *University of Rochester Medical Center, Rochester, New York*

I. PARKINSON'S DISEASE

A. Clinical Features

Parkinson's disease (PD) is a progressive illness with broad impact on motor function and activities of independent living. Although largely a result of dopaminergic neuron loss, PD is attended by multiple neurochemical abnormalities (1). The consequences are not limited to the classic triad of rigidity, tremor, and bradykinesia described by James Parkinson in 1817 (2). Depression, cognitive decline, and a broader spectrum of movement disorders are now recognized. This disease is not rare; nearly 1 million individuals are affected in North America, a prevalence of 1:300 persons. The average age at onset is about 60 years; however, improved symptomatic treatment has been associated with prolongation of life to nearly normal expectancy. Cognitive impairment and psychiatric disturbances have increasingly become disabling problems, in part related to the increased longevity of patients with PD. In this chapter, we review the neuropsychological impairments of Parkinson's disease and related diseases, their pathophysiology, and their current treatments.

B. Neuropsychological Profile

Early descriptions of PD tended to ignore or minimize cognitive dysfunction as part of the illness (3). Several authors described features consistent with depression and dementia, speculating that these might be a fundamental part of Parkinson's disease. Not until the late 1960s, however, were attempts made to investigate dementia as a separate entity (4). Over the past two decades, both dementia and depression have been documented commonly in PD (5,6).

Cognitive dysfunction has been reported to occur in 4–94% of patients with PD. This wide range in prevalence is a result of differences in cognitive assessment techniques, diagnostic accuracy, and patient selection factors. Few studies have been able to control for age, gender, duration of illness, drug treatment, severity of dementia, and coexistent medical and psychiatric variables. More recent estimates of the prevalence of dementia in PD range between 40 and 60% (7,8). It remains unclear whether dementia is an inevitable consequence of advanced PD. The various types of cognitive impairment may represent distinct neuropathological entities, or they may reflect varied expression of a protean neurodegenerative process.

Three general patterns of cognitive impairment are commonly observed (Table 1). Most often patients with idiopathic (or typical) PD show mild impairment of memory and visuospatial skills, while retaining normal language and analytic abilities. This pattern may develop at any time in the course of illness and usually is not seriously disabling for the patient (9). Another pattern of cognitive impairment in PD disturbs the planning and execution of cognitive operations that are the hallmark of frontal lobe function. These tasks may be referred to as *executive skills,* which encompass the ability to process competing or conflicting information, shift among sets or concepts, and carry out analysis despite ambiguity. This mental flexibility allows planning and execution of complex motor plans. The Stroop (10) Test and Wisconsin Card-Sorting Test (11) (WCST) assess such skills. The Stroop requires subjects to identify words or colors belonging to different sets despite conflicting information. The WCST requires formation, maintenance, and shifting of sets. Altered frontal lobe function in a variety of neurological conditions as well as PD results in decreased performance on these tests

TABLE 1 Patterns of Altered Cognition in Parkinson's Disease

1. Mild impairment of short-term memory and visuospatial skills
2. Abnormal frontal "executive" skills
3. Coexistent with Alzheimer's dementia

(12). The third and most severe dementing process results from the apparent coexistence of PD with a more global and "cortical dementia" of the Alzheimer type (AD) (13). However, the mental operations that are most typically impaired in PD are those of a "subcortical dementia."

The concept of *subcortical dementia* has evolved to describe the type of intellectual failure characteristic of PD, Huntington's disease (HD), progressive supranuclear palsy (PSP), and other conditions in which cortical functions have been relatively spared (14–16). Although imprecise for neuropathological correlates, subcortical dementia is distinguished by slowed central processing, memory deficits, and affective disturbances from the more typical apraxia, aphasia, agnosia, and more global amnesia of AD. This concept may not adequately represent current appreciation of anatomical linkage of cortex and basal ganglia (17).

Testing by the Wechsler Adult Intelligence Scale (WAIS) reveals inconsistent performance deficits when PD patients are compared with controls. The most frequently abnormal subtests include block design, memory, and picture completion (7,18,19). Performance IQ may be impaired in part due to the motor disturbance of PD, since some subtests have time constraints.

Patients with PD often have difficulty with recent memory or with the ability to store and recall newly learned information (20). Immediate recall (e.g., digit span) seems spared in PD, and remote memory (i.e., recalling distant events) seems impaired only in patients who have more global cognitive impairment. Memory in PD patients is very sensitive to proactive interference in recall testing. Presentation of a second task calling upon short-term memory markedly worsens recall on the first task. Early in the course of PD, memory impairment may have little effect on day-to-day function. With progression of PD, memory performance typically deteriorates in proportion to other markers of cognitive decline (e.g., visuospatial skills), but this is not necessarily linked to motor declined (6,9).

It has been suggested that at least two types of learning exist. *Procedural knowledge* refers to the acquisition of a motor skill or cognitive routine in specific settings. Once acquired, problem-solving strategies become more of a habit than memory (21–24). *Declarative knowledge* refers to storage and recall or recognition of visual or verbal material (24). Dysfunction of declarative knowledge is associated with "pure" amnestic disorders such as Korsakoff's syndrome and the broader problems of AD. Procedural knowledge is most impaired in PD, even when allowances are made for slowed movement. The learning problems are felt to reflect difficulty in acquiring and executing motor sequences as automatic cognitive sequences.

Language function is usually preserved in PD. Naming, comprehension, and repetition are similar to age-matched control subjects (25). Verbal fluency, as measured by number of items generated in word categories, often decreases in proportion to bradykinesia. Most disturbances of speech, such as palilalia, occur independently of other language operations. When paraphasic errors or problem with comprehension emerge, concomitant AD or focal vascular lesions may be present.

Visuospatial skills are frequently abnormal in PD (7,19,20,26,27). Poor performance on block design, Raven's Progressive Matrices, figure ground discrimination, and other measures of visuospatial abilities may not be solely due to spatial problems. Faulty executive function appears responsible for some visuospatial problems when timed response is not a limiting factor.

Patients with PD perform poorly on a variety of attentional tasks that are dependent on reaction time (28). Correction for movement time reveals persistent deficits, possibly attributable to delays in motor preparation. Since planning and execution of automatic motor and cognitive sequences are impaired in PD, executive function abnormalities may be responsible for apparent attentional deficits.

Three types of perseveration have been defined operationally by Sanson and Albert (29). *Recurrent perseveration* represents recurrence of a previous response to a subsequent stimulus within the context of an established set. *Stuck-in-set perseveration* refers to inappropriate maintenance of a category or framework of activity. *Continuous perseveration* reflects abnormal prolongation or continuation without cessation of a current behavior. Patients with PD may show stuck-in-set perseveration, possibly owing to disturbance of mesolimbic dopaminergic projections to the frontal lobes.

A compounding effect of age has been noted in PD patients with dementia. Dubois and colleagues studied PD patients with onset before 45 years and compared them to PD patients with onset after 65 years, matched for disease severity and duration (30). The young-onset patients had minor cognitive changes, as found in earlier studies (e.g., memory only), whereas the older-onset patients had more global dysfunction, particularly for frontal, "executive" tasks. They postulate that this older group lacks the cognitive capacity required to compensate for the PD-imposed deficits. Such compensation may be provided by nondopaminergic systems (e.g., acetylcholine or norepinephrine).

Slowing of cognition, whether seen with impaired sequencing, reaction time, prolongation, or stuck-in-set perseveration, may be viewed as more discrete components of the older concept of bradyphrenia. Bradyphrenia was used originally to represent a cognitive analogue to the bradykinesia of PD. Given the emerging knowledge of neuroanatomical substraits (e.g., complex loops from frontal cortex to caudate and thalamus to supplemental motor area) (17), bradyphrenia is inadequate for describing the spectrum of cognitive impairments in PD.

C. Pathophysiology

From an anatomical perspective, the dementia of PD reflects at least three patterns of pathology (Table 2). Idiopathic or typical PD corresponds to a predominant degeneration of neurons in the substantia nigra (SN), with subsequent reductions of dopamine in the SN and its projection sites (e.g., striatal, limbic) and hypothalamic regions. Lewy bodies are found in the degenerated SN, thalamus, locus coeruleus, hypothalamus, and temporal lobes (31). Although dementia has been described in the setting of isolated SN degeneration (32), it is usually attended by more widespread neuropathological abnormalities. The second anatomical category of PD dementia results when neurofibrillary tangles (NFT) and neuritic plaques (NP) of AD coexist with nigrostriatal pathology (33). The distribution of NFT and NP are variable in PD patients. Precise clinical criteria defining coexistent PD and AD are lacking. The third category involves PD pathology in association with multiple cerebral infarctions, usually involving small vessels. The clinician is frequently faced with the evaluation of a patient whose cognitive decline occurs in the setting of multiple white matter lesions detected by computed tomography (CT) or magnetic resonance imaging (MRI). The origin of these subcortical changes on neuroimaging may well reflect small-vessel ischemic disease (SVID).

Support for the concept that certain cognitive operations depend on dopaminergic neurotransmission has been proven from observations of methylphenyltetrahydropyridine (MPTP)-induced neurotoxicity. Stern and colleagues studied six individuals who had been exposed to relatively low levels of MPTP, but had not developed the motor features of PD (34). Positron emission tomography (PET) demonstrated reduced uptake of labeled 6-fluorodopa in their striatal regions, compared with healthy individuals. Neuropsychologic performance in these motorically normal individuals was similar to patients with manifest MPTP-induced PD. The authors argue that cognitive impairment may develop at a lower level of dopamine depletion than is required for onset of motor signs. The pattern of deficits was consistent with their proposed model that the corticostriatal system aids in planning and modulating ongoing activity in the absence of external guidance of automatic learning. It will be of interest to follow these

TABLE 2 Pathology of PD Dementia

1. Isolated degeneration of substantia nigra with Lewy bodies
2. PD with NFT and NP of Alzheimer's disease
3. PD with multiple small vessel infarctions

presymptomatic individuals to determine the pattern and extent of deterioration and dopaminergic responsiveness.

A simple model of dopamine deficiency producing cognitive dysfunction is probably overly simplistic. Several studies have indicated that bradykinesia, the hallmark of dopamine deficiency, is not statistically correlated with impairment on subtests of cognitive performance. Levin et al. note that only 2 of their 17 cognitive measures were correlated to motor impairment (19). They speculate that other neurotransmitter systems, (e.g., cholinergic, noradrenergic, and serotonergic) may be involved. Alternatively, the nigrostriatal, mesolimbic, and mesocortical systems may be influenced differentially by the effects of dopamine depletion (35,36). For example, the mesolimbic dopamine supply comes from the ventral tegmental area (VTA) (37). Loss of dopaminergic neurons in the VTA occurs in PD, but this is not tightly linked to the nearby SN dopaminergic neuronal loss. Relative sparing or depletion of VTA dopaminergic neurons may result in variable degrees of cognitive or affective problems.

Cholinergic deficiency may contribute to dementia in PD. Variably reduced levels of choline acetyltransferase (ChAcT) in the nucleus basalis and cortex have been reported in PD patients with dementia (38,39). When cholinergic deficits are superimposed upon DA deficiency, cognitive dysfunction is presumed to be more severe.

Noradrenergic deficiency has been linked to locus coeruleus lesions in PD dementia (40,41). The NE content in the locus coeruleus is subnormal in brains from PD patients who were demented, but normal in those without dementia (40). Decreased NE levels can be due to primary noradrenergic cell loss (with associated Lewy body formation) or may occur indirectly as noradrenergic activity is partially dependent upon adequate DA levels.

Commonly used antiparkinsonian therapies can improve or worsen cognitive performance (42). Replacement therapy with levodopa can improve performance on memory tasks, although this may be state-dependent. Patients treated with levodopa during both learning and recall did better than those receiving levodopa during only learning or only recall (43). Excess dopaminergic stimulation can produce psychiatric and attentional problems that interfere with a variety of neuropsychological variables. Anticholinergics generally worsen cognition in PD patients, as they do in normal individuals and patients with AD (44).

1. Electrophysiological Studies

Three electrophysiological methods have been applied to the study of dementia in PD; electroencephalography (EEG), evoked potentials (EP), and movement-related potentials (MRP). Although not usually helpful in making clinical decisions, these techniques have aided our general understanding of PD.

Routine EEG is abnormal in approximately 40% of unselected populations of PD patients, a prevalence higher than in unaffected aged individuals (45). The abnormalities consist most often of slowing of background activity, increased theta and delta patterns, and occasional intermittent focal slowing. The EEG slowing, both focal and diffuse, increases with advancing disease, especially with coexistent dementia (46). This slowing appears unrelated to drug effects, and levodopa, dopamine agonists, and anticholinergics may actually improve abnormally slow tracings. Although abnormal EEGs are more common among PD patients with dementia, specific EEG patterns do not distinguish discrete types of cognitive impairment.

Evoked potential studies in PD generally show normal early conduction velocity and wave morphology, especially brain stem auditory-evoked responses (BAER) and visual-evoked responses (VER). Dopaminergic medications may occasionally normalize preexisting VER abnormalities. Particular interest in EP stems from abnormalities found with late potentials, particularly the P_3 component. This positive wave occurs approximately 300 msec after novel stimuli when repeated trials are averaged. Demented patients with PD often have prolongation of the P_3 (47). This finding is not specific to PD and occurs with AD aand other dementias.

Movement-related potentials (MRP) comprise a large array of investigative techniques correlating averaged scalp potentials with various motor tasks. In general, these methods reveal slowing or cortical activity associated with movement initiation in PD patients and corresponding asymmetries of abnormalities in hemiparkinsonian patients (48–50). Dopaminergic medications may normalize the MRP (51).

2. *Neuroimaging*

Specific radiographical markers for cognitive decline in PD have been sought using CT, MRI, and PET. Computed tomography does not distinguish the various PD–dementia subtypes, nor even PD from AD in early disease stages. Later stages of PD may have disproportionate subcortical atrophy on CT or MR images. Some PD variants (e.g., progressive supranuclear palsy and olivoponto cerebellar atrophy) may be distinguishable radiographically by MRI. Decreased signal intensity is found in the basal ganglia on T_2-weighted MR images. These changes correlate with increased iron content in the affected region and are due to the paramagnetic effect of the metal. These findings have been used to differentiate PD from other parkinsonian states (52). Correlation between MRI abnormalities and histopathology has been reported for two such states—Hallervorden–Spatz

(53) disease and striatonigral degeneration (54). The relationship of other common radiographic findings in this aged group (e.g., multiple small areas of increased signal on T_2-weighted MRI images or generalized atrophy on CT) to cognition in PD is not defined.

The use of PET imaging reveals the underlying DA deficiency in the SN and striatum when labeled fluorodopa, a presynatpic marker of nigrostriatal neurotransmission, is used (55). Fluorodeoxyglucose, a glycolytic marker, reveals hypometabolism of the frontal cortex and striatum consistent with the proposed model linking cognitive operations in the striatum and frontal cortex. Clinical application of these techniques awaits definition.

D. Affective Disorders

Between 20 and 50% of PD patients are affected by depression (56–58). Gotham and coauthors presented data comparing PD patients with age-matched controls and individuals with chronic arthritis (59). Moderate to severe depression (as measured by the Beck Depression Inventory) was present in 29% of the PD group, 30% of the arthritis group, and 6% of the controls. Self-rated performance on the activities-of-daily-living scale correlated best with depression in PD and arthritis groups. This study differs from previous studies in that parkinsonians were not more depressed than the chronically ill, as reported by others (60).

Depression occurs both early and late in the course of PD, and it may antedate the onset of motor impairment (57). Starkstein et al. reported an association between severity of cognitive impairment and depression in patients whose onset of PD was 55 years or less, in contrast with patients with onset older than 55 years in whom depression was associated with decline in activities of daily living (ADL) (56). Gibb and Lees report a similar prevalence of depression among young-onset (median, 38 years) and older-onset (73 years) PD patients when early severe dementia was excluded (61).

Asymmetric involvement of cortical and subcortical structures in hemiparkinsonian patients may correlate with distinct affective and cognitive disturbances. In one study, patients with predominately left nigrostriatal disease (postulated on the basis of right hemiparkinsonism) have a higher frequency of depression, compared with those with right hemisphere involvement) (56). Others report no such correlation (62).

Neurochemical investigations of depressed PD patients reveal abnormalities in dopamine, norepinephrine, and serotonin systems. Dopamine deficiency and low homovanillic acid (HVA) levels, although correlating with some motoric deficits of PD, do not reliably account for differences in depressed and nondepressed PD patients (41,57). The mesolimbic and mesocortical dopamine projections from cell beds in the ventral tegmental area may play an important role in affective disturbances (63).

Cerebrospinal fluid (CSF) concentrations of serotonin (5-HT) and its metabolite, 5-hydroxyindoleactic acid (5-HIAA) are reduced in depressed PD patients (64). They are also diminished in PD patients with other psychiatric symptoms, especially hallucinations. Not all studies reveal these CSF abnormalities (41). Although major methodological problems remain, a link between low serotonin levels and depression may allow more precise treatment strategies.

Norepinephrine and its metabolite 3-methoxy-4-hydroxyphenylglycoaldehyde are reduced in demented PD patients (40). This deficit, linked to lesions in the locus coeruleus, has been proposed as one explanation for intellectual impairment in PD. Noradrenergic deficiencies have been described in depressed patients without PD and provides a theoretical basis for treatment with tricyclic antidepressants and monoamine oxidase (MAO) inhibitors. It is not clear whether distinct features of depression or dementia in PD can be specifically attributed to NE and 5-HT deficiencies.

Depression may mimic cognitive impairment, resulting in a "pseudodementia" that is ameliorated with appropriate antidepressant therapies. Treatment of depression can lead to marked improvement in daily function. Treatment strategies must take into account psychosocial factors, PD severity, treatment side effects, and drug interactions. Underlying causes of depression must be considered. For example, neuropsychological impairment with depression can be seen with hypothyroidism or vitamin B_{12} deficiency, two conditions that occur commonly in the older-aged group. The possibility of drug-induced depression (e.g., caused by benzodiazepines or beta-blockers) should be explored. If antidepressant medications are to be used, the optimal neurochemical profile should be considered. Significant benefits accrue from even low doses of tricyclic antidepressants, the anticholinergic "side effects" of which may actually be useful in ameliorating tremor. The modest sedation of amitriptyline (10–50 mg at bedtime) may reduce insomnia. Nortriptyline (10–25 mg twice daily) may produce a daytime stimulator effect. Emphasis must be placed on careful monitoring of drug response. The PD patients are susceptible to anticholinergic-induced delirium, urinary retention, and of course, orthostatic hypotension. Antidepressant drugs that predominantly affect serotonergic mechanisms, such as fluoxetine, have not yet been systematically evaluated in PD.

Electroconvulsive therapy (ECT) may be an effective treatment for refractory or psychotic depression; it also exerts short-term antiparkinsonian benefits (65). The mechanism for this improvement presumably derives from mobilization of dopamine and increased sensitization of dopamine receptors. Although prolonged benefit has been reported, a gradual return to pre-ECT motor function usually occurs after weeks or months. Dopaminergic medications may require reduction during and immediately following ECT to minimize dyskinesais and other features of heightened dopamine responsiveness.

Psychosis may occur in parkinsonian patients. Drug-induced hallucinations, delusions, and paranoid ideation have been associated with dopaminergic therapies, including levodopa, dopamine agonists, and MAO inhibitors (66). Delirium and hallucinations are also associated with anticholinergic medications (67). Levodopa-induced hallucinations are well documented; they can be quite vivid and may occur in patients without obvious dementia. Levodopa-induced hallucinations may be seen more frequently in patients with prior psychiatric problems. Overactivity of mesolimbic dopamine has been implicated in schizophrenia and psychosis, giving support to a neurochemical basis for psychosis in PD. Hallucinosis usually resolves with reductions in levodopa or other dopaminergic agents.

On balance, it appears that depression in PD is common, potentially disabling, and often responsive to therapy. The etiology is complex, comprising reactive and endogenous factors. Clearly, affected individuals are "at-risk" for depression given the neurochemical deficiencies and the progression of their physical disability.

II. AKINETIC RIGID SYNDROMES

The more commonly recognized atypical forms of parkinsonism are listed in Table 3. These disorders represent a broad variety of pathological changes within the basal ganglia, brain stem, and subcortical projection systems. Postsynaptic dopaminergic neurons are involved, along with the presynaptic nigral neurons. Most of the syndromes are associated with

TABLE 3 Most Commonly Recognized Atypical Forms of Parkinsonism

Multisystem atrophy
Striatonigral degeneration (SND)
Shy-Drager syndrome
Olivopontocerebellar atrophy (OPCA)
Progressive supranuclear palsy (PSP)
Multiinfarct state
Corticobasal degeneration (CBD)
Diffuse Lewy body disease (DLBD)
Postinfectious parkinsonism

some degree of cognitive dysfunction, although no consensus exists on whether there is a unique dementia for each illness.

Progressive supranuclear palsy (PSP) is clinically defined as an akinetic rigid syndrome associated with limitations in vertical gaze, particularly downward. Neuronal loss and gliosis are found in the SN, globus pallidus, subthalamic nuclei, locus coeruleus, and periaqueductal gray matter (68). Many PSP patients show apparent difficulty with cognition; however, dementia may be overestimated owing to bradykinesia and slowed oculomotor functions. Attempts to define a deficit in central-processing time, while correcting for motor components, was carried out by Dubois et al. (69). They concluded that cognitive slowing was related to insufficient activation of the frontal lobes by the striatum. That this "frontal deafferentation" is truly unique to PSP is unlikely given similar striatal to frontal disruptions implicated in Huntington's disease, among others.

The dementia–parkinsonism–amyotrophic lateral sclerosis complex has been described in people from Guam and elsewhere (70,71). Dementia may be an early manifestation. A PET scan reveals hypometabolism in the frontal lobes. Neuropathological change consists of widespread NFT in subcortical and nigral areas. The NFT appear immunocytologically similar to those found in AD (72). The exact mechanism of this neurodegenerative process is unknown.

Akinetic–rigid patients with widespread autonomic dysfunction (e.g., orthostatic hypotension, bladder incontinence) fall under the heading of multisystem atrophies (MSA) (73). The Shy–Drager variant is included. Striatonigral degeneration (SND) and the olivopontocerebellar atrophies (OPCA) are also types of MSA. Striatonigral degeneration is a prototypic postsynatpic striatal condition. The OPCAs show a mixture of pathological changes in brain stem, cerebellum, and cortices. Multisystem atrophy has been reviewed recently by Quinn, who concludes that dementia is not an integral feature (74). Although inappropriate laughter or crying may occur in MSA, clearcut dementia is suggestive of an alternative diagnosis, such as diffuse Lewy body disease (see following discussion).

Corticobasal degeneration (CBD) is an uncommon, but disabling problem. Clinical and pathological descriptions were first provided in 1968 by Rebeiz and associates (75). Since then, a variety of names for this or similar conditions have emerged including "corticodentatonigral degeneration with neuronal achromasia," "corticobasal ganglionic degeneration," and "corticobasal degeneration" (76). Patients manifest focal or asymmetric features of apraxia, rigidity, bradykinesia, limb dystonia, and corticosensory deficit, in association with gait instability. The apraxia, dystonia, and corticosensory deficit may produce a striking "alien limb" phenomena.

TABLE 4 Differential Diagnosis of Cognitive Decline in PD

Depression
Drug-induced (e.g., benzodiazepines, anticholinergics, beta-blockers)
Concurrent neurodegenerative processes (e.g., Alzheimer's)
Atypical PD (e.g., DLBD)
Systemic metabolic abnormality (e.g., hypothyroidism)
Multi-infarct state
Cognitive decline secondary to PD

Onset is nearly always unilateral, and the asymmetry of dysfunction persists throughout most of the course of the illness. Diagnosis is based on clinical characterization, although MRI may reveal hemispheric atrophy, particularly in the parietal region contralateral to the affected limb. Treatment with dopaminergic medications, tricyclic antidepressants, anticholinergics, and benzodiazepines alone or in combination has produced limited benefit.

Diffuse Lewy body disease (DLBD) is more distinct pathologically than clinically. Burkhart and colleagues, who reviewed 34 postmortem cases, found that 82% presented clinically with a neurobehavior syndrome (77). Memory impairment progressed relentlessly to dementia, with rigidity and psychosis frequently present. Men were affected twice as often as women, and the average age at onset was between 50 and 80 years of age. Lewy bodies, the hallmark of idiopathic PD were more widespread in DLBD with involvement in cortical, limbic, hypothalamic, and brain stem regions. No specific therapies have been of benefit in DLBD.

III. DIFFERENTIAL DIAGNOSIS AND RESEARCH GOALS

Table 4 outlines the differential diagnosis of cognitive decline in the setting of PD. The goals of future research in PD and cognition are many: 1. Clinicians must be provided with accurate prognostic indicators for patients and families. 2. Specific neuroanatomical and neurochemical substrates of dementia and depression in PD require identification. 3. The apparent subtypes of PD–dementia require more precise definition. 4. New promising therapies (78) must be examined as they influence neuropsychological function. 5. Ultimately, prevention of cognitive decline may be possible.

ACKNOWLEDGMENT

Supported by a Veola S. Kerr Fellowship from the Parkinson's Disease Foundation, New York (CFO) and United States Public Health Service (USPHS) Grant NS-24778.

REFERENCES

1. Agid Y, Cervera P, Hirsch E, Javoy-Agid F, Lehericy S, Raisman R, Ruberg M. Biochemistry of Parkinson's disease 28 years later: a critical review. Mov Disord 1989; 4(Suppl 1):S126–144.
2. Parkinson J. An essay on the shaking palsy. London: Sherwood, Neely and Jones, 1817.
3. Hoehn MM, Yahr MD. Parkinsonism: onset, progression and mortality. Neurology 1967; 17:427–442.
4. Pollock M, Hornabrook RW. The prevalence, natural history and dementia of Parkinson's disease. Brain 1966; 89:429–448.
5. Mjones H. Paralysis agitans, a clinical and genetic study. Acta Psychol Neurol 1949; Suppl 54:1–195.
6. Pirozzolo FJ, Hnasch ED, Mortimer JA, Webster DD, Kuskowski MI. Dementia in Parkinson's disease: a neuropsychological analysis. Brain Cogn 1982; 1:71–83.
7. Lichter DG, Corbett AJ, Fitzgibbon GM, Davidson OR, Ayton Hope JK, Goddard GV, Sharples KJ, Pollock M. Cognitive and motor dysfunction in Parkinson's disease: clinical, performance and computed tomographic correlations. Arch Neurol 1988; 45:854–860.
8. Portin R, Rinne UK. Predictive factors for cognitive deterioration and dementia in Parkinson's disease. Adv Neuro 1986; 45:413–416.
9. Hietanen M, Teravainen H. Cognitive performance in early Parkinson's disease. Acta Neurol Scand 1986; 73:151–159.
10. Stroop JR. Studies of interference in serial verbal reactions. J Exp Psychol 1935; 18:643–662.
11. Grant DA, Berg EA. A behavioral analysis of degree of reinforcement and ease of shifting to new responses in a Weigl-type card-sorting problem. J Exp Psychol 1948; 38:401–411.
12. Taylor AE, Saint-Cyr JA, Lang AE. Frontal lobe dysfunction in Parkinson's disease. Brain 1986; 109:845–883.
13. Yoshimura M. Pathological basis for dementia in elderly patients with idiopathic Parkinson's disease. Eur Neurol 1988; 28(suppl):29–35.
14. McHugh PR, Folstein MF. Psychiatric syndromes of Huntington's chorea: a clinical and phenomenologic study. In: Benson DF, Blummer D, eds. Psychiatric aspects of neurologic disease. New York: Grune & Stratton, 1975: 267–286.
15. Mayeux R, Stern Y, Rosen J, Benson DF. Is "subcortical dementia" a recognizable clinical entity? Ann Neurol 1983; 14:278–283.
16. Whitehouse PJ. The concept of subcortical and cortical dementia: another look. Ann Neurol 1986; 19:1–6.
17. Albin RL, Young AB, Penney JB. The functional anatomy of basal ganglia disorders. Trends Neurosci 1989; 12:366–375.
18. Girotti F, Soliveri P, Carella F, Geminiani G, Aiello G, Caraceni T. Role of motor performance in cognitive processes in parkinsonian patients. Neurology 1988; 38:537–540.

19. Levin BE, Llabre MM, Weiner WJ. Cognitive impairments associated with early Parkinson's disease. Neurology 1989; 39:557–561.
20. Huber SJ, Shuttleworth EC, Paulson GW. Dementia in Parkinson's disease. Arch Neurol 1986; 43:987–990.
21. Saint-Cyr JA, Taylor AE, Lang AE. Procedural learning and neostriatal dysfunction in man. Brain 1988; 111:941–959.
22. Mishkin M, Malmut B, Bachevalier J. Memories and habits: two neural systems. In: Lynch G, McGaugh JL, Weinberger NM, eds. Neurobiology of learning and memory. New York: Guilford Press, 1984:65–77.
23. Cohen NJ, Squire LR. Preserved learning and retention of pattern-analyzing skill in amnesia: dissociation of knowing how and knowing that. Science 1980; 210:207–210.
24. Squire LR. Mechanisms of memory. Science 1986; 232:1612–1619.
25. Cummings JL, Darkins A, Mendez M, Hill MA, Benson DF. Alzheimer's disease and Parkinson's disease: comparison of speech and language alterations. Neurology 1988; 38:680–684.
26. Huber SJ, Shuttleworth EC, Freidenberg DL. Neuropsychological differences between the dementias of Alzheimer's and Parkinson's diseases. Arch Neurol 1989; 46:1287–1291.
27. Stern Y, Mayeux R. Intellectual impairment in Parkinson's disease. Adv Neurol 1986; 45:405–408.
28. Girotti F, Grassi MP, Carella F, Soliveri P, Musicco M, Lamerti E, Caraceni T. Possible involvement of attention processes in Parkinson's disease. Adv Neurol 1986; 45:425–429.
29. Sandson J, Albert ML. Perseveration in behavioral neurology. Neurology 1987; 37:1736–1741.
30. Dubois B, Pillon B, Sternic N, Lhermitte F, Agid Y. Age-induced cognitive disturbances in Parkinson's disease. Neurology 1990; 40:38–41.
31. Gibb WR. The pathology of Parkinsonian disorders. In: Quinn NP, Jenner PG, eds. Disorders of movement. London: Academic Press, 1989.
32. Oyanagi K, Nakashima S, Ikuta F. An autopsy case of dementia and parkinsonism with severe degeneration exclusively in the substantia nigra. Acta Neuropathol 1986; 70:190–192.
33. de la Monte SM, Wells SE, Hedley-Whyte ET, Growdon JH. Neuropathologic distinction between Parkinson's dementia and Parkinson's plus Alzheimer's disease. Ann Neurol 1989; 26:309–320.
34. Stern Y, Tetrud JW, Martin WRW, et al. Cognitive change following MPTP exposure. Neurology 1990; 40:261–264.
35. Eggertson DE, Sima AAF. Dementia with cerebral Lewy bodies: a mesocortical dopaminergic defect? Arch Neurol 1986; 43:524–527.
36. Rinne JO, Rummukainen J, Palijarvi L, Rinne UK. Dementia in Parkinson's disease is related to neuronal loss in the medial substantia nigra. Ann Neurol 1989; 26:47–50.
37. Bjorkland A, Lindvall O. Dopamine containing systems in the CNS. In: Bjorkland A, Hokfelt T, eds. Handbook of chemical neuroanatomy, vol. 2: classical transmitters in the CNS, Part 1. Amsterdam: Elsevier, 1984:55–122.

38. Dubois B, Ruberg M, Javoy-Agiel F, Ploska A, Agid Y. A subcorticocortical cholinergic system is affected in Parkinson's disease. Brain 1983; 288:213–218.
39. Perry EK, Curtis M, Dick DJ, Candy JM, Atack JR, Bloxham CA, Blessed G, Fairbairn A, Tomlinson BE, Perry RH. Cholinergic correlates of cognitive impairment in Parkinson's disease: comparisons with Alzheimer's disease. J Neurol Neurosurg Psychiatry 1985; 48:413–421.
40. Cash R, Dennis T, L'Heureus R, Raisman R, Javoy-Agid F, Scatton B. Parkinson's disease and dementia: norepinephrine and dopamine in locus ceruleus. Neurology 1987; 37:42–46.
41. Zubenko GS, Moossy J, Kopp U. Neurochemical correlates of major depression in primary dementia. Arch Neurol 1990; 47:209–214.
42. Gotham AM, Brown RG, Marsden CD. "Frontal" cognitive function in patients with Parkinson's disease "on" and "off" levodopa. Brain 1988; 111:299–321.
43. Huber SJ, Shulman HG, Paulson GW, Shuttleworth EC. Dose-dependent memory impairment in Parkinson's disease. Neurology 1989; 39:438–440.
44. Dubois B, Danze F, Pillon B, Cusimano G, Lhermitte F, Agid Y. Cholinergic-dependent cognitive deficits in Parkinson's disease. Ann Neurol 1987; 22:26–30.
45. Sirakov AA, Mezan IS. EEG findings in parkinsonism. Electroencephalogr Clin Neurophysiol 1963; 15:321.
46. Nufeld MY, Inzelberg R, Korczyn AD. EEG in demented and non-demented parkinsonian patients. Acta Neurol Scand 1988; 78:1–5.
47. Goodin DS, Aminoff MJ. Electrophysiological differences between demented and nondemented patients with Parkinson's disease. Ann Neurol 1987; 21:90–94.
48. Deecke L, Englitz HG, Kornhuber HH, Schmitt G. Cerebral potentials preceding voluntary movement in patients with bilateral or unilateral Parkinson akinesia. Prog Clin Neurophysiol 1977; 1:151–163.
49. Simpson JA, Khuraibet AJ. Readiness potential of cortical area 6 preceding self paced movement in Parkinson's disease. J Neurol Neurosurg Psychiatry 1987; 50:1184–1191.
50. Barrett G, Shibasaki H, Neshige R. Cortical potential shifts preceding voluntary movement are normal in parkinsonism. Electroencephalogr Clin Neurophysiol 1986; 63:340–348.
51. Dick JPR, Cantello R, Buruma O, Gioux M, Benecke R, Day BL, Rothwell JC, Thompson PD, Marsden CD. The bereitschaftspotential, *l*-dopa and Parkinson's disease. Electroencephalogr Clin Neurophysiol 1987; 66:263–274.
52. Rutledge JN. Magnetic resonance of movement disorders. In: Jankovic J, Tolosa E, eds. Parkinson's disease and movement disorders. Baltimore: Urban & Schwarzenbert, 1988:441–459.
53. Schaffert DA, Johnsen SD, Johnson PC, Drayer BP. Magnetic resonance imaging in pathologically proven Hallervorden–Spatz disease. Neurology 1989; 39:440–442.
54. O'Brien C, Sung JH, McGeachie RE, Lee MC. Striatonigral degeneration: clinical, MRI, and pathologic correlation. Neurology 1990; 40:710–711.

55. Leenders KL. The neurochemistry of Parkinson's disease as revealed by PET scanning. In: Quinn NP, Jenner PG, eds. Disorders of movement. London: Academic Press 1989:115–124.
56. Starkstein SE, Preziosi TJ, Bolduc PL, Robinson RG. Depression in Parkinson's disease. J Nerv Ment Dis 1990; 178:27–31.
57. Sano M, Stern Y, Williams J, Cote L, Rosenstein R, Mayeux R. Coexisting dementia and depression in Parkinson's disease. Arch Neurol 1989; 46:1284–1286.
58. Mayeux R, Stern Y, Rosen J, Leventhal J. Depression, intellectual impairment, and Parkinson's disease. Neurology 1981; 31:645–650.
59. Gotham AM, Brown RG, Marsden CD. Depression in Parkinson's disease: a quantitative and qualitative analysis. J Neurol Neurosurg Psychiatry 1986; 49:381–389.
60. Robins AH. Depression in patients with parkinsonism. Br J Psychiatry 1976; 128:141–145.
61. Gibbs WR, Lees AJ. A comparison of clinical and pathologic features of young- and old-onset Parkinson's disease. Neurology 1988; 38:1402–1406.
62. Direnfeld LK, Albert ML, Volicer L, Langlais PJ, Marquis J, Kaplan E. Parkinson's disease. The possible relationship of laterality to dementia and neurochemical findings. Arch Neurol 1984; 41:935–941.
63. Javoy-Agid F, Agid Y. Is the mesocortical dopaminergic system involved in Parkinson's disease? Neurology 1980; 30:1326–1330.
64. Mayeux R, Stern Y, Sano M, Williams JBW, Cote LJ. The relationship of serotonin to depression in Parkinson's disease. Mov Disord 1988; 3:237–244.
65. Douyon R, Serby M, Klutchko B, Rotrosen J. ECT and Parkinson's disease revisited: a "naturalistic" study. Am J Psychiatry 1989; 146:1451–1455.
66. Nausieda PA, Glanta R, Weber S, Baum R, Klawans HL. Psychiatric complications of levodopa therapy of Parkinson's disease. In: Hassler R, Christ J, eds. Adv Neurol 1984; 40:271–277.
67. DeSmet Y, Ruberg M, Serdaru M, Dubois B, Lhermitte F, Agid Y. Confusion, dementia and anticholinergics in Parkinson's disease. J Neurol Neurosurg Psychiatry 1982; 45:1161–1164.
68. Golbe L, Davis P. Progressive supranuclear palsy. In: Jankovic J, Tolosa E, eds. Parkinson's disease and movement disorders. Baltimore: Urban & Schwarzenberg, 1988:121–130.
69. Dubois B, Pillon B, Lagault F, Agid Y, Lhermitte F. Slowing of cognitive processing in progressive supranuclear palsy. Arch Neurol 1988; 45:1194–1199.
70. Rodgers-Johnson P, Garruto RM, Yanagihara R, Chen KM, Gajdusek DC, Gibbs CJ. Amyotrophic lateral sclerosis and parkinsonism–dementia on Guam: a 30-year evaluation of clinical and neuropathologic trends. Neurology 1986; 36:7–13.
71. Schmitt HP, Emser W, Heimes C. Familial occurrence of amyotrophic lateral sclerosis, parkinsonism and dementia. Ann Neurol 1984; 16:642–648.
72. Shankar S, Yanagihara R, Garruto RM, Grundke-Iqbal I, Kosik KS, Gajdusek DC. Immunocytochemical characterization of neurofibrillary tangles in

amyotrophic lateral sclerosis and parkinsonism–dementia of Guam. Ann Neurol 1989; 25:146–151.
73. Polinsky RJ. Multiple system atrophy: clinical aspects, pathophysiology, and treatment. Neurol Clin 1984; 2:487–498.
74. Quinn N. Multiple system atrophy—the nature of the beast. J Neurol Neurosurg Psychiatry 1989; 52:78–89.
75. Rebeiz J, Kolodny E, Richardson E. Corticodentatonigral degeneration with neuronal achronasia. Arch Neurol 1968; 18:20–33.
76. Gibb WRG, Luthert PJ, Marsden CD. Corticobasal degeneration. Brain 1989; 112:1171–1192.
77. Burkhardt CR, Filley CM, Kleinschmidt-DeMasters BK, et al. Diffuse Lewy body disease and progressive dementia. Neurology 1988; 38:1520–1528.
78. Parkinson Study Group. Effect of deprenyl on the progression of disability in early Parkinson's disease. N Engl J Med 1989; 321:1364–1371.

10

Vascular Dementias

G. Webster Ross and Jeffrey L. Cummings *West Los Angeles Veterans Affairs Medical Center and UCLA School of Medicine, Los Angeles, California*

Cerebrovascular disease is a common cause of disability in the elderly. Although the annual incidence of stroke has decreased since 1945, the American Heart Association estimates that there are 500,000 new stroke victims each year (1). Cognitive impairment frequently results from stroke, and cerebrovascular disease may lead to a dementia syndrome. Cerebrovascular dementia (CVD) is associated with a stepwise deteriorating course, patchy distribution of deficits, focal neurological signs and symptoms, and evidence from history, physical examination, or laboratory tests of cerebrovascular disease (2). This disease is the second most common cause of dementia in the elderly and is responsible for approximately half of acute hospitalizations for dementia (3). This chapter addresses the classification, clinical and diagnostic attributes, pathophysiology, and treatment of CVD. In addition, therapeutic strategies directed toward arresting disease progression and ameliorating associated behavioral disturbances are discussed.

I. DEMOGRAPHY

The annual incidence of stroke in the United States is approximately 89 cases per 100,000 population (4). Stroke risk is markedly age-related: between ages 65 and 74 the incidence is 510 cases per 100,000, and from ages 75 to 84, the incidence increases to 957 cases. Approximately 25% of patients with stroke will develop CVD, and the prevalence of CVD may be as high as 70–80% among patients with lacunar state (5,6).

The exact prevalence of CVD is difficult to ascertain owing to variations in the definition of dementia and in the design of epidemiological studies. In a community study of 8000 Finnish patients, Sulkava and associates (7) found the prevalence of severe CVD in the population over 30 years of age to be 0.7%. This rose to 2.7% in the population over aged 65. Alzheimer's disease (AD) accounted for 50% of persons with dementia in the study, whereas CVD and combined dementia (CVD plus AD) constituted 39%. Other studies have also shown CVD to be the second most common cause of dementia with relative prevalence figures, ranging from 8 to 34% of cases (6).

The mean age of diagnosis of patients with CVD is usually younger than that of AD, 74 years and 79 years, respectively (7). Cerebrovascular disease is slightly more common in men than in women (5). The 50% survival duration from onset of CVD is 5–7 years compared with 6–8 years for AD (6,9). Death of patients with CVD is most often due to pneumonia, recurrent stroke, or myocardial infarction (8,10).

II. CLASSIFICATION

Cerebrovascular disease is a heterogeneous disorder that may be classified by anatomical location of strokes, clinical syndrome, or etiology. In most cases, CVD is a product of thromboembolic vascular occlusion, although intracerebral hemorrhage may also cause intellectual impairment. In thromboembolic disorders, the anatomical distribution of strokes and the pattern of neurobehavioral deficits are determined by the vessels that are occluded (Table 1). Cortical infarctions result from atherosclerotic thrombosis or embolic occlusion of the anterior, middle, or posterior cerebral arteries. Thrombosis may be a consequence of atherosclerosis, hypercoaguable states, hematological disorders, or inflammatory vascular diseases, such as temporal arteritis. Emboli may arise from the heart in patients with cardiac rhythm disturbances (especially atrial fibrillation), valvular heart disease, cardiomyopathy, or atrial myxoma. Ulcerated atherosclerotic plaques located in the carotid or vertebral arteries are also a common source of cerebral emboli.

Lacunar infarctions are small areas of ischemic damage that involve the subcortical brain regions including the basal ganglia, thalamus, internal capsule, and subcortical white matter. Lacunes are 2–15 mm in diameter and result from occlusion of small penetrating lenticulostriate branches of the an-

TABLE 1 Classification of Vascular Dementia Syndromes

Syndrome	Typical location of infarctions	Vessels involved	Pathogenesis
Lacunar state	Basal ganglia, internal capsule, thalamus	Deep lenticulostriate branches of middle cerebral and thalamoperforant branches of posterior cerebral arteries	Vascular microatheroma, fibrosis, and lipohyalinosis
Binswanger's disease	Subcortical white matter	Deep penetrating arteries and arterioles	Lipohyalinosis and fibrosis of vessels, ischemic demyelination of periventricular white matter
Large vessel	Vascular borderzone regions	Carotid arteries	Hypotension, carotid occlusion
Medium-sized vessels	Specific vascular territory	Anterior cerebral artery, middle cerebral artery, posterior cerebral artery	Thrombosis or embolism
Mixed syndromes	Cortical and subcortical	Mixed	Mixed

terior and middle cerebral arteries or thalamoperforant branches of the posterior cerebral arteries (11). The vascular pathology is variable, but microatheroma, lipohyalinosis, and fibrinoid necrosis secondary to severe hypertension are the usual causes of vessel occlusion (12). Lacunar state is defined as a chronic progressive disorder associated with multiple lacunes. It typically progresses to include dementia, dysarthria, and gait disturbance (11).

Binswanger's disease is another subcortical vascular syndrome characterized pathologically by multiple lacunar infarctions, ventricular dilatation (hydrocephalus ex vacuo), and diffuse ischemic demyelination and gliosis of the periventricular white matter. The long, deep-penetrating vessels supplying these regions are thickened with lipohyalinosis and fibrosis (13). The cortex and subcortical arcuate association fibers receive an independent blood supply from short penetrating vessels and are typically spared in Binswanger's disease. Lacunar state and Binswanger's disease often co-occur.

Infarction in the cerebral borderzones located between the major vascular territories of the anterior, middle, and posterior cerebral arteries occurs as a result of carotid stenosis or occlusion, systemic hypotension, or cardiac arrest (14).

Intracerebral hemorrhage or subarachnoid hemorrhage may cause direct brain damage or lead to vascular spasm resulting in cerebral infarction. Hypertensive hemorrhages occur most commonly in the putamen, thalamus, caudate nucleus, and pons. Cerebral amyloid angiopathy is a rare cause of cerebral hemorrhage in the elderly. It is associated with recurrent lobar hemorrhages in demented patients. The patients often also have neuritic plaques and neurofibrillary tangles typical of AD (15).

The relative incidence of the CVD syndromes is difficult to ascertain owing to the differences in etiological classification among authors. Meyer et al. (10) found lacunar state and Binswanger's disease to be the most common CVD syndromes, comprising 44% of patients. Multiple cerebral emboli occurred in 30% of patients with CVD, and borderzone infarctions in patients with extracranial occlusive disease occurred in 26% (10). Erkinjuntii divided patients into cortical and subcortical CVD based on computed tomographic (CT) scan findings (3). Cortical infarctions (with or without subcortical infarctions, but will little evidence of white matter disease) accounted for 82%, and isolated subcortical infarctions with extensive white matter changes were observed in 18%.

III. CLINICAL FEATURES

The clinical signs and symptoms of CVD are variable depending on the location and extent of tissue injury. There are common features in the history and examination, however, that distinguish CVD from other forms of dementia. Typical clinical characteristics reflect the occurrence of multiple strokes and the accumulation of deficits with each ischemic insult. Hachinski and associates (16) devised a scale assigning a value of 1 or 2 points to each of 13 characteristics common in CVD. These are abrupt onset (2 points), stepwise deterioration (1), fluctuating course (2), nocturnal confusion (1), relative preservation of personality (1), depression (1), somatic complaints (1), emotional incontinence (1), history of hypertension (1), history of strokes (2), evidence of associated atherosclerosis (1), focal neurological symptoms (2), and focal neurological signs (2). A score of 7 or more supports a diagnosis of CVD, whereas a score of 4 or fewer suggests a degenerative disorder. Most of the elements of this scale were supported by an autopsy-based confirmation study (17), and it has been found to be useful for distinguishing patients with CVD from those with AD by most investigators. Patients with mixed CVD–AD syndromes, however, cannot be reliably differentiated from those with CVD using the ischemia scale.

Hypertension, the most common risk factor for CVD, is present in 65–80% of CVD patients (18,19). Other associated risk factors are heart disease, cigarette smoking, hyperlipidemia, diabetes, and peripheral vascular disease (3,10,20,21).

Lacunar state and Binswanger's disease share many clinical features and commonly coexist (10,13,22). The pattern of cognitive deterioration resembles that of a subcortical dementia (6). Speech is agrammatic, dysarthric, and hypophonic, whereas language function is usually intact. Memory function is characterized by impaired recall and retrieval deficits that are improved with clues. Patients exhibit loss of executive function or dilapidation in planning, organizing, and initiating tasks. They often exhibit considerable psychomotor retardation. Insight may remain intact until late in the course of the illness. Patients may manifest typical lacunar syndromes, such as pure motor hemiparesis, pure hemisensory deficit, or clumsy hand–dysarthria syndrome (11); or, they may have unilateral or bilateral pyramidal tract dysfunction. Less common is an extrapyramidal syndrome marked by rigidity, masked face, and bradykinesia, bearing similarities to Parkinson's disease (22). Urinary incontinence may occur early in the course. The gait disorder of Binswanger's disease is typified by a widened base and slow, shuffling steps (23). Cortical signs such as aphasia, apraxia, and amnesia are absent until the late stages of the illness, unless there is concomitant cortical infarction. Pseudobulbar palsy is common.

The deficits of CVD resulting from multiple cortical infarctions reflect the vascular territories involved. Occlusions of the left middle cerebral artery cause aphasia and apraxia (24), whereas lesions in the territory of the right middle cerebral artery cause disturbances of visuospatial function and prosody (25). Hemiparesis and hemisensory deficit may or may not be present. Lesions in the area of the angular gyrus supplied by the posterior division of the left middle cerebral artery give rise to a dementia syndrome characterized by transcortical sensory aphasia, alexia, Gerstmann syndrome (acalculia, dysgraphia, finger agnosia, and right–left disorientation), and constructional disturbances (26). This syndrome may be difficult to distinguish from AD. Occlusions of the posterior circulation are associated with unilateral neglect, amnestic disorders, and visual perception disturbances (27–29). Hemianopias, hemiparesis, and hemisensory loss are commonly associated with these lesions.

Infarction of the cerebral border zones typically causes weakness that is more severe in the proximal extremities. Border zone infarctions of the left hemisphere may result in transcortical aphasic syndromes that may be distinguished from the perisylvian syndromes by preservation of repetition (14,24).

Neuropsychiatric disturbances are common in patients with CVD. Delusions are present in half the patients at some time in the course of their illness. There are usually loosely held, uncomplicated paranoid beliefs of theft or infidelity (30). Visual or auditory hallucinations may be present. Visual hallucinations are usually associated with sensory loss arising from ocular abnormalities or visual field defects. Auditory hallucinations occur with diminished hearing or in conjunction with paranoid delusions (30).

Disorders of mood are also frequently encountered in CVD. The prevalence of depression is approximately 25% (31), and it appears to be more common in patients with subcortical infarctions, compared with those with cortical injury (3). Depression after a single stroke occurs most commonly in patients with infarctions of the left frontal lobe, whereas mania, although rare, has been associated more commonly with right hemisphere lesions (32). Other behavioral disturbances include irritability, agitation, and aggressive behavior.

IV. PATHOPHYSIOLOGY

Cognitive loss in CVD is due to multiple cerebral infarctions. Both the quantity of tissue damage and the location of infarction are important determining factors in the occurrence of intellectual decline. Chronic cerebral ischemia may also play a limited role in cognitive compromise.

Tomlinson and associates (33) first investigated the importance of quantity of tissue damage in CVD. They found that the mean volume of infarcted tissue in CVD patients examined at autopsy was 50 ml, and all patients with greater than 100 ml of infarcted brain tissue were demented. Erkinjuntii et al. (34) examined the brains of 23 patients with CVD and found the mean volume of macroscopic infarctions to be 39 ml, with a range of 1–229 ml. There was a tendency for the total volume of tissue loss to increase with increasing severity of dementia.

The wide range of quantity of tissue damage in CVD and the frequent presence of infarctions in elderly people who are not demented suggest that the amount of tissue damage is not the sole determinant of CVD. Topography is also important. Patients with CVD tend to have more bilateral infarctions, more left hemisphere lesions, and more thalamic lesions, when compared with stroke patients without dementia (34–36). Patients with dementia caused by lacunar state have most of their lacunes concentrated in the periventricular white matter of the frontal lobes and caudate nucleus (37). Furthermore, dementia syndromes may result from infarction in small, but strategic, areas of the hemispheres. Examples include the angular gyrus syndrome (26) and dementia syndromes resulting from branch occlusions of the posterior cerebral artery with thalamic infarction (27–29).

Subcortical lesions produce local damage and may disconnect regions of intact cortical tissue, rendering them nonfunctional. For example, one well-studied patient with multiple cerebral infarctions showed decreased metabolism in the left frontal lobe on fluorodeoxyglucose positron emission tomography (PET). The patient died soon after the scan was performed, and postmortem examination revealed the left frontal cortex to be structurally intact. A lacune in the genu of the left internal capsule interrupted afferent and efferent pathways to the frontal lobe, compromising its functional integrity and diminishing its glucose utilization (38).

Cerebral blood flow (CBF) studies have helped elucidate the pathophysiology of CVD. The CBF measured by xenon-133 inhalation is reduced in CVD patients 2 years before the onset of dementia. This contrasts with studies in AD in which CBF does not fall until after the appearance of intellectual changes (21). It is theorized that the early bilateral, irregular patchy reductions in CBF seen in CVD are secondary to atherosclerotic vessel narrowing that increases the risk for later infarction, whereas the more diffuse reduction in CBF found in AD patients occurring after the onset of dementia follows a decline in cerebral metabolic activity. In CVD, changes in CBF vary concordantly with observed clinical improvement and deterioration; whereas AD patients have a steadily progressive decline in CBF and cognition (39). Oxygen-15 PET studies of CVD patients demonstrate a pattern of focal areas of decreased oxygen utilization, located primarily in the distribution of the middle cerebral arteries (40).

Further evidence for a vascular etiology of CVD is provided by studies of cerebral vasomotor responsiveness. The response of normal cerebral vessels to 100% inhaled oxygen is vasoconstriction, resulting in decreased CBF. Cerebral vasomotor responsiveness is calculated as the percentage difference between CBF while breathing room air and while inhaling 100% oxygen. Studies have shown that cerebral vasoresponsiveness diminishes diffusely with age owing to age-related changes in cerebral vessel structure and function (41–44). In AD patients, there is a diffuse symmetric decline in vasomotor responsiveness that is not significantly different from that of age-matched controls. Cerebral vasomotor responsiveness in CVD, however, is highly abnormal showing asymmetric patchy reductions mixed with regions of absent vasomotor responsiveness and even areas of paradoxical flow increases (42). These focal areas of abnormality reflect impaired metabolic and vascular function related to previous vascular injury and tissue infarction. Focal areas of abnormal cerebral vasomotor responsiveness correspond to areas of cerebral infarction seen on CT scans (44). Furthermore, there is a direct correlation between the degree of cognitive impairment in CVD patients and the severity of impairment of cerebral vasomotor responsiveness (41).

The contribution of chronic cerebral ischemia to cognitive impairment in CVD is controversial. It is known that patients with CVD secondary to multiple embolic strokes have a greater volume of infarcted tissue than those with multiple lacunes or bilateral carotid occlusion. However, CVD patients with muliple embolic strokes show higher rates of CBF than patients with carotid occlusive disease or multiple lacunes. Meyer and associates (19) have hypothesized that the more marked change in perfusion associated with multiple lacunes or carotid occlusive disease cannot be attributed entirely to brain infarction and must reflect an additional element of diffuse cerebral ischemia. Similarly, the observation that cognition fluctuates in concert with fluctuations in CBF suggests that varying cerebral ischemia contributes to cognitive impairment (39). Most PET studies, however, have not shown an increase in the oxygen extraction ratio or an uncoupling of CBF and oxygen extraction that would be expected in chronic ischemic states. These observations suggest that any contribution of chronic ischemia to CVD must be of limited magnitude (40).

V. EVALUATION

Neuroimaging studies are the best antemortem means of distinguishing CVD from AD and differentiating among the subtypes of CVD.

Computed tomographic scanning identifies focal, low-density areas consistent with cerebral infarction as well as cortical atrophy, ventricular dilatation, and leukoaraiosis (low-density areas in periventricular white matter). Approximately 75% of patients with CVD have at least one cerebral infarction visible on CT, with or wihout atrophy; 20% have atrophy only; and 5% have a normal CT scan (35). Leukoaraiosis is found in 97% of CVD patients, compared with 55% of patients with AD and is more severe in those with CVD (45).

Magnetic resonance imaging (MRI) is replacing CT as the imaging technique of choice in the evaluation of dementia. It is more sensitive in detecting focal vascular lesions and diffuse white matter changes, especially when T_2-weighted images are obtained (Fig. 1). Essentially all patients with CVD have white matter changes present on MRI (46–48). In one study, only 36% of AD patients had such changes, and the degree of white matter pathology was mild compared with the moderate to severe degree of change seen in all the CVD patients (46). The presence of white matter alterations on MRI is not as useful in distinguishing CVD patients from nondemented patients with cerebrovascular disease. One study found that

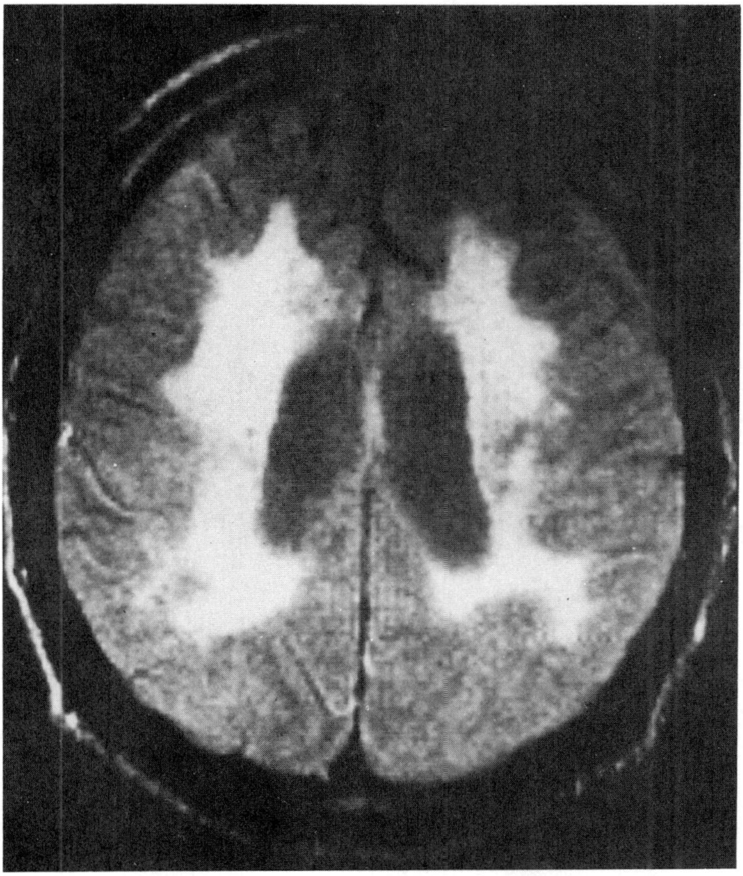

Figure 1 MRI scan of patient with vascular dementia showing prominent hemispheric white matter changes and ventriculomegaly.

60% of nondemented patients had white matter changes, compared with 100% of demented patients. The severity of change did not differ between the two groups (47). Ventricular size distinguished the two groups: enlarged ventricles were found in 58% of demented patients, compared with 6% of nondemented patients (47). Careful clinical judgment should be used in interpreting the white matter lesions on MRI; demyelinating or neoplastic lesions may have an appearance similar to vascular lesions. Binswanger's disease is becoming a common radiological diagnosis, but this diagnosis should be based on clinical characteristics and, when available, neuropathological findings, rather than on white matter changes and enlarged ventricles on MRI scans.

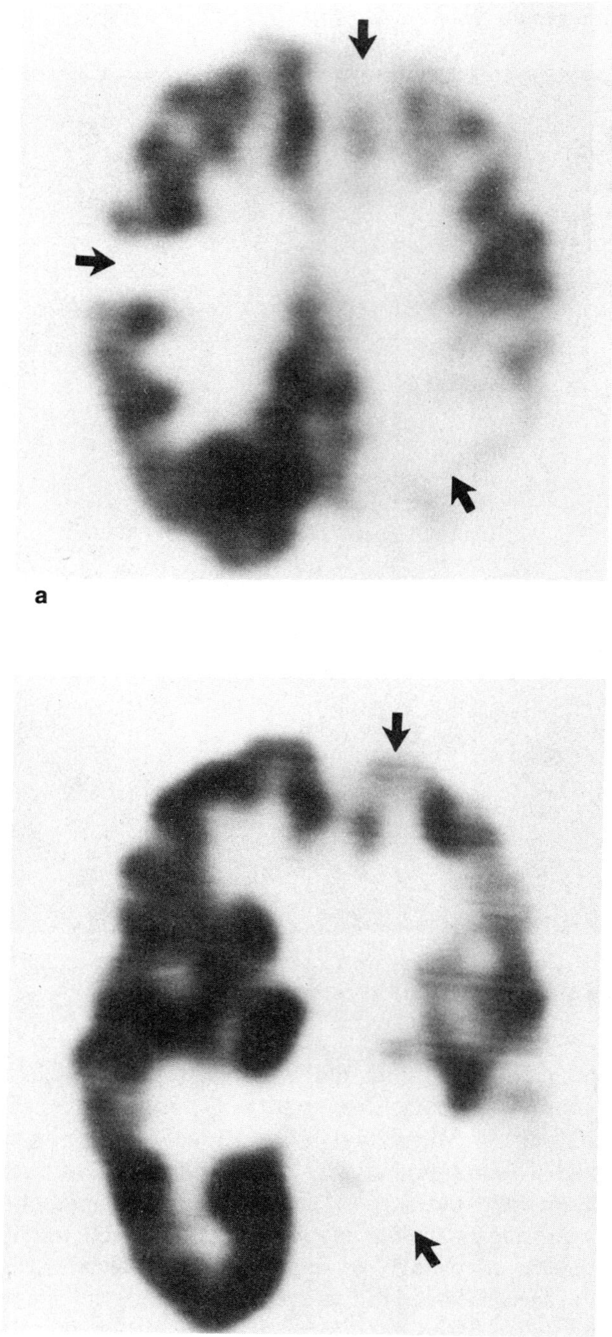

a

b

Figure 2 PET scan of patient with vascular dementia showing multiple areas of focal hypometabolism (arrows).

Functional imaging techniques such as single-photon emission computed tomography (SPECT) and PET scanning measure cerebral perfusion and brain metabolism. In patients with CVD, they reveal a pattern of scattered, focal defects in perfusion or metabolism (40) (Fig. 2).

The laboratory evaluation of patients with CVD should be directed toward investigation of stroke etiology and coexisting vascular abnormalities, such as ischemic retinopathy, heart disease, renal failure, and peripheral vascular disease. Complete blood count, platelet count, clotting studies, and erythrocyte sedimentation rate; syphilis serology; renal function tests; and levels of electrolytes, glucose, blood urea nitrogen, and serum cholesterol and lipids should be obtained for all patients with CVD. Further testing may be indicated by the clinical findings and results of baseline tests. These might include antinuclear antibody, anticardiolipin antibodies, lupus anticoagulant, and rheumatoid factor for patients with suspected inflammatory or rheumatic disease; hypercoagulation screen for patients with recurrent venous thrombosis; or hemoglobin electrophoresis for patients at risk for sickle cell anemia.

A chest x-ray study should be obtained to evaluate heart size and the presence of pulmonary disease. An electrocardiogram reveals cardiac arrhythmias in 24–50% of patients with CVD and evidence of myocardial infarction in 22% (3,18). Echocardiography should be performed for patients with a history suggestive of cardiac embolic disease or evidence of overt heart disease.

Seizures occur in approximately 15% of patients with CVD. Electroencephalography reveals focal abnormalities in 40–75% of patients with CVD, generalized slowing in 15–65%, and normal cerebral rhythms in 10–35% (49–51).

Lumbar puncture need not be routinely performed in patients with CVD, but should be pursued in patients with possible inflammatory or infectious etiologies of their infarctions, or when there is diagnostic uncertainty about the dementia syndrome. Mild protein elevations may occur in the cererbrospinal fluid of patients with uncomplicated CVD (13).

VI. TREATMENT

Treatment of CVD emphasizes halting the progression of the disease and allowing spontaneous improvement through control of risk factors and minimizing the underlying vascular pathology (Table 2).

Control of systolic blood pressure in the range of 135–150 mmHg has been shown to increase cerebral blood flow and improve cognitive performance in a group of CVD patients. In the same study, cognitive deterioration occurred when the treated mean systolic blood pressure declined to 128 mmHg (52). Overtreatment of blood pressure may lead to decreased

TABLE 2 Treatment of Cerebrovascular Dementia

Risk factor control	*Behavioral complications*
Eliminate hypertension	Depression
Eliminate smoking	Antidepressants
Control serum lipids	Psychosis
Control diabetes mellitus	Neuroleptics
Platelet antiaggregants	Agitation
Aspirin	Neuroleptics
Ticlopidine	Benzodiazepines
Experimental cognitive enhancers	Propranolol
Ergoloid mesylates (Hydergine)	Trazodone
Pentoxifylline	Carbamazepine
Nootropics	*General measures*
Piracetam	Occupational therapy
Oxiracetam	Physical therapy
Nimodipine	Speech therapy
	Adequate nutrition
	Adequate hydration
	Skin care

CBF because of impaired cerebral autoregulation and diminished lumen size in chronically hypertensive patients (53).

Cigarette smoking decreases cerebral blood flow and accelerates the development of atherosclerosis (54). Cessation of smoking has been shown to increase CBF in elderly patients (55). One small study of normotensive CVD patients has demonstrated an improvement in cognitive performance following cessation of cigarette use (52). Recent evidence has suggested that passive smoking may be a risk factor for cerebrovascular disease; therefore, household members of patients with CVD should be urged to discontinue smoking (56).

Lowering serum lipids may also reduce the risk for further strokes and prevent progression of dementia. One study using the triglyceride-lowering agent gemfibrozil in hyperlipidemic CVD patients showed a reduction in serum triglycerides and slight improvement in cognitive performance in patients taking the drug compared with no change in triglyceride levels and a slight decline in cognitive performance in untreated controls (10).

The use of aspirin as a platelet antiaggregant has been shown to reduce the risk of recurrent stroke by 15–30%, and it is now an accepted therapy in most patients with cerebrovascular disease (57). One 325-mg tablet a day is probably as effective as larger doses in preventing stroke (58). There have been few studies of aspirin therapy in CVD. In one study comparing aspirin and placebo in CVD patients, the treated patients showed improvement in cognitive function, whereas the untreated patients evidenced a slight decline in performance (59).

Ticlopidine, an agent that prevents platelet aggregation through a direct effect on the platelet membrane, was recently shown to be more effective than aspirin in the prevention of stroke in high-risk patients (60). Its use in CVD has not been studied, but application in CVD is likely to follow its approval for use in stroke.

Dipyridamole, another platelet antiaggregant, has not been shown to decrease the incidence of stroke or to provide additional benefit when given with aspirin (58,61) and is not currently recommended for use in CVD patients.

Anticoagulants such as warfarin may be useful in the prevention of recurrent stroke in patients with transient ischemic attacks, atrial fibrillation, or a source of cardiac emboli (58). Maintaining the clotting parameters at 1.3–1.5 times normal control values is probably as effective as traditionally higher levels and is safer (62). The risk of hemorrhagic complications is high in elderly demented patients. Anticoagulants should be administered with caution and only to selected CVD patients. The elderly may be receiving medications that alter the action of warfarin derivatives, and clotting studies should be otained frequently.

Carotid endarterectomy for stroke prevention remains controversial. There may be a subset of patients with high-grade carotid stenosis and recurrent transient ischemic attacks, recalcitrant to medical therapy, who benefit from this procedure. The efficacy of endarterectomy in CVD is doubtful. A few studies with nondemented patients have demonstrated improvement on neuropsychological testing postoperatively (63,64), but long-term studies of CVD patients who have undergone endarterectomy are not available. Carotid endarterectomy and surgical revascularization procedures are not recommended in the treatment of CVD.

Medications that might enhance cognitive function are presently being investigated in CVD. These include cerebral vasodilators and nootropics. The evidence supporting the use of cerebral vasodilators in CVD is inconclusive. Hydergine, a trade name for the ergoloid mesylates (a combination of four ergot alkaloids), is a commonly used vasodilator–nootropic agent. The mechanism of action of this compound is thought to include cerebral vasodilatation as well as direct effects on brain metabolism. Modest improvement has been documented in patients taking 3–6 mg/day (65).

Pentoxifylline is a xanthine derivative that reduces blood viscosity and has a direct vasodilatory effect. It is marketed for the treatment of intermittent claudication. Small, preliminary trials with pentoxifylline have shown a slight benefit in cognitive function in CVD patients; there were few adverse side effects. Further studies are needed before pentoxifylline can be recommended routinely in the treatment of CVD (66–68).

Piracetam and oxiracetam are nootropic agents that may enhance brain metabolism by increasing ATP synthesis and carbohydrate metabolism. Several short-term studies with oxiracetam have shown modest improvement in cognitive function and behavior in treated CVD patients compared with untreated controls (69,70).

Nimodipine, a calcium channel blocker used to treat vasospasm following subarachnoid hemorrhage, has been shown to improve cognition and behavior in preliminary investigations (71). In one study, 44% of patients treated with this agent improved substantially, 33% had mild improvements, 18% showed no change, and 5% were minimally worse (72).

Neuropsychiatric disturbances associated with CVD may be successfully treated with a variety of medications, but drug intervention should be balanced with an awareness of potential deleterious side effects. Depressed patients frequently respond to tricyclic antidepressants, such as nortriptyline or desipramine (73). Newer antidepressants such as trazodone, fluoxetine, and bupropion, are associated with fewer cardiac and anticholinergic side effects (74,75) and may become the agents of choice in depressed CVD patients. Psychosis may be treated with small doses of neuroleptics, such as haloperidol or thioridazine. Hyperactivity, agitation, or violent behavior may respond to small doses of neuroleptic agents, benzodiazepines, trazodone, carbamazepine, or propranolol (76–80).

Occupational and physical therapy are aimed at improving and maintaining functional capabilities. Speech and swallowing therapy may benefit patients with aphasic syndromes, dysarthria, or dysphagia.

Cerebrovascular dementia patients require constant surveillance and treatment of coexisting complications of vascular disease, such as heart conditions, renal failure, retinal ischemia, and peripheral vascular disease. In advanced stages of the illness the patients are vulnerable to dehydration, malnutrition, urinary tract infection, aspiration pneumonia, and decubitus ulcers.

VII. SUMMARY

Cerebrovascular dementia is a heterogeneous disorder that may present with cortical, subcortical, or mixed features, depending on the location of ischemic injury. Clinical, neuropathological, and neuroimaging studies indicate that cognitive decline results primarily from completed cerebral infarction. Both the quantity of tissue damage and the location of infarction are important determinants of dementia severity and type of neuropsychological deficits. Chronic cerebral ischemia may play a limited role in the dementia in some patients.

Treatment is directed at control of vascular risk factors, such as hypertension, smoking, hyperlipidemia, and cardiac disease and prevention of recurrent stroke primarily with platelet antiaggregants. Associated behavioral disturbances may respond to treatment with psychotropic medications. Cognitive enhancing agents are being investigated for amelioration of the dementia and may play a larger role in future management regimens.

ACKNOWLEDGMENTS

This project was supported by the Department of Veterans Affairs, the French Foundation for Alzheimer Research, and NIA training grant AG00172-02.

REFERENCES

1. Wolf PA, Kannel WB, McGee DL. Epidemiology of strokes in North America. In: Barnett HJM, Stern BM, Mohr JP, Yatsu FM, eds. Stroke: pathophysiology, diagnosis and management. New York: Churchill-Livingstone, 1986:19–29.
2. American Pyschiatric Association. Diagnostic and statistical manual of mental disorders, 3rd ed, revised. Washington, DC: American Psychiatric Press, 1987.
3. Erkinjuntii T. Types of multi-infarct dementia. Acta Neurol Scand 1987; 75:391–399.
4. Garraway WM, Whisnant JP, Drury I. The continuing decline in the incidence of stroke. Mayo Clin Proc 1983; 58:520–523.
5. Mirsen T, Hachinski V. Epidemiology of vascular and multi-infarct dementia. In: Meyer JS, Lechner H, Marshall J, Toole JF, eds. Vascular and multi-infarct dementia. Mount Kisco, NY: Futura Publishing, 1988:61–79.
6. Cummings JL, Benson DF. Dementia: a clinical approach. Boston: Butterworths, 1983.
7. Sulkava R, Wikstrom J, Aromaa A, Raitasalo R, Lehtinen V, Lahtela K, Palo J. Prevalence of severe dementia in Finland. Neurology 1985; 35:1025–1029.
8. Molsa PK, Marttila RJ, Rinne UK. Survival and cause of death in Alzheimer's disease and multi-infarct dementia. Acta Neurol Scand 1986; 74:103–107.
9. Barcay LL, Zemcov A, Blass JP, Sansone J. Survival in Alzheimer's disease and vascular dementia. Neurology 1985; 35:834–840.
10. Meyer JS, McClintic K, Sims P, Rogers RL, Mortel KF. Etiology, prevention, and treatment of vascular and multi-infarct dementia. In: Meyer JS, Lechner H, Marshall J, Toole JF, eds. Vascular and multi-infarct dementia. Mount Kisco, NY: Futura Publishing, 1988:129–147.

11. Fisher CM. Lacunar strokes and infarcts: a review. Neurology 1982; 32:871–876.
12. Mohr JP. Lacunes. Neurol Clin 1983; 1:201–221.
13. Babikian V, Ropper AH. Binswanger's disease: a review. Stroke 1987; 18:2–12.
14. Bogousslavsky J, Regli F. Unilateral watershed cerebral infarcts. Neurology 1986; 36:373–377.
15. Gilbert JJ, Vinters HV. Cerebral amyloid angiopathy: incidence and complications in the aging brain. I. Cerebral hemorrhage. Stroke 1983; 14:915–922.
16. Hachinski VC, Iliff LD, Zilhka E, Du Boulay GH, McAllister VL, Marshall J, Russell RW, Symon L. Cerebral blood flow in dementia. Acta Neurol 1975; 32:632–637.
17. Rosen WG, Terry RD, Fuld PA, Katzman R, Peck A. Pathological verification of ischemic score in differentiation of dementias. Ann Neurol 1980; 7:486–488.
18. Tresch DD, Folstein MF, Rabins PV, Hazzard WR. Prevalence and significance of cardiovascular disease and hypertension in elderly patients with dementia and depression. J Am Geriatr Soc 1985; 33:530–537.
19. Meyer JS, McClintic KL, Rogers RL, Sims P, Mortel KF. Aetiological considerations and risk factors for multi-infarct dementia. J Neurol Neurosurg Psychiatry 1988; 51:1489–1497.
20. Meyer JS, Rogers RL, Mortel KF, Judd MA. Hyperlipidemia is a risk factor for decreased cerebral perfusion and stroke. Acta Neurol 1987; 44:418–422.
21. Rogers RL, Meyer JS, Mortel KF, Mahurin RK, Judd BW. Decreased cerebral blood flow precedes multi-infarct dementia, but follows senile dementia of Alzheimer type. Neurology 1986; 36:1–6.
22. Roman GC. Senile dementia of the Binswanger type: a vascular form of dementia in the elderly. JAMA 1987; 258:1782–1788.
23. Thompson PD, Marsden CD. Gait disorder of subcortical arteriosclerotic encephalopathy: Binswanger's disease. Mov Disord 1987; 2:1–8.
24. Benson DF. Aphasia, alexia, and agraphia. New York: Churchill-Livingstone, 1979.
25. Heilman KM, Bowers D, Valenstein E, Watson RT. The right hemisphere: neuropsychological functions. J Neurosurg 1986; 64:693–704.
26. Benson DF, Cummings JL, Tsai SY. Angular gyrus syndrome simulating Alzheimer's disease. Arch Neurol 1982; 39:616–620.
27. Guberman A, Stuss D. The syndrome of bilateral paramedian thalamic infarction. Neurology 1983; 33:540–546.
28. Katz DI, Alexander MP, Mandell AM. Dementia following strokes in the mesencephalon and diencephalon. Arch Neurol 1987; 44:1127–1133.
29. De Renzi E, Zambolin A, Crisi G. The pattern of neuropsychological impairment associated with left posterior cerebral artery infarcts. Brain 1987; 110:1099–1116.
30. Cummings JL, Miller B, Hill MA, Neshkes R. Neuropsychiatric aspects of multi-infarct dementia and dementia of the Alzheimer type. Arch Neurol 1987; 44:389–393.

31. Cummings JL. Depression in vascular dementia. Hillside J Clin Psychiatry 1988; 10:209–231.
32. Robinson RG, Kubos KL, Starr LB, Rao K, Price TR. Mood disorders in stroke patients. Brain 1984; 107:81–93.
33. Tomlinson BE, Blessed G, Roth M. Observations on the brains of demented old people. J Neurol Sci 1970; 11:205–242.
34. Erkinjuntii T, Haltia M, Palo J, Sulkava R, Paetau A. Accuracy of the clinical diagnosis of vascular dementia: a prospective clinical and post-mortem neuropathological study. J Neurol Neurosurg Psychiatry 1988; 51:1037–1044.
35. Ladurner G, Iliff LD, Lechner H. Clinical factors associated with dementia in ischemic stroke. J Neurol Neurosurg Psychiatry 1982; 45:97–101.
36. Loeb C, Gandolfo C, Bino G. Intellectual impairment and cerebral lesions in multiple cerebral infarcts: a clinical–computed tomography study. Stroke 1988; 19:560–565.
37. Ishii N, Nishihara Y, Imamura T. Why do frontal lobe symptoms predominate in vascular dementia with lacunes? Neurology 1986; 36:340–345.
38. Metter EJ, Mazziotta JC, Itabashi HH, Mankovich NJ, Phelps ME, Kuhl DE. Comparison of glucose metabolism, x-ray CT, and postmortem data in a patient with multiple cerebral infarcts. Neurology 1985; 35:1695–1701.
39. Meyer JS, Rogers RL, Judd BW, Mortel KF, Sims P. Cognition and cerebral blood flow fluctuate together in multi-infarct dementia. Stroke 1988; 19:163–169.
40. Frackowiak RSJ, Pozzilli C, Legg NJ, Du Boulay GH, Marshall J, Lenzi GL, Jones T. Regional cerebral oxygen supply and utilization in dementia: a clinical and physiological study with oxygen-15 and positron tomography. Brain 1981; 104:753–778.
41. Judd BW, Meyer JS, Rogers RL, Ganchi S, Tanahashi N, Mortel KF, Tawaklna T. Cognitive performance correlates with cerebrovascular impairments in multi-infarct dementia. J Am Geriatr Soc 1986; 34:355–360.
42. Amano T, Meyer JS, Okabe T, Shaw T, Mortel KF. Cerebral vasomotor responses during oxygen inhalation. Acta Neurol 1983; 40:277–282.
43. Rogers RL, Meyer JS, Mortel KF, Mahurin RK, Thornby J. Age-related reductions in cerebral vasomotor reactivity and the law of initial value: a four year prospective longitudinal study. J Cereb Blood Flow Metabol 1985; 5:79–85.
44. Nakajima S, Meyer JS, Amano T, Shaw T, Okabe T, Mortel KF. Cerebral vasomotor responsiveness during 100% oxygen inhalation in cerebral ischemia. Arch Neurol 1983; 40:271–276.
45. Aharon-Peretz J, Cummings JL, Hill MA. Vascular dementia and dementia of the Alzheimer type: cognition, ventricular size, and leuko-araiosis. Arch Neurol 1988; 45:719–721.
46. Erkinjuntii T, Ketonen L, Sulkava R, Sipponen J, Vuorialho M, Iivanainen M. Do white matter changes on MRI and CT differentiate vascular dementia from Alzheimer's disease? J Neurol Neurosurg Psychiatry 1987; 50:37–42.
47. Hershey LA, Modic MT, Greenough G, Jaffe DF. Magnetic resonance imaging in vascular dementia. Neurology 1987; 37:29–36.

48. Brant-Zawadzki M, Fein G, Van Dyke C, Kieran R, Davenport L, de Groot J. MR imaging of the aging brain: patchy white-matter lesions and dementia. Am J Neuroradiol 1985; 6:675–681.
49. Bucht G, Adolfsson R, Winblad B. Dementia of the Alzheimer type and multi-infarct dementia: a clinical description and diagnostic problems. J Am Geriatr Soc 1984; 32:491–498.
50. Roberts MA, McGeorge AP, Caird FI. Electroencephalography and computerised tomography in vascular and non-vascular dementia in old age. J Neurol Neurosurg Psychiatry 1978; 41:903–906.
51. Striano S, Vacca G, Bilo L, Meo R. The electroencephalogram in dementia. Acta Neurol 1982; 3:727–734.
52. Meyer JS, Judd BW, Tawakina T, Rogers RL, Mortel KF. Improved cognition after control of risk factors for multi-infarct dementia. JAMA 1986; 256:2203–2209.
53. Strandgaard S. Autoregulation of cerebral blood flow in hypertensive patients. Circulation 1976; 53:720–727.
54. Rogers RL, Meyer JS, Shaw TG, Mortel KF, Hardenberg JP, Zaid RR. Cigarette smoking decreases cerebral blood flow suggesting increased risk for stroke. JAMA 1983; 250:2796–2800.
55. Rogers RL, Meyer JS, Judd BW, Mortel KF. Abstention from cigarette smoking improves cerebral perfusion among elderly chronic smokers. JAMA 1985; 253:2970–2974.
56. Donnan GA, Adena MA, O'Malley HM, McNeil JJ, Doyle AE, Neill GC. Smoking as a risk factor for cerebral ischemia. Lancet 1989; 2:643–647.
57. The Canadian Cooperative Study Group. A randomized trial of aspirin and sulfinpyrazone in threatened stroke. N Engl J Med 1978; 299:53–59.
58. Grotta JC. Current medical and surgical therapy for cerebrovascular disease. N Engl J Med 1987; 317:1505–1516.
59. Meyer JS, Rogers RL, McClintic K, Mortel KF, Lotfi J. Randomized clinical trial of daily aspirin therapy in multi-infarct dementia: a pilot study. J Am Geriatr Soc 1989; 37:549–555.
60. Hass WK, Easton JD, Adams HP, Pryse-Phillips W, Molony BA, Anderson S, Kamm B, for the ticlopidine aspirin stroke study group. A randomized trial comparing ticlopidine hydrochloride with aspirin for the prevention of stroke in high risk patients. N Engl J Med 1989; 321:501–507.
61. Acheson J, Danta G, Hutchinson EC. Controlled trial of dipyridamole in cerebral vascular disease. Br Med J 1969; 1:614–615.
62. Hirsh J, Levine M, Therapeutic range for control of oral anticoagulant therapy. Arch Neurol 1986; 43:1162–1164.
63. Hemmingsen R, Mejsohlm B, Vorstrup S, Lester J, Engell HC, Boysen G. Carotid surgery, cognitive function, and cerebral blood flow in patients with transient ischemic attacks. Ann Neurol 1986; 20:13–19.
64. Kelly MP, Garron DC, Javid H. Carotid artery disease, carotid endarterectomy, and behavior. Arch Neurol 1980; 37:743–748.
65. Cook P, James I. Cerebral vasodilators. N Engl J Med 1981; 305:1508–1513.

66. Ghose K. Oxypentifylline in dementia: a controlled study. Arch Gerontol Geriatr 1987; 6:19–26.
67. Dominguez D, de Cayaffa CL, Gomensoro J, Aparicio NJ. Modification of psychometric, practical and intellectual parameters in patients with diffuse cerebrovascular insufficiency during prolonged treatment with pentoxifylline: a double-blind, placebo controlled trial. Pharmatherapeutica 1977; 1:498–506.
68. Harwart D. The treatment of chronic cerebrovascular insufficiency. A double-blind study with pentoxifylline. Curr Med Res Opin 1979; 6:73–84.
69. Dysken MW, Katz R, Stallone F, Kuskowski M. Oxiracetam in the treatment of multi-infarct dementia and primary degenerative dementia. J Neuropsychol 1989; 1:249–251.
70. Villardita C, Parini J, Grioli S, Quattropani M, Lomeo C, Scapgnini U. Clinical and neuropsychological study with oxiracetam versus placebo in patients with mild to moderate dementia. J Neural Transm 1987 (suppl);24:293–298.
71. Tobares N, Pedromingo N, Bigona J. Nimodipine treatment improves cognitive function in vascular dementia. In: Gergener M, Reisberg B, eds. Diagnosis and treatment of senile dementia. New York: Springer-Verlag, 1989:360–365.
72. Fischkof PK, Wagner G, Littschauer L, Ruther E, Apecechea M, Hiersemenzel R, Robinel J, Hoffmeister F, Schmage N. Therapeutic results from nimodipine in primary degenerative dementia and mulit-infarct dementia. In: Bergener M, Reisberg B, eds. Diagnosis and treatment of senile dementia. New York: Springer-Verlag, 1989:350–359.
73. Lipsey JR, Robinson RG, Pearlson GD, Rao K, Price TR. Nortriptyline treatment of post-stroke depression: a double-blind study. Lancet 1984; 1:297–300.
74. Redding M, Haycox J. Blass J. Depression in patients referred to a dementia clinic. Arch Neurol 1985; 42:894–896.
75. Baldessarini RJ. Drugs and the treatment of psychiatric disorders. In: Gilman AG, Goodman LS, Rall TW, Murad F, eds. The pharmacological basis of therapeutics. New York: Macmillan Publishing, 1985;387–445.
76. Cummings JL. Clinical neuropsychiatry. Orlando, Fla: Grune & Stratton, 1985.
77. Yudofsky SC, Stevens L, Silver J, Barsa J, Williams D. Propranolol in the treatment of rage and violent behavior in patients with chronic brain syndromes. Am J Psychiatry 1981; 138:218–220.
78. Smeraski PJ. Clonazepam treatment of multi-infarct dementia. J Geriatr Psychiatry Neurol 1988; 1:47–48.
79. Pinner E, Rich CL. Effects of trazodone on aggressive behavior in seven patients with organic mental disorders. Am J Psychiatry 1988; 145:1295–1296.
80. Salzman C. Treatment of the elderly agitated patient. J Clin Psychiatry 1987; 48(suppl 5):19–22.

11

Age-Associated Memory Impairment

Glenn J. Larrabee* and William J. McEntee *Memory Assessment Clinics, Inc., Sarasota, Florida*

Thomas H. Crook III *Memory Assessment Clinics, Inc., Bethesda, Maryland*

I. INTRODUCTION

Clinicians frequently encounter healthy, nondemented older patients who complain of memory problems. Upon formal evaluation, these older patients may perform at the level of other persons their age on various memory and neuropsychological measures, leading some clinicians to make reassuring statements that memory is "normal" for the patient's age. Others may employ the descriptive term *benign senescent forgetfulness* to characterize memory problems in healthy, nondemented older adults (1).

Determination of "normality" of memory function obviously depends upon the normative reference group. The reference group chosen by patients themselves typically is internal; that is, patients complain that their memory abilities have declined from what they once were. Indeed, it is unusual for elderly persons to complain that their memory abilities are worse than the average person of 60 or 70 years of age. Hence, as in the case for the majority of age-related changes, the concern of most elderly individuals is not that they are less robust than their peers, but that they are less robust than they once were. Accordingly, the reference group by which older persons typically define memory problems is composed of young, healthy adults. By contrast, the clinician typically defines normality by comparing the performance of the older patient with that of other persons

**Current affiliation:* private practice, Hill View Park Medical Complex, Sarasota, Florida

of the same age. Alternatively, the group implicitly referenced may be composed of patients suffering from such conditions as Alzheimer's disease (AD), depression, or multi-infarct dementia (2–4).

Until recently, there has been no generally accepted terminology or criteria for describing older persons who have experienced memory loss, but who are clearly not demented. Persons falling in the area between normal aging and dementia have been characterized as suffering *benign senescent forgetfulness* (1) or *senescent forgetfulness* (5). Unfortunately, there are no clearly defined behavioral or performance characteristics for formulating a diagnosis of benign senescent forgetfulness. Moreover, there are no guidelines for delineating the clinical, behavioral, and performance characteristics for the much larger group of healthy elderly manifesting normal, age-related decline in memory functions.

In addition to these clinical considerations, further specification of the boundaries of normal and abnormal aging has important implications for the development of effective treatments for memory impairment in later life. In this respect, it is noteworthy that age-related memory changes seen in nonhuman mammalian species have been pharmacologically ameliorated (6). Unfortunately, drugs demonstrated to be effective for improving memory in healthy aged animals have been clinically evaluated subsequently only in neurologically diseased aged adults (7). Thus, it is not surprising that the results of clinical trials have been disappointing. However, it is quite possible that compounds found effective in reducing age-related memory deficits in animals may also be effective in reducing analogous deficits in neurologically normal aged humans. For such trials to be undertaken it is necessary to carefully define and operationalize the clinical phenomenon under study (8).

The clinical and research significance of defining and operationalizing a condition marked by diminished memory abilities in healthy older patients led the National Institute of Mental Health (NIMH) to form a work group of experts to consider diagnostic terminology and criteria. This work group, which comprised neurologists, psychiatrists, pharmacologists, neuropsychologists, and psychologists, considered age-related literature in comparative psychobiology, pharmacology, neuropathology, experimental psychology, and psychometrics in formulating the original criteria for age-associated memory impairment (AAMI; 7). The interested reader is referred to this original paper for the relevant literature reviews.

The following sections of this chapter will present the AAMI criteria as originally specified (7). This will be followed by consideration of pharmacologic treatment strategies focusing on noradrenergic, serotonergic, and cholinergic neurotransmitter systems. The final section of the chapter will focus on neuropsychological aspects of AAMI, including data on behavioral remediation, and further descriptive characteristics of this age-associated cognitive disorder.

II. PROPOSED DIAGNOSTIC TERMINOLOGY FOR AGE-ASSOCIATED MEMORY IMPAIRMENT

A. Diagnostic Terminology

The diagnostic term proposed by the NIMH work group was *age-associated memory impairment* (AAMI; 7). The clinical entity is characterized by complaints of memory impairment in tasks of daily life, substantiated by evidence of such impairment on psychological performance tests with adequate normative data. The performance tests employed should assess recent memory for verbal and nonverbal material. The term AAMI is applied to people over 50 years of age, although this does not imply that such impairment is qualitatively different from that seen (less frequently) in younger adults. The term is also nonspecific relative to etiology and does not necessarily imply that the disorder is nonprogressive (although deterioration beyond a specified point would exclude individuals from a diagnosis of AAMI).

B. Proposed Research Diagnostic Criteria

1. Inclusion Criteria

1. Men and women at least 50 years of age.

2. Complaints of memory loss reflected in such everyday problems as difficulty remembering names of individuals following introduction, misplacing objects, difficulty remembering multiple items to be purchased or multiple tasks to be performed, problems remembering telephone numbers or mailing codes, and difficulty recalling information quickly or following distraction. Onset of memory loss must be described as gradual, without sudden worsening in recent months. The Memory Complaint Questionnaire (MAC-Q; available from the authors) has been devised to quantify complaints of age-associated memory decline for selection of subjects for drug studies. The subject rates their current ability on five everyday tasks (e.g., "Remembering the name of a person just introduced to you") in comparison with their perceived ability level when they were in high school or college. Ratings are on a 5-point scale (range: "Much better now," worth 1 point, to "Much poorer now," worth 5 points). Additionally, there is a global item, "In general, how would you describe your memory as compared with when you were in high school." There are five rating anchors for this item. These anchors and associated score values are: "Much better

now," 2 points; "Somewhat better now," 4 points; "About the same," 6 points; "Somewhat poorer now," 8 points; and "Much poorer now," 10 points. The subject must score at least 25 on the MAC-Q to qualify for investigation of AAMI, in addition to meeting the following psychometric criteria in item 3.

3. Memory test performance that is at least 1 standard deviation (SD) below the mean established for young adults on a standardized test of secondary (recent) memory for which adequate normative data are available. Tests that have been employed in recent AAMI clinical trials include the Benton Visual Retention Test (number correct, administration A, cutoff of 6 or less; 9), Logical Memory Subtest of the Wechsler Memory Scale (cutoff of 6 or less; WMS; 10), and the Associate Learning subtest of the WMS (cutoff of 13 or less).

4. Evidence of adequate intellectual function as determined by a scaled score of at least 9 (raw score of at least 32) on the vocabulary subtest of the Wechsler Adult Intelligence Scale (WAIS; 11).

5. Absence of dementia. This was originally given an operational definition of a score of 24 or higher on the Mini-Mental State Examination (12). Many investigators have chosen a score of 27, rather than 24, to exclude questionable cases of dementia. Indeed, published scores for "normal" individuals in the later decades supports the latter approach (13).

2. *Exclusion Criteria*

1. Evidence of delirium, confusion, or other disturbances of consciousness.
2. Any neurological disorder that could produce cognitive deterioration as determined by history, clinical neurological examination, and, if indicated, neuroradiological examination. Such disorders include AD, Parkinson's disease, stroke, intracranial hemorrhage, focal brain lesions including tumors, and normal pressure hydrocephalus.
3. History of any infective or inflammatory brain disease including those of viral, fungal, or syphilitic causes.
4. Evidence of significant cerebral vascular pathology operationally defined by a Hachinski Ischemia Score (modified version; 14) of 4 or more, or by neuroradiological examination.
5. History of repeated minor head injury (as in boxing) or a single injury resulting in a period of unconsciousness for 1 hr or more.
6. Current psychiatric diagnosis according to *DSM-III* criteria (15) of depression, mania, or any major psychiatric disorder.
7. Current diagnosis or history of alcoholism or drug dependence.
8. Evidence of depression operationally defined by a Hamilton Psychiatric Rating Scale for Depression (16), score or 13 or more.

9. Any medical disorder that could produce cognitive deterioration, including renal, respiratory, cardiac, and hepatic disease; diabetes mellitus, unless well controlled by diet or oral hypoglycemics; endocrine, metabolic, or hematological disturbances; and malignancy not in remission for more than 2 years. Determination should be based on complete medical history, clinical examination (including electrocardiogram), and appropriate laboratory tests.
10. Use of any psychotropic drug or any other drug that may substantially affect cognitive function during the month before psychometric testing.

These criteria are certainly seen as modifiable in drug studies, depending upon characteristics of the compound under study or specific concerns of the investigators.

III. PHARMACOLOGIC TREATMENT STRATEGIES

In previous papers, we have reviewed strategies for pharmacologic treatment of AAMI, including transmitter-based approaches, neuropeptides, and nootropics (17–19). In the following section, we briefly review the literature relevant to memory improvement consequent to pharmacologic manipulation of catecholamines, serotonin, and acetylcholine. The reader is referred to a more extensive series of recent reviews for more detailed discussion (20–22). In considering AAMI treatment strategies, the ideal drug should be safe for long-term use with minimal side effects, have a long duration of action, pass readily into the brain, and have a wide therapeutic window (22).

A. Catecholamines

McEntee and Crook (20) recently reviewed the relationship of AAMI to catecholamine (CA) function. Catecholamine systems show age-related declines in humans and animals, although little is known about the relationship between CA activity and cognitive function in normal elderly humans. However, CA systems are related to spatial memory performance in aged monkeys (23) and to memory function in humans suffering from Korsakoff's disease (24,25). Arnsten and Goldman-Rakic (23) demonstrated improved delayed response in aged monkeys after administration of clonidine, an α_2-noradrenergic agonist. Consistent with this pattern of improvement, McEntee and Mair found enhanced performance of Korsakoff's patients on multiple measures of memory following administration of clonidine (26).

In considering extensions of these studies to age-related memory disorders, McEntee and Crook noted that preliminary studies of the effects of clonidine on cognition in patients with AD have provided mixed results (20). They observe, however, that clonidine has side effects of hypotension and sedation, which might be limiting factors in treatment of memory-impaired elders. Another α_2-agonist, guanfacine, appears to have more potent memory-enhancing results in old monkeys, without significant sedating or hypotension effects (27). Guanfacine had no treatment effect in a recent trial with five AD patients (28). However, the drug is now being evaluated in multicenter clinical trials in both AD and AAMI.

B. Serotonin

In contrast with the preponderance of data reflecting an age-associated decline in brain CA activity, evidence for age-associated changes in brain serotonin (5-HT) function in humans and animals is inconsistent (21). Overall, no clear picture emerges of changes in brain 5-HT function with age, but the data do suggest that turnover of 5-HT is increased (29,30) and the numbers of 5-HT receptors are decreased (31,32) in the brain consequent to aging.

In general, stimulation of 5-HT neurotransmission impairs memory performance in animals, whereas interference with 5-HT function enhances memory performance (33). The deficits in passive avoidance–retention characteristic of middle-aged and aged rats are attenuated by posttraining administration of the 5-HT antagonists, ketanserin and mianserin (34). Consistent with these findings, several 5-HT receptor agonists can produce a dose-related impairment of performance on a radial maze task (35). These data suggest that treatment trials of 5-HT antagonists may be worthwhile in memory-impaired humans. The 5-HT antagonist approach may be refined to include 5-HT receptor subtype-specific antagonists, given the recent identification of multiple 5-HT receptor subtypes (36).

Drugs that inhibit 5-HT uptake may also play a role in improving serotonergic-mediated memory performance. Administration of the 5-HT uptake inhibitors, alaproclate and zimeldine, improved memory performance in mice (37). This improvement was blocked by quipazine, a putative 5-HT agonist, and tended to be potentiated by cyproheptadine, a 5-HT antagonist. These somewhat paradoxical findings prompted the speculation that 5-HT uptake blockers may indirectly interfere with, rather than potentiate, 5-HT transmission (38).

C. Acetylcholine

The association of cholinergic mechanisms with memory function is well-established (see Ref. 39 for review). This, plus the demonstration of reduced presynaptic markers for acetylcholine (ACh) activity in the brains of patients dying of AD (40–42) generated the cholinergic hypothesis of aging and dementia, leading to a multitude of clinical trials of cholinomimetic drugs in treating this disorder. In general, the studies have produced mixed results. This may be the result of several factors, including evidence that noncholinergic neurochemical deficiencies are also important (43) and that brain cholinoreceptive function is lost in AD (44).

In spite of the uncertain outcome of cholinergic trials in AD, the possibility remains that cholinergic dysfunction may also underlie the relatively mild memory impairments associated with normal aging (45).

Decker (46) concluded that there is no reliable degeneration of cholinergic innervation of the hippocampus or cortex in normal aging, unlike AD. However, he did observe that function of brain cholinergic systems is disturbed with advancing age, as reflected by reduced ACh synthesis, reduced stimulation-induced release of ACh, and decreased responsivity of postsynaptic neurons to ACh.

As noted earlier in this chapter, the ideal drug for effective treatment of AAMI should be safe for long-term use with minimal side effects, have a long duration of action, pass readily into the brain, and have a wide therapeutic window. However, as McEntee and Crook note in a recent review (22), other than ACh precursors, no available cholinomimetic drugs come close to meeting these criteria. Treatment trials with the ACh precursor, choline, or its principal dietary source, lecithin (phosphatidylcholine; PC), have not consistently demonstrated beneficial effects on cognition in demented or nondemented aged subjects (47). Since these trials were conducted before the definition of AAMI, it may be worthwhile to reexamine choline treatment in subjects with psychometrically defined AAMI.

Indirectly related to consideration of ACh treatment strategies is the growing interest in testing phospholipids, known for their potential for normalizing cell membrane fluidity, for treatment of dementia and AAMI. Phosphatidylserine (PS), a normal component of cell membranes, is the most studied phospholipid in this respect. Amaducci and colleagues (48) suggest that sustained PS treatment limits cognitive deterioration in AD patients. Moreover, rats treated with PS show improvement in spatial memory and in shock-motivated avoidance behavior (49).

It is possible that these improvements may, in part, be due to pharmacologic actions of PS on cholinergic mechanisms. Treatment with PS causes increased release of ACh from the rat cortex (50) and specifically reverses the reduction of stimulus-induced release and synthesis of ACh in the cortex of aged rats (51). The enhanced synthesis of ACh by PS in aged rat cortex may be the result of an endogenous increase in brain choline through conversion of PS to PC by *N*-methylation. It has been suggested that the small increase in brain choline resulting from conversion of PS to

PC may be used more efficiently for ACh synthesis than the larger amounts available from exogenous dietary sources (52).

D. Interactions of Neurotransmitters

Although the typical treatment strategy focuses on modification of one neurotransmitter system, multiple neurotransmitter systems change with age and in dementing disorders such as AD. Several animal experiments suggest that central cholinergic function depends, at least in part, on an intact forebrain noradrenergic system (53–59). Depletion of central CA by α-methyl-p-tyrosine blocks the facilitation of memory in mice produced by the muscarinic agonist, oxotremorine (54). Phospholipids have potential for normalizing cell membrane fluidity, which is linked to disturbance of cell functions, such as enzyme activity (60), signal transmission (61), or ion transport (62). Consequently, treatment with agents that reverse abnormalities of membrane fluidity may improve function of several different neurotransmitter systems.

Although multiple transmitter abnormalities may be involved in AAMI, pharmacologic research on this condition is still in its early stages and promising single drugs should be investigated before proceeding with more complex experiments designed to modify the balance of activity across multiple neurotransmitter systems. Currently, several ongoing clinical trials of the effects of single compounds on AAMI are nearing completion, and one hopes that these will begin to lay the groundwork for more complex multisystem research.

IV. NEUROPSYCHOLOGICAL AND PSYCHOLOGICAL RESEARCH

Research on AAMI has focused on treatment (63,64), diagnostic, and descriptive studies (65–69).

A. Treatment Studies

Sheikh et al. (63) reviewed the literature on normal age-associated cognitive decline and noted AAMI changes of about 30% compared with young normals. These authors observed that performance increases of the same order of magnitude are not uncommon immediately following memory training. In their own study, Sheikh and colleagues focused on long-term cognitive training in subjects with AAMI deficits. They found that a visual interactive imagery mnemonic, coupled with active pretraining (either verbal judgment and imagery training, imagery training, or relaxation) improved posttest memory for names and faces. Moreover, the posttest gains were maintained over a 6-month period and reflected percentages of improvement ranging from 73 to 111% of baseline performance. The authors concluded that active pretreatment led to maintenance of mnemonic training effects over time in AAMI.

One limitation of traditional visual imagery-training techniques is that they may not be used outside of the laboratory. Consequently, West and Crook (64) evaluated the efficacy of videotape imagery training for recall of names and faces, grocery list learning, and object location recall. By using a wait list control group, these authors demonstrated improved performance on relevant tasks in a computerized everyday memory battery (70–72) when the videotape was used by subjects themselves outside the laboratory. The videotape was particularly useful in this training paradigm, since the image training could be linked with the computer-graphic display employed in the everyday memory battery.

Given the successes of these two studies in behaviorally reversing some of the effects of AAMI, one can expect additional behavioral approaches to treatment of AAMI. A particularly promising treatment strategy might be the combination of behavioral training with pharmacologic intervention.

B. Diagnostic and Descriptive Studies

Larrabee and Crook (65) presented data suggesting that AAMI comprises at least two groups of subjects: those with memory impairment when compared with younger adults (AAMI), and those with memory impairment when compared with their aged peers (senescent forgetfulness). Specifically, Larrabee and Crook conducted cluster analyses on the adjusted and unadjusted performance scores of 158 normal subjects on a battery of computer-simulated everyday memory tests (70–72). Cluster analysis of unadjusted performance scores yielded a group of subjects with poor performance, who had the lowest self-rated memory and the oldest mean age when compared with other subjects. Of course, this finding is consistent with the operational definition of AAMI.

A second cluster analysis was conducted using age-adjusted performance scores. Age adjustment basically resulted in all subjects being compared as "age peers" by removing from their performance scores the effects of memory decline associated with the aging process. In this cluster analysis, the group with the poorest performance also showed a trend toward being the oldest, which is a pattern suggestive of senescent forgetfulness (1,5). Of particular interest was that 84% of these subjects appeared in the AAMI cluster in the unadjusted performance score analysis. These cross-sectional data suggest that 1. forgetfulness is not uniform across the adult-aged range, and 2. that AAMI comprises subjects with normal age-related decline, compared with young normals, as well as subjects manifesting senescent forgetfulness, compared with their-aged peers.

At present, data on the long-term prognosis of AAMI are limited. Reisberg and colleagues (66) conducted a longitudinal follow-up over 3–4 years of subjects using the Global Deterioration Scale (GDS; 73) as the principal assessment instrument. They concluded that persons initially rated as GDS stage 4 (moderate cognitive decline) displayed the earliest signs of Alzheimer-type dementia. Seventy-three percent of these subjects manifested further decline on follow-up, whereas there was no notable progression in 95% of GDS stage 2 patients (very mild cognitive decline). Persons between these two stages, at GDS stage 3, showed a 16.7% negative outcome (operationally defined as a 2-point GDS increment, institutionalization, or death). Reisberg and his colleagues concluded that GDS stage 2 and most of the GDS stage 3 patients had performance and complaint patterns consistent with AAMI. From the perspective of the Larrabee and Crook (65) cluster analyses, the GDS stage 2 subjects likely reflect decline relative to younger persons, whereas the GDS stage 3 subjects likely manifest decline relative to their-aged peers (senescent forgetfulness).

Recently, Lane and Snowdon (67) reported on the prevalence and incidence of AAMI and dementia with 2 years of follow-up in subjects over 65 years of age living in a suburban area of Sydney, Australia. Lane and Snowdon employed the GDS, Beck Depression Inventory (74), Hamilton Depression Scale (16), Mini-Mental State (12), WAIS vocabulary (11), the Guild Memory Test (75), and the original AAMI criteria (7) in defining their AAMI sample. To qualify as AAMI, subjects had to complain (on an interviewer rating scale) of memory decline, obtain Guild Memory Test scores of 2 and 3, score at least 24 on the Mini-Mental State, score at least 32 raw score points on WAIS vocabulary, obtain a GDS score less than 4, and Beck Depression Inventory score less than 13. Using these criteria, Lane and Snowdon established an AAMI prevalence of nearly 40%, with an incidence of 6.63% per annum. By contrast, at baseline, 22% had possible dementia; 21% were excluded owing to reduced WAIS vocabulary; 7% had possible depression; 8% scored within the normal range on the Guild and GDS; 3% had no subjective memory complaint; and another 3% had histories of stroke, head trauma, Parkinson's disease, or use of a psychotropic drug. Of the 51 cases initially classified as AAMI, 26 remained substantially unchanged 2 years later, 3 were excluded at follow-up because of possible criterion artifacts, 7 improved their Guild Memory Test to the normal range, 2 stopped complaining about their memory, and 13 were lost to follow-up (4 died, 2 relocated, and 7 refused the follow-up). Lane and Snowdon's data are the first to examine the prevalence of AAMI, although a large epidemiological study is now underway in Italy in which a true random sample of the normal population is being tested. Their data are also consistent with Reisberg et al. (66) in documenting a benign prognosis for AAMI over the course of 2 years.

Data on the discrimination of AAMI from mild to moderate AD are presented by Youngjohn and associates (68). This study contrasted 127 AD subjects meeting the NINCDS–ADRDA criteria (76) for probable AD and with Mini-Mental State scores of 23 and below (mean, 18.79; SD, 3.27) with 386 subjects meeting the criteria for AAMI (7) and obtaining a Mini-Mental State score of 24 or greater (mean, 28.46; SD, 1.55). With use of a computer-simulated everyday memory battery (70–72), self-report, and family ratings of everyday memory (77), 94.66% of AD and AAMI subjects were correctly classified (AD misclassification rate was 11.0%; AAMI misclassification rate was 3.5%). This high degree of group separation on variables not employed in the original diagnoses of AD and AAMI speaks to the discriminative validity of the original AAMI criteria.

Modifications to the original AAMI criteria were recommended recently in a paper by Blackford and La Rue (69). The authors suggested that standardized memory complaint questionnaires be used to establish the presence of memory complaint. They also recommended that the age range be restricted to 50–79 years. Other recommended changes included demonstration of verbal and performance IQs in the range of 90–130, and a forward digit span of greater than 5, to exclude delirium. Moreover, in an interesting suggestion, the authors recommended using a minimum of four or more tests of secondary memory, and differentiating three categories of subjects: AAMI (performance at least 1 SD below the mean established for young adults on one or more tests); age consistent memory impairment (ACMI; performance within ± 1 SD of the mean established for age on 75% or more of the tests administered); and late-life forgetfulness (LLF; performance between 1 and 2 SD below the mean established for age on 50% or more of the tests administered). The authors noted that the LLF group would be consistent, generally, with Kral's definition of benign senescent forgetfulness. This group would also be consistent with the subgroups identified by Larrabee et al. (5) and Larrabee and Crook (65) and with subjects in the GDS stage 3 category (66).

V. SUMMARY

In the present chapter, we discussed a new diagnostic category for age-related memory decline, AAMI. Individuals in this category have experienced memory loss, relative to their young adult years, and are concerned about this loss. However, they are not demented and are not likely to become demented. Diagnostic criteria for AAMI are reviewed, as are strategies for pharmacologic remediation through noradrenergic, serotonergic, and cholinergic neurotransmitter systems. Behavioral remediation of AAMI through memory retraining is also considered, as well as data on the incidence and prevalence of the condition, its prognosis, and discrimination of AAMI from AD. This research gives reason to hope that an important behavioral deficit associated with aging may be modified through drug and behavioral treatment. Further research on the neurochemical aspects of AAMI may also lead to additional advances in treatment of the more severe impairments associated with Alzheimer-type dementia.

REFERENCES

1. Kral VA. Senescent forgetfulness: benign and malignant. J Can Med Assoc 1962; 86:257–260.
2. Cummings JL, Benson DF. Dementia. A clinical approach. Boston: Butterworths, 1983.
3. Haase GR. Diseases presenting as dementia. In: Wells CE, ed. Dementia, 2nd ed. Philadelphia: FA Davis, 1977:27–67.
4. Reisberg B, Ferris SH, Borenstein J, Sinaiko E, de Leon MJ, Buttinger C. Assessment of presenting symptoms. In: Poon LW, Crook T, Davis KL, Eisdorfer C, Gurland BJ, Kaszniak AW, Thompson LW, eds. Handbook for clinical memory assessment of older adults. Washington, DC: American Psychological Association, 1986:108–128.
5. Larrabee GJ, Levin HS, High WM. Senescent forgetfulness: a quantitative study. Dev Neuropsychol 1986; 2:373–385.
6. Bartus RT, Dean RL, Beer B, Lippa AS. The cholinergic hypothesis of geriatric memory dysfunction. Science 1982; 217:408.
7. Crook T, Bartus RT, Ferris SH, Whitehouse P, Cohen GD, Gershon S. Age-associated memory impairment: proposed diagnostic criteria and measures of clinical change—report of a National Institute of Mental Health workgroup. Dev Neuropsychol 1986:261–276.
8. Leber P. Establishing the efficacy of drugs with psychogeriatric indications. In: Crook T, Bartus RT, Ferris S, Gershon S, eds. Treatment development strategies for Alzheimer's disease. Madison, CT: Mark Powley Associated, 1986:1–14.
9. Benton AL. Revised visual retention test: clinical and experimental applications. New York: Psychological Corporation, 1974.
10. Wechsler DA. A standardized memory scale for clinical use. J Psychol 1945; 19:87–95.
11. Wechsler D. Manual for the Wechsler Adult Intelligence Scale. New York: Psychological Corporation, 1955.
12. Folstein MF, Folstein SE, McHugh PR. Mini-Mental State: a practical method for grading the cognitive state of patients for the clinician. J Psychiatr Res 1975; 12:189–198

13. Bleecker ML, Bolla-Wilson K, Kawas C, Agnew J. Age-specific norms for the Mini-Mental State exam. Neurology 1988; 38:1565–1568.
14. Rosen WG, Terry RD, Fuld PA, Katzman R, Peck A. Pathological verification of ischemic score in differentiation of dementias. Ann Neurol 1980; 7:486–488.
15. American Psychiatric Association. Diagnostic and statistical manual of mental disorders, 3rd ed. Washington, DC: American Psychiatric Association, 1980.
16. Hamilton M. A rating scale for depression. J Neurol Neurosurg Psychiatry 1960; 23:56–62.
17. Crook T, Larrabee GJ. Age-associated memory impairment: diagnostic criteria and treatment strategies. Psychopharmacol Bull 1988; 24:509–514.
18. Crook TH, Larrabee GJ. Age-associated memory impairment. In: Barclay L, ed. Clinical geriatric neurology. Philadelphia: Lea & Febiger (in press).
19. Crook T. Diagnosis and treatment of normal and pathologic memory impairment in later life. Semin Neurol 1989; 9:20–31.
20. McEntee WJ, Crook TH. Age-associated memory impairment: a role for catecholamines. Neurology 1990; 40:526–530.
21. McEntee WJ, Crook TH. Serotonin, memory, and the aging brain. Psychopharmacology 1991; 103:143–149.
22. McEntee WJ, Crook TH. Cholinergic function in the aged brain: implications for treatment of memory impairments associated with aging. (submitted).
23. Arnsten AFT, Goldman-Rakic PS. Catecholamines and cognitive decline in aged nonhuman primates. Ann NY Acad Sci 1985; 444:218–234.
24. McEntee WJ, Mair RG, Langlais PJ. Neurochemical pathology in Korsakoff's psychosis: implications for other cognitive disorders. Neurology 1984; 34:648–652.
25. Mair RG, McEntee WJ, Zattore RJ. Monoamine activity correlates with psychometric impairments in Korsakoff's disease. Behav Brain Res 1985; 15:247–254.
26. McEntee WJ, Mair RG. Memory enhancement in Korsakoff's psychosis with clonidine: further evidence for a noradrenergic deficit. Ann Neurol 1980; 7:466–470.
27. Arnsten AFT, Cai JX, Goldman-Rakic PS. The alpha-2 adrenergic agonist guanfacine improves memory in aged monkeys without sedative or hypotensive side-effects: evidence for alpha-2 subtypes. J Neurosci 1988; 8:4287–4298.
28. Schlegel J, Mohr E, Williams J, Mann U, Gearing M, Chase TN. Guanfacine treatment of Alzheimer's disease. Clin Neuropharmacol 1989; 12:124–128.
29. Moretti A, Carfagna N, Trunzo F. Effect of aging on monoamines and their metabolites in the rat brain. Neurochem Res 1987; 12:1035–1039.
30. Brunello N, Riva M, Rovescalli AC, Galimberti R, Racasni G. Age-related changes in rat serotonergic and adrenergic systems and in receptor responsiveness to subchronic desipramine treatment. Pharmacol Toxicol 1988; 63: 150–155.
31. Allen SJ, Benton JS, Goodhardt MJ, Hann EA, Sims NR, Smith CCT, Spillane JA, Bowen DM, Davison AN. Biochemical evidence of selective

nerve cell changes in the normal ageing human and rat brain. J Neurochem 1983; 41:256–265.

32. Middlemiss DN, Palmer AM, Edel N, Bowen DM. Binding of the novel serotonin agonist 8-hydroxy-2(di-*n*-propylamino)tetralin in normal and Alzheimer brain. J Neurochem 1986; 46:993–996.
33. Altman HJ, Normile HJ. Enhancement of the memory of a previously learned aversive habit following pre-test administration of a variety of serotonergic antagonists in mice. Psychopharmacology 1986; 90:24–27.
34. Altman HJ, Normile HJ. What is the nature of the role of the serotonergic nervous system in learning and memory: prospects for development of an effective treatment strategy for senile dementia. Neurobiol Aging 1988; 9:627–638.
35. Winter JC, Petti DT. The effects of 8-hydroxy-2-(di-*n*-propylamino)tetralin and other serotonergic agonists on performance in a radial maze: a possible role for 5-HT_{1A} receptors in memory. Pharmacol Biochem Behav 1987; 27:625–628.
36. Schmidt AW, Peroutka SJ. 5-Hydroxytryptamine receptor families. FASEB J 1989; 3:2242–2249.
37. Altman HJ, Nordy DA, Ogren SO. Role of serotonin in memory: facilitation by alaproclate and zimeldine. Psychopharmacology 1984; 84:496–502.
38. Altman HJ, Stone WS, Ogren SO. Evidence for a possible functional interaction between serotonergic and cholinergic mechanisms in memory retrieval. Behav Neural Biol 1987; 48:49–62.
39. Collerton D. Cholinergic function and intellectual decline in Alzheimer's disease. Neuroscience 1986; 19:1–28.
40. Bowen DM, Smith CB, White P, Davison AN. Neurotransmitter-related enzymes and indices of hypoxia in senile dementia and other abiotrophies. Brain 1976; 99:459–496.
41. Davies P, Malone AJF. Selective loss of central cholinergic neurons in Alzheimer's disease. Lancet 1976; 2:1403.
42. Perry EK, Perry RH, Blessed G, Tomlinson BE. Necropsy evidence of cholinergic deficits in senile dementia. Lancet 1977; 1:189.
43. Rossor M, Iversen LL. Non-cholinergic neurotransmitter abnormalities in Alzheimer's disease. Br Med Bull 1986; 42:70–74.
44. Pomara N, Bagne CA, Stanley M, Yarbrough GG. Prospective strategies for cholinergic interventions in Alzheimer's disease. Neuropsychopharmacol Biol Psychiatry 1986; 10:553–570.
45. Bartus RT, Dean RL, Beer B, Lippa AS. The cholinergic hypothesis of geriatric memory dysfunction. Science 1982; 217:408–417.
46. Decker MW. The effects of aging on hippocampal and cortical projections of the forebrain cholinergic system. Brain Res Rev 1987; 12:423–438.
47. Bartus RT, Dean RL, Beer B. Cholinergic precursor therapy for geriatric cognition: its past, its present and a question of its future. In: Ordy MM, Harman D, Alfin-Slater R, eds. Nutrition in gerontology. New York: Raven Press, 1984:191–225.

48. Amaducci L, SMID group. Phosphatidylserine in the treatment of Alzheimer's disease: results of a multicenter study. Psychopharmacol Bull 1988; 24:130–134.
49. Zanotti A, Valzelli L, Toffano G. Chronic phosphatidylserine treatment improves spatial memory and passive avoidance in aged rats. Psychopharmacology 1989; 99:316–321.
50. Cassamenti F, Mantovani P, Amaducci L, Pepeu G. Effect of phosphatidylserine on acetylcholine output from the cerebral cortex of the rat. J Neurochem 1979; 32:529–533.
51. Vannucchi MG, Pepeu G. Effect of phosphatidylserine on acetylcholine release and content in cortical slices from aging rats. Neurobiol Aging 1987; 8:403–407.
52. Rotrosen J. Membrane lipids: can modification reduce symptoms or halt progression of Alzheimer's disease? In: Crook T, Bartus RT, Ferris S, Gershon S, eds. Treatment development strategies for Alzheimer's disease. Madison CT: Mark Powley Associated, 1986:519–537.
53. Mason ST, Fibiger HC. Possible behavioral function for noradrenaline–acetylcholine interaction in brain. Nature 1979; 277:396–397.
54. Huygens P, Baratti CM, Gardella JL, Filinger E. Brain catecholamines modification. The effects on memory facilitation induced by oxotremorine in mice. Psychopharmacology 1980; 69:291–294.
55. Waterhouse BD, Moises HC, Woodward DJ. Noradrenergic modulation of somatosensory cortical neuronal responses to iontophoretically applied putative neurotransmitters. Exp Neurol 1980; 69:30–49.
56. Waterhouse BD, Moises HC, Woodward DJ. alpha-Receptor-mediated facilitation of somatosensory cortical neuronal responses to excitatory synaptic inputs and iontophoretically applied acetylcholine. Neuropharmacology 1981; 20:907–920.
57. Decker MW, Gallagher M. Scopolamine-disruption of radial arm maze performance: modification by noradrenergic depletion. Brain Res 1987; 417:59–69.
58. Haroutunian V, Kanof PD, Tsuboyama GK, Campbell GA, Davis KL. Animal models of Alzheimer's disease: behavior, pharmacology, transplants. Can J Neurol Sci 1986; 13:385–393.
59. Haroutunian V, Kanof PD, Tsuboyama G, Davis KL. Restoration of cholinomimetic activity by clonidine in cholinergic plus noradrenergic lesioned rats. Brain Res (in press).
60. Farias RN, Bloj B, Morero RD, Sineriz F, Trucco RE. Regulation of allosteric membrane-bound enzymes through changes in membrane lipid composition. Biochim Biophys Acta 1975; 415:231–251.
61. Hirata F, Axelrod J. Phospholipid methylation and biological signal transmission. Science 1980; 209:1082–1090.
62. Kimmelberg HK. Alterations in phospholipid-dependent ($Na^+ + K^+$)-ATPase activity due to lipid fluidity effects of cholesterol and Mg^{2+}. Biochim Biophys Acta 1975; 413:143–156.
63. Sheikh JI, Hill RD, Yesavage JA. Long-term efficacy of cognitive training for

age-associated memory impairment: A six-month follow-up study. Dev Neuropsychol 1986; 2:413–424.

64. West RL, Crook TH. Video training of imagery for mature adults. Appl Cogn Psychol (in press).
65. Larrabee GJ, Crook TH. Performance subtypes of everyday memory function. Dev Neuropsychol 1989; 15:267–283.
66. Reisberg B, Ferris SH, Franssen E, Kluger A, Borenstein J. Age-associated memory impairment: the clinical syndrome. Dev Neuropsychol 1986; 2:401–412.
67. Lane F, Snowdon F. Memory and dementia: a longitudinal survey of suburban elderly. In: Lovibond P, Wilson P, eds. Clinical and abnormal psychology. Amsterdam: Elsevier North-Holland, 1989:365–376.
68. Youngjohn JR, Larrabee GJ, Crook TH. Discriminating age-associated memory impairment and Alzheimer's disease. J Clin Exper Neuropsychol 1991; 13:71.
69. Blackford RC, La Rue A. Criteria for diagnosing age-associated memory impairment: proposed improvements from the field. Dev Neuropsychol 1989; 5:295–306.
70. Crook TH, Larrabee GJ. Interrelationships among everyday memory tests: stability of factor structure with age. Neuropsychology 1988; 2:1–12.
71. Larrabee GJ, Crook T. A computerized everyday memory battery for assessing treatment effects. Psychopharmacol Bull 1988; 24:695–697.
72. Larrabee GJ, Crook TH. Dimensions of everyday memory in age-associated memory impairment. Psychol Assess J Consult Clin Psychol 1989; 1:92–97.
73. Reisberg G, Ferris SH, de Leon MJ, Crook T. The Global Deterioration Scale for assessment of primary degenerative dementia. Am J Psychiatry 1982; 139:1136–1139.
74. Beck AT, Ward CH, Mendelson M, Mock J, Erbaugh J. An inventory for measuring depression. Arch Gen Psychiatry 1961; 4:53–63.
75. Crook TH, Gilbert JG, Ferris SH. Operationalizing memory impairment for elderly persons: The Guild Memory Test. Psychol Rep 1980; 47:1315–1318.
76. McKhann G, Drachman D, Folstein M, Katzman R, Price D, Stadlan EM. Clinical diagnosis of Alzheimer's disease: report of the NINCDS–ADRDA work group under the auspices of Department of Health and Human Services Task Force on Alzheimer's Disease. Neurology 1984; 34:939–944.
77. Crook TH, Larrabee GJ. A self-rating scale for evaluating memory in everyday life. Psychol Aging 1990; 5:48–57.

IV

PHARMACOLOGICAL TREATMENT: FUTURE POSSIBILITIES AND THEIR EVALUATION

12

Pharmacological "Prospectives"

Walter H. Moos *Chiron Corporation, Emeryville, California*

Robert E. Davis *Parke-Davis Pharmaceutical Research Division, Warner-Lambert Co., Ann Arbor, Michigan*

Elkan R. Gamzu *Cambridge NeuroScience, Inc., Cambridge, Massachusetts*

I. INTRODUCTION

Pharmacology deals with the origin, nature, chemistry, effects, and uses of drugs. In this chapter, we review through historical perspective the direction that pharmacology is taking in cognitive disorders. Brief reviews of material presented in greater detail elsewhere in this book are included where necessary for background.

Cognitive disorders are widespread, but it is especially those cognitive disorders of the burgeoning elderly population that force a commitment to discovering and developing *cognition activators*. Regrettably, the hope of enhancing human cognitive function in a meaningul way by pharmacologic means remains unfulfilled; hence, the proposition is one of high risk. Fortunately, ". . .the great efforts being made in basic and applied research warrant cautious optimism" (1).

Numerous reports covering various aspects of cognition activators and cognitive decline have appeared in the recent literature (2–5). Given the vast new literature on cognitive disorders, updated commentaries from different perspectives (or "prospectives") are constantly needed. For leading references, readers are referred to the aforementioned reviews.

As in the past, we will refer generically to the spectrum of cognitive disorders found in the elderly as *senile cognitive decline* (SCD). Moreover, we introduce here the term *cognetics* to refer generically to the many past, present, and future cognition activators or cognition enhancers.

A. Dementia and Senile Cognitive Decline

Dementia is a clinical syndrome involving reduced intellectual functioning, with acquired impairment in memory and other cognitive domains such as language and visuospatial skills (6). The dementias and related disorders of the elderly often involve short-term working memory loss, and a decrease in attention span and motivation.

The most frequently encountered cognitive disorders, especially Alzheimer's disease (AD), age-associated memory impairment (AAMI; see Chap. 11) (7), and multi-infarct dementia (MID; see Chap. 10) present the greatest challenges because they are currently untreatable. Alzheimer's disease remains a focus of much clinical research on cognitive disorders because it is currently the best-characterized as well as the most common disorder producing cognitive dysfunction.

B. Alzheimer's Disease

Alois Alzheimer's commonly cited 1907 report (8) describes a 56-year-old woman who had died following a 5 to 6-year illness characterized by disorientation, memory loss, and personality changes. Postmortem microscopic examination of her brain tissue, using the then newly available silver stains, revealed a high density of lesions called neuritic plaques and neurofibrillary tangles. These microscopic changes, now accepted as the pathological hallmark of AD, had previously been observed only in brains of people over 70 years of age. The relationship between normal aging and AD is still unresolved.

Alzheimer's disease was a medical curiosity for many years. In fact, the magnitude of its occurrence and effect on society was not appreciated until the 1970s (Table 1). It is now the most prevalent accepted form of SCD, although AAMI may ultimately represent a larger patient popula-

TABLE 1 Alzheimer's Disease and Related Dementias (US Estimates)

AD responsible for	$\geq$ 50% of all dementias
Cases of AD	$\approx$ 2–4 million
Cost of illness to society ($)	$>$ 50 billion (9)
Potential market ($)	$\approx$ 1 billion
Effective therapy	None marketed at this writing

tion. With an expected 100,000 deaths per year, AD indirectly constitutes the fourth leading cause of death in the United States (10). Data from population studies suggest at least a tenfold increase in the prevalence of AD between ages 60 and 80. Indeed, prevalence may exceed 50% among those 95 and over (11). The prevalence of AD can only increase in the coming years as the geriatric segment of the population grows (12–15). For example, in the United States alone, the segment of the population presently over age 65 is estimated at 11% (25 million people); over the next 50 years this figure should grow to 20% of the population (55 million people) (16).

Currently, AD is diagnosed using *DSM-III* (*DSM-III-R*; 6) or NINCDS–ADRDA criteria (17). The clinical diagnosis of AD is approximately 70–90% accurate. Multi-item scales and neuropsychological tests are useful for assessing the degree of dementia (see, e.g., 18). Other possible causes of dementia are excluded based upon clinical history or laboratory data (see Chap. 8 for additional discussion).

TABLE 2 Possible Factors in the Pathogenesis of Alzheimer's Disease

Abnormal proteins (e.g., A-68) (see 20)
Disorders of membrane metabolism
Genetic aspects [e.g., familial AD, Down (21), chromosome 21, dementia of Guam, Parkinson's dementia, and β-amyloid]
Infectious agents (e.g., prions)
Multifactorial dysfunction (e.g., genetic predisposition plus environmental toxins)
Neurotransmitter deficits (e.g., cholinergic deficit hypothesis of aging and dementia)
Toxins (e.g., aluminum; 22)

The etiology and pathogenesis of AD are unclear. However, many factors could be involved (19). A nonexhaustive list is presented in Table 2. Important and fundamental assessments that may provide clues to the etiology and pathogenesis have appeared, including reviews of the neurochemistry of dementia (23,24) and antemortem markers in AD (25).

Although beyond the scope of this chapter, the role of amyloid, plaques, neurofibrillary tangles, chromosomal abnormalities, and programmed cell death (apoptosis), all are areas of competitive and rapidly developing research (26,27).

C. Animal Models

To develop new therapeutic agents in a rational and efficient manner, satisfactory biological models are needed (Table 3). Unfortunately, appro-

TABLE 3 Examples of Classes of Animal Models

Assays of function or dysfunction that mimic symptoms (e.g., disrupted memory)
Models of biological disruption that parallel known disease pathology (e.g., nucleus basalis lesions)
Models of the disease state itself (possibly overidealistic)

priately validated animal models do not yet exist, and many considerations are important in developing effective animal models (28).

The earliest cognetics were developed almost entirely through leads discovered during the course of functional behavior testing. Newer agents represent a shift to better-defined mechanisms of action. For example, consider the cholinergic hypothesis of aging and dementia, which has been proposed to explain the pathology and symptoms of geriatric memory dysfunction (29). Much research was guided by this rationale in the 1980s. If indeed the cholinergic deficits observed in AD cause the observed cognitive decline, then, in principle, symptomatic treatment should be possible with several types of cholinergic agents. However, because multiple neurotransmitter deficiencies are present, activation of just one neurotransmitter system may not be sufficient to improve symptoms in AD. (It should be noted that certain alternative hypotheses with little resemblance to the cholinergic hypothesis could also have merit, e.g., calpain-related phenomena, 30).

To the extent that a biochemically based mechanism is the target of a drug development process, biological questions are best addressed at an early stage through in vitro biochemical studies. This approach is both useful and efficient in light of the high testing throughput and minimal complicating pharmacokinetic and metabolic factors inherent to such studies. Regardless of in vitro biochemical specificity, however, whole-animal biology remains a sine qua non of drug development. Table 4 lists possible in vitro and in vivo assays for one mechanistic approach. Table 5, which lists some additional whole-animal assays, is followed here by a brief discussion of a few of the models.

Ethylcholine mustard aziridinium (AF-64A), a neurotoxic choline analogue, produces long-lasting hypofunction of central cholinergic systems in mice, and it reduces presynaptic cholinergic markers in the rat hippocampus without affecting postsynaptic muscarinic receptor binding. Moreover, maze performance is impaired following AF-64A treatment, but successful use of AF-64A depends upon its careful preparation (33). The interest in this area is considerable, because lesions caused by alkylating agents, such as the aziridiniums, may eventually provide a suitable animal

TABLE 4 Possible Mechanistic Screens for a Cholinergic Approach

In Vitro	
Muscarinic receptor binding	High-affinity choline uptake
Acetylcholine release	Choline acetyltransferase activity
Inhibition of cholinesterase	Phosphatidylinositol turnover
Cyclase activity	Ion flux
In Vivo	
Electroencephalography (EEG)	Local cerebral blood flow (LCBF)
Reversal of anticholinergic-induced behavior	

TABLE 5 Some In Vivo Assays

Genetically inbred strains
Hippocampally deficient mouse (31)
Senescence-accelerated mouse (SAM) (32)
Trisomy 16 mouse
Aged animals
Aged rats and monkeys
Chemical lesions/deficits
Anticholinergics (e.g., scopolamine)
Aziridiniums (e.g., AF-64A, BM-123, BM-130)
Benzodiazepines (e.g., diazepam)
Excitatory toxins (e.g., ibotenic acid, kainic acid)
False transmitters (e.g., *N*-aminodeanol)
Neurotransmitter synthesis inhibitors (e.g., BW-813U)
Miscellaneous (e.g., trialkyltin halides, electrolytic lesions)
Other deficits
Electroconvulsive shock (ECS)
Oxygen deficits (i.e., hypoxia, anoxia)

model of AD. However, adequate behavioral evidence to completely validate these models is still lacking. Anticholinergic-induced cognitive deficits have also been used as a model of age-related impairments, with agents tested for their ability to reverse the deficits. Benzodiazepine-induced amnesia (34), first described as a result of clinical experience, has been used as an animal model of amnesia. Unfortunately, the results of such studies have been subject to overinterpretation. Thus, the extension of various preclinical and clinical findings toward the development of clinically useful agents is not always straightforward (35).

Electroconvulsive shock (ECS) has been used to produce severe retrograde amnesia, an effect that is well documented at the clinical level and extensively studied in animals. The effects of agents on impaired memory in depressed patients undergoing ECS therapy are under study (36). Since many cognetics were discovered and developed based upon activity against ECS-induced amnesia, these studies will test the predictive value of the preclinical ECS model.

Are the animal models valid? Unfortunately, this question cannot now be answered. Perhaps the models are valid, but greater preclinical efficacy is needed. Certainly, drugs with more robust preclinical effects are needed. Perhaps side effects, a short duration of action, or a narrow active dose range mask the clinical efficacy of useful drugs. Here, agents with fewer side effects, longer duration, or wider active dose ranges are required.

II. DRUG STRATEGIES

The efficacy of drugs used to treat AD in the recent past is questionable. Early therapeutic strategies used agents that were claimed to either improve cerebral blood flow or have mild psychostimulant properties. In the United States, the metabolic enhancer dihydroergotoxine; the vasodilators papaverine, isoxsuprene, and cyclandelate; and the psychostimulants methylphenidate and pentylenetetrazole, have been used to treat SCD. Dihydroergotoxine, a mixture of several hydrogenated ergot alkaloids, has until recently been a worldwide market leader. Despite more than 100 clinical trials of cerebral vasodilators and psychostimulants in the dementias, the effectiveness of these drugs remains uncertain (see Ref. 37 for review). In fact, not one of these agents has been demonstrated to improve cognition unequivocally in AD patients, although dihydroergotoxine may have a small positive effect on mood.

Compounds that improve CBF through vascular mechanisms have also been employed internationally to treat AD. These compounds include nafronyl, pentoxifylline, suloctidil, vincamine, and calcium channel blockers (e.g., nimodipine). The use of these agents is questionable because a vascular origin for AD is no longer widely accepted. Current best-selling international products include idebenone, pentoxifylline, vinpocetine, dihydroergotoxine, and citicoline. Unfortunately, none of these compounds has shown convincing, reproducible efficacy in AD under appropriately blinded, placebo-controlled conditions (see, e.g., 38,39). The leading international market remains Japan (over 1 billion dollars in sales of nootropics and related compounds), followed by France, Germany, and Italy.

The most widely studied drug classes, vasodilators, metabolic enhancers, nootropics, and psychostimulants, are considered in more detail in the following.

A. Vasodilators and Metabolic Enhancers

The original justification for the use of vasodilators in treating AD was the assumption that narrowing of cerebral vessels ("hardening of the arteries") was responsible for dementia. Agents that increased cerebral blood flow would, therefore, reverse cognitive decline. The apparent failure to show true effectiveness with these drugs probably reflects the lack of a vascular origin for AD. More recent clinical studies with vasodilators and metabolic enhancers have focused on populations with MID and MIX (mixed AD and MID).

Agents that affect cellular metabolism by mechanisms distinct from direct action on cerebral vasculature have been classified as metabolic enhancers, and a number of alkaloid derivatives fall into this class (Table 6).

B. Nootropics

The term *nootropic,* from the Greek, means "acting upon the mind" (40). Nootropics (41,42) are a unique class of drugs (Table 7), affecting mental function through as yet unknown mechanisms. Predominant among the nootropics are the pyrrolidones, the forerunner being piracetam, a cyclic relative of γ-aminobenzoic acid (GABA). Interestingly, 2-pyrrolidinone and succinimide are endogenous to several mammalian species. The *therapeutic window* concept, or inverted U-shaped dose–response function, characteristic of nootropic agents like pramiracetam, has been demonstrated in a wide variety of models. Although piracetam and related nootropics facilitate learning and memory in animal models, human studies continue to give mixed results, except perhaps in dyslexia (43,44). (It is

TABLE 6 Representative Vasodilators and Metabolic Enhancers

Bromvincamine	Cyclandelate	Dihydroergocristine
Dihydroergotoxine (ergoloid mesylates)	Isoxsuprene	Nafronyl
	Nimodipine	Papaverine
Nicergoline	Suloctidil	Vinburnine
Pentoxifylline	Vindeburnol	Vinpocetine
Vincamine		

TABLE 7 Representative Nootropics

Aniracetam	BMY 21502	CI-933
Dupracetam	Etiracetam	Oxiracetam
Piracetam	Pramiracetam	Rolziracetam

important to note that the potential therapeutic effects of piracetam and related compounds encompass many clinical indications, such as dyslexia, that are only remotely related to SCD).

C. Psychostimulants

A recent reconsideration of the use of psychostimulants in general psychiatry concluded that there is some evidence to support the judicious use of psychostimulants in selected clinical instances of several adult psychiatric syndromes, but importantly *not* in senile organic brain syndrome (45). The administration of psychostimulants (e.g., methylphenidate, amphetamine, pemoline) can affect certain aspects of learning disabilities in adolescents as well as attentional deficits in adults, but such treatment may be of limited use. In contrast, individuals with AD are generally unresponsive to these drugs.

D. Mechanism-Based Strategies

Although nootropics and variations of older compounds have not been abandoned, the focus of much research has now shifted to biochemical, neurochemical, and peptide-based approaches in the hope of identifying agents that improve the behavioral endpoints of learning and memory by better defined mechanisms of action.

1. Cholinergic Agents

The most widely accepted biochemical hypothesis for the cognitive deficit in AD, at present, involves the cholinergic system (46). However, although the cholinergic rationale remains a viable explanation for memory deficits in AD, it is unlikely to account for the entire range of biochemical, pathological, anatomical, and pharmacological deficits in dementia. Clinical studies in AD with muscarinic acetylcholine receptor (mAChR) agonists, cholinesterase (ChE) inhibitors, and cholinergic releasing agents have shown significant, albeit weak, activity, but cholinergic precursors such as choline (Ch) or lecithin have little or no effect by themselves.

a. Cholinesterase Inhibitors (Table 8; 47). Physostigmine has been the subject of more clinical trials than any other cholinergic agent. It is believed to have a small positive effect on the symptoms of SCD. Heptylphysostigmine has been developed to improve upon physostigmine's poor oral availability and half-life.

Cholinesterase inhibitors related to miotine have a longer duration of action and greater central selectivity than physostigmine. The potential of galantamine and the huperzines, longer-acting anticholinesterases, has also been studied in a preliminary fashion. Recently, there has been a renewed interest in so-called *ir*reversible ChE inhibitors (e.g., methanesulfonyl fluoride, metrifonate).

TABLE 8 Acetylcholinesterase Inhibitors

Amiridin (NIK-247)	E-2020	Galantamine
Huperzine A	Methanesulfonyl fluoride (MSF)	Metrifonate
Miotine (RA-2)	Physostigmine	SM-10888
Suronacrine (HP-128)	Tacrine (THA)	Velnacrine (HP-029)

TABLE 9 Muscarinic Receptor Agonists

AF-series (i.e., AF-30; AF-102)	Arecoline
BM-5	CI-979 (PD 129409)
McN-A-343	Oxotremorine
Pilocarpine series (e.g., PD 133315)	RS-86
SDZ-210-086 (SDZ-210-BOP)	

A meta-analysis of the literature has suggested that all cholinergic treatments produce some improvement in memory function provided that dosages are individualized. Treatments combining a precursor (e.g., lecithin) with an anticholinesterase appear to offer the greatest promise for clinically useful results (48). Indeed, with individualized doses and preloading with lecithin, one study of 1,2,3,4-tetrahydro-9-acridinamine (tacrine) claimed activity in AD patients (49). Well-designed Phase III trials assessing the therapeutic potential of tacrine in AD under more controlled conditions are nearing completion. Hydroxy derivatives (velnacrine, HP-029; suronacrine, HP-128) of tacrine have also entered clinical trials (50,51).

b. Muscarinic Receptor Agents. (Table 9; 2,52,53) Reductions in receptor number for the M_2 receptor subtype and in choline acetyltransferase (ChAcT) activity are observed in cortical samples from AD patients and from rats cholinergically denervated with ibotenic acid; receptors of the M_1 subtype are unchanged. The M_2 receptors may act presynaptically to regulate ACh release, with M_1 receptors facilitating postsynaptic cellular excitation (54). Thus, selective presynaptic (M_2) antagonists or postsynaptic (M_1) agonists might provide useful therapy in AD.

As a screening technique, antagonist/agonist-binding ratios have been proposed as predictors of efficacy at muscarinic receptors (55). This method works with a variety of agonist and antagonist ligands, and coupled with computer-assisted drug design, has been used to uncover new classes of agonists, such as the tetrahydropyridine oximes (e.g., CI-979).

Rigid muscarinic agents have been prepared to explore the muscarinic receptor pharmacophore; rigidity may reflect drug specificity. Both AF-30 and AF-102 are rigid muscarinic agonists reported to have a degree of M_1-

selectivity. Related oxadiazoles show high potency and efficacy. However, no unequivocally selective agonists yet exist. RS-86 is the most extensively studied muscarinic acetylcholine receptor agonist in humans. It penetrates the blood–brain barrier, has high central receptor affinity, and is reported to show no specific toxicity other than dose-related cholinergic effects. Unfortunately, the clinical efficacy of RS-86 is equivocal, perhaps owing to its weak partial agonist characteristics or high degree of peripheral parasympathetic effects.

c. Other Cholinergic Agents. (Table 10) Although several agents interact negatively with allosteric sites on muscarinic receptors (e.g., the inhibitor gallamine), no allosteric activator has yet been reported. Many agents influence ACh release, including some new ureas like PD 121323 and related compounds like DuP 996. 4-Aminopyridine and 3,4-diaminopyridine alter ACh metabolism and behavior during hypoxia, and an exploratory study of 4-aminopyridine in AD was mildly positive (58).

Most research on cognition and the cholinergic system has focused on muscarinic receptors. However, nicotinic receptors are increasingly of interest, as evidence accumulates for changes in both muscarinic and nicotinic receptors in AD. For example, a parallel and marked reduction in the number of nicotine (59) and presynaptic ACh-binding sites is found in the frontal cortex of AD brains, compared with age-matched controls.

The cholinergic system interacts with several other neurochemical receptor and enzyme systems, including norepinephrine, serotonin, excitatory amino acids, adenosine, adenylate cyclase, and phosphodiesterase. The potential exists, therefore, for many classes of agents to alleviate indirectly the cholinergic deficit in AD.

d. Neurotrophic Factors. Neurotrophic factors (60,61), especially nerve growth factor (NGF) and the gangliosides, represent a possible new

TABLE 10 Other Cholinergic Agents

Acetylcholine release and storage modulators	
4-Aminopyridine (4-AP)	3,4-Diaminopyridine (3,4-DAP)
Linopirine (DuP 996 (56,57))	
Nicotinamide	
Substituted ureas (e.g., PD 121323)	Vesamicol (AH-5183)
Allosteric modifiers of cholinergic functioning	
Gallamine	McN-A-343
Bisquaternary pyridinium oximes	
Nonspecific "cholinergic agents"	
Minaprine	Bifemelane (MCI-2016)
Salbutiamine	

direction for research on the etiology and treatment of SCD. The degeneration of cholinergic neurons of the mammalian basal forebrain in AD could result from a dysfunction of the trophic interactions that support cholinergic connections. However, this is unlikely to result from a simple decrease in NGF, because NGF levels are not reduced in AD (see Chap. 13).

2. *Biogenic Amines* (5)

Adrenergic systems are involved in the modulation of memory storage and selective attention as they relate to memory retrieval, thus a role in age-related memory dysfunction is not surprising (62). For example, epinephrine facilitates memory, and its effects are attenuated by adrenoceptor antagonists. Clonidine and guanfacine have been reported to ameliorate cognitive deficits in aged monkeys (63,64). In other studies, however, clonidine impaired performance in both aged monkeys and normal humans (65,66). In all studies, clonidine induces significant sedation that must be overcome to show significant improvements in cognitive function.

Data from postmortem brain, CSF, and serotonin receptor studies indicate significant impairment of the serotonergic system in AD. Alaproclate, a specific inhibitor of neuronal serotonin (5-HT) reuptake, may have a positive effect on emotional functions in AD (67); others report little effect in MID and AD (68). Zimeldine, another 5-HT reuptake blocker, has no effect on memory or reaction time in AD (69).

Selegiline (deprenyl), a monoamine oxidase (MAO) inhibitor that is selective for MAO-B at low doses, was noted to enhance performance on an episodic memory and learning task requiring complex information processing and sustained conscious effort. Knowledge memory, intrusions, and other cognitive functions relevant to AD were not altered (70). Although no conclusive trial has been conducted in AD with selegiline, studies in Parkinson's disease (71,72) have drawn attention to the possibility of decreasing the rate of decline in progressive neurological disorders.

3. *Neuropeptide Systems* (Table 11; 5)

A somatostatinergic deficit occurs in AD, but the somatostatin analogue L-363,586 did not improve memory impairment in AD patients (73). Behavioral measurements indicate that vasopressin (VP) enhances memory, probably not by central mechanisms, but possibly through peripheral reinforcement and central modulation of arousal. A recent paper demonstrated that DGAVP (Org 5667) is without therapeutic benefit in AD (74). Results of studies with ORG 2766, a synthetic analogue of ACTH 4-9 that received considerable attention at one time, partly because cerebrospinal fluid (CSF) levels of corticotropin (ACTH) are low in AD, have been disappointing.

TABLE 11 Neuropeptides of Interest in Senile Cognitive Decline

Angiotensin-related agents		
Captopril	Enalapril	Quinapril
Somatostatin analogues		
L-363,586		
Vasopressin (VP) analogues		
DDAVP	DGAVP	
Adrenocorticotropin (ACTH) analogues		
ACTH 4-9	ORG 2766	
Opiate-related peptides		
Dynorphin	β-Endorphin	β-Lipotropin
Thyrotropin-releasing hormone (TRH) analogues		
CG-3509	MK-771	
Other peptides		
Neuropeptide Y	Neurotensin	
Cholecystokinin-8 (CCK-8)	Saralasin	
Vasoactive intestinal polypeptide (VIP)		

The CSF levels of β-endorphin are low in AD and MID. Indeed, β-endorphin produces a retrograde amnesia in animals that is blocked by opiate antagonists (e.g., naloxone) and by cholinergic agents (e.g., oxotremorine, physostigmine), but dynorphin 1-13 does not cause retrograde amnesia. Despite the animal data, opiate antagonists do not appear to be effective in treating dementia (75,76).

Various other neuropeptide systems have been investigated sporadically in this field. Protease modulators (i.e., inhibitors or activators) are also of interest [e.g., angiotensin-converting enzyme (ACE) inhibitors and prolyl endopeptidase (PEP) inhibitors]. For example, protease inhibitors might block the processing of amyloid precursors, thereby retarding the progression of AD. Alternatively, protease activators might speed the breakdown of plaques and tangles.

4. *Excitatory Amino Acids*

Excitatory amino acids (EAAs; 77) appear to be intimately involved in synaptic mechanisms and neurological function. An increasing body of knowledge supports a possible role for EAAs in SCD (78). Some investigators have reported decreased L-glutamate binding in Alzheimer's and Huntington's diseases. Others, however, have found no evidence of a deficiency of glutamate, aspartate, or taurine in the AD brain (79). The distribution of *N*-methyl-D-aspartate (NMDA) receptors corresponds to the predilection for neuritic plaques and neurofibrillary tangles to be present in hippocampal subfields in AD. A marked loss of NMDA receptors in the hippocampus and cerebral cortex of patients dying with AD has been observed, and phencyclidine (PCP)-related analogues have been found to bind to a site whose regional distribution is highly correlated with that of NMDA receptor sites. Moreover, paired helical filaments of the Alzheimer type are induced in cultured human neurons by glutamate and aspartate (80), and selective impairment of learning and blockade of long-term potentiation (LTP) has been reported with the NMDA receptor antagonist AP-5 (81). Interestingly, the EAA agent MK-801 has had positive effects in residual attentional deficit disorder (ADD) (82). Clinical trials of EAA antagonists in AD have not yet been carried out.

E. Other Agents

Many other agents (Table 12) have been investigated in animals and in humans for cognetic properties. Some of the following compounds may in fact be better classified otherwise (e.g., as vasodilators; 83), but their

TABLE 12 Representative Other Cognetics

Benzodiazepines (BDZ) and BDZ receptor agents		
β-Carbolines (e.g., ZK93426)	Razobazam	
Dopaminergic agents		
Fipexide	Memantine	
Excitatory amino acids and related agents		
MK-801	AP-5	
Glycinergic agents		
Milacemide		
Monoamine oxidase inhibitors		
Phenelzine	Selegiline	Tranylcypromine
Noradrenergic agents		
Clonidine	Guanfacine	
Opiates		
Naloxone	Naltrexone	
Phosphodiesterase inhibitors		
Pentoxifylline	Rolipram	
Serotonergic agents		
Alaproclate	Buspirone	Citalopram
Fluoxetine	Minaprine	Zimeldine
Steroids		
Dehydroepiandrosterone	Estradiol	Hydrocortisone
Lazaroids (aminosteroids)		
Miscellaneous		
Acetylcarnitine	Buflomedil	Cyclandelate
Dihydroxyphenylserine	Exifone	Glucose
Idebenone	Indeloxazine	Phosphatidylserine
Pyritinol	Sabeluzole	Sulfoxazine

mechanisms have not yet been fully elucidated. Although a number of these agents have been successfully marketed, unequivocal efficacy remains to be demonstrated.

III. CONCLUSION

The search for a cognetic with clinically relevant efficacy and an adequate margin of safety continues. This search is most likely to be successful if the basic mechanisms underlying the disease state are understood. Attention to pharmacology, pharmacokinetics, and issues of trial design are necessary to adequately demonstrate the cognitive enhancing potential of a given agent.

REFERENCES

1. Gamzu ER, Gracon SI. Drug improvement of cognition: hope and reality. Psychiatr Psychobiol 1988; 3(spec B):115S–124S.
2. Pavia MR, Davis RE, Schwarz RD. Cognition enhancers. Annu Rep Med Chem 1990; 25:21–29.
3. Moos WH, Hershenson, FH. Potential therapeutic strategies for senile cognitive disorders. Drug News Perspect 1989; 2:397–409.
4. Fröstl W, Maître L. The families of cognition activators. Pharmacopsychiatry 1989; 22(suppl):54–100.
5. Moos WH, Davis RE, Schwarz RD, Gamzu ER. Cognition activators. Med Res Rev 1988; 8:353–391.
6. American Psychiatric Association. Diagnostic and statistical manual of mental disorders. 3rd ed. Washington, DC: American Psychiatric Association, 1980.
7. Crook T, Bartus RT, Ferris SH, Whitehouse P, Cohen GD, Gershon S. Age-associated memory impairment: proposed diagnostic criteria and measures of clinical change—report of a National Institute of Mental Health work group. Dev Neuropsychol 1986; 2:261–276.
8. Wilkins RH, Brody IA. Alzheimer's disease. Arch Neurol 1969; 21:109–110.
9. Huang, LF, Cartwright WS, Hu TW. The economic cost of senile dementia in the United States. Public Health Rep 1988; 103:3–7.
10. Robertson A. The politics of Alzheimer's disease: a case study in apocalyptic demography. Int J Health Serv 1990; 20:429–442.
11. Evans DA, Funkenstein HH, Albert MS, Scherr PA, Cook NR, Chown MJ, Hebert LE, Hennekens CH, Taylor JO. Prevalence of Alzheimer's disease in a community population of older persons. JAMA 1989; 262:2551–2556.
12. Jorm AF, Korten AE, Henderson AS. The prevalence of dementia: a quantitative integration of the literature. Acta Psychiatr Scand 1987; 76:465–479.
13. O'Connor DW, Pollitt PA, Hyde JB, Fellows JL, Miller ND, Brook CPB, Reiss BB, Roth M. The prevalence of dementia as measured by the Cambridge Mental Disorders of Elderly Examination. Acta Psychiatr Scand 1989; 79:190–198.

14. Pieri L, Cumin R, Hinzen DH. Nosological and epidemiological aspects of Alzheimer's disease. Drug News Perspect 1989; 2:248–253.
15. Regier DA, Boyd JH, Burke JD Jr, Rae DS, Myers JK, Kramer M, Robins LN, George LK, Karno M, Locke BZ. One-month prevalence of mental disorders in the United States. Arch Gen Psychiatry 1988; 45:977–986.
16. Schneider EL, Guralnik JM. The aging of America. JAMA 1990; 263:2335–2355.
17. McKhann G, Drachman D, Folstein M, Katzman R, Price D, Stadlan EM. Clinical diagnosis of Alzheimer's disease: report of the NINCDS–ADRDA work group under the auspices of Department of Health and Human Services Task Force on Alzheimer's Disease. Neurology 1984; 34:939–944.
18. Galasko D, Klauber MR, Hofstetter CR, Salmon DP, Lasker B, Thal LJ. The Mini-Mental State Examination in the early diagnosis of Alzheimer's disease. Arch Neurol 1990; 47:49–52.
19. Wurtman RJ. Alzheimer's disease. Sci Am 1985; 252:62–74.
20. Ghanbari HA, Miler BE, Haigler HF, Arato M, Bissette G, Davies P, Nemeroff CB, Perry EK, Perry R, Ravid R, Swaab DR, Whetsell WO, Zemlan FP. Biochemical assay of Alzheimer's disease—associated protein(s) in human brain tissue. JAMA 1990; 263:2907–2910.
21. Greene JJ. Common ground in the molecular biology of Down syndrome and Alzheimer's disease? Clin Biotechnol 1990; 2:6–8.
22. Birchall JD, Chappell JS. The chemistry of aluminum and silicon in relation to Alzheimer's disease. Clin Chem 1988; 34:265–267.
23. Gottfries CG. Neurochemical aspects of dementia disorders. Dementia 1990; 1:56–64.
24. Whitehouse PJ, Unnerstall JR. Neurochemistry of dementia. Eur Neurol 1988; 28(suppl 1):36–41.
25. Hollander E, Mohs RC, Davis KL. Antemortem markers of Alzheimer's disease. Neurobiol Aging 1986; 7:367–387.
26. Nelson RB, Siman R. Clipsin, a chymotrypsin-like protease in rat brain which is irreversibly inhibited by α-1-antichymotrypsin. J Biol Chem 1990; 265:3836–3843.
27. Roberts GW, Lofthouse R, Allsop D, Landon M, Kidd M, Prusiner SB, Crow TJ. CNS amyloid proteins in neurodegenerative diseases. Neurology 1988; 38:1534–1540.
28. Smith G. Animal models of Alzheimer's disease: experimental cholinergic denervation. Brain Res Rev 1988; 13:103–118.
29. Bartus RT, Dean RL III, Beer B, Lippa AS. The cholinergic hypothesis of geriatric memory dysfunction. Science 1982; 217:408–417.
30. Lynch G, Baudry M. The biochemistry of memory: a new and specific hypothesis. Science 1984; 224:1057–1063.
31. Symons JP, Davis RE, Marriott JG. Water-maze learning and effects of cholinergic drugs in mouse strains with high and low hippocampal pyramidal cell counts. Life Sci 1988; 42:375–383.
32. Miyamoto M, Kiyota Y, Yamazaki N, Nagaoka A, Matsuo T, Nagawa Y,

Takeda T. Age-related changes in learning and memory in the senescence-accelerated mouse (SAM). Physiol Behav 1986; 38:399–406.
33. Moos WH, Davis RE, Schwarz RD. A simplified procedure for preparing the cholinergic neurotoxin 1-ehtyl-1-(2-hydroxyethyl)aziridinium ion (AF64A). Org Prep Proc Int 1989; 21:315–319.
34. Gamzu ER. The role of benzodiazepines in amnesia: laboratory predictors. J Clin Psychiatry 1987; 5:8–13.
35. Gamzu ER, Birkhimer LJ, Hoover T, Gracon ST. Early human trials in the assessment of cognition activators. Pharmacopsychiatry 1990; 23:44–48.
36. Ezzat DH, Ibraheem MM, Makhawy B. The effect of piracetam on ECT-induced memory disturbances. Br J Psychiatry 1985; 147:720–721.
37. Yesavage JA, Tinklenberg JR, Hollister LE, Berger PA. Vasodilators in senile dementias: a review of the literature. Arch Gen Psychiatry 1979; 36:220–223.
38. Thal LF, Salmon DP, Lasker B, Bower D, Klauber MR. The safety and lack of efficacy of vinpocetine in Alzheimer's disease. J Am Geriatr Soc 1989; 37:515–520.
39. Thompson TL, Filley CM, Mitchell WD, Culig KM, LoVerde M, Byyny R. Lack of efficacy of Hydergine in patients with Alzheimer's disease. N Engl J Med 1990; 323:445–448.
40. Gamzu ER, Hoover TM, Gracon SI, Ninteman, MV. Recent developments in 2-pyrrolidinone-containing nootropics. Drug Dev Res 1989; 18:177–189.
41. Müller WE. Nootropics, the therapy of dementia between aspiration and reality. Drug News Perspect 1989; 2:295–300.
42. Nicholson CD. Pharmacology of nootropics and metabolically active compounds in relation to their use in dementia. Psychopharmacology 1990; 101:147–159.
43. Wilsher CR. The nootropic concept and dyslexia. Ann Dyslexia 1986; 118–137.
44. Wilsher CR, Bennett D, Chase C, Connors CK, DiIanni M, Feagans L, Hanvik LJ, Helfgott E, Koplewicz H, Overby P, Reader MJ, Rudel RG, Tallal P. Piracetam and dyslexia: effects on reading tests. J Clin Psychopharmacol 1987; 7:230–237.
45. Chiarello RJ, Cole JO. The use of psychostimulants in general psychiatry. Arch Gen Psychiatry 1987; 44:286–295.
46. DeFeudis FV. Cholinergic systems and Alzheimer's disease. Drug Dev Res 1988; 14:95–109.
47. Becker RE, Giacobini E. Mechanisms of cholinesterase inhibition in senile dementia of the Alzheimer type: clinical, pharmacological, and therapeutic aspects. Drug Dev Res 1988; 12:163–195.
48. Jorm AF. Effects of cholinergic enhancement therapies on memory function in Alzheimer's disease: a meta-analysis of the literature. Aust NZ J Psychiatry 1986; 20:237–240.
49. Summers WK, Majovski LV, Marsh GM, Tachiki K, Kling A. Oral tetrahydroaminoacridine in long-term treatment of senile dementia, Alzheimer type. N Engl J Med 1986; 315:1241–1245.
50. Shutske GM, Pierrat FA, Cornfeldt ML, Szewczak MR, Huger FP, Bores

GM, Haroutunian V, Davis KL. (±)-9-Amino-1,2,3,4-tetrahydroacridin-1-ol. A potential Alzheimer's disease therapeutic of low toxicity. J Med Chem 1988; 31:1278–1279.
51. Shutske GM, Pierrat FA, Kapples KJ, Cornfeldt ML, Szewczak MR, Huger FP, Bores GM, Haroutunian V, Davis KL. 9-Amino-1,2,3,4-tetrahydroacridin-1-ols: synthesis and evaluation as potential Alzheimer's disease therapeutics. J Med Chem 1989; 32:1805–1813.
52. Mei L, Roeske WR, Yamamura HI. Molecular pharmacology of muscarinic receptor heterogeneity. Life Sci 1989; 45:1831–1851.
53. Palacios JM, Spiegel R. Muscarinic cholinergic agonists: pharmacological and clinical perspectives. Prog Brain Res 1986; 70:485–498.
54. Mash DC, Flynn DD, Potter LT. Loss of M_2 muscarine receptors in the cerebral cortex in Alzheimer's disease and experimental cholinergic denervation. Science 1985; 228:1115–1117.
55. Freedman SB, Beer MS, Harley EA. Muscarinic M_1, M_2 receptor binding. Relationship with functional efficacy. Eur J Pharmacol 1988; 156:133–142.
56. Cook L, Nickolson VJ, Steinfels GF, Rohrback KW, DeNoble VJ. Cognition enhancement by the acetylcholine releaser DuP 996. Drug Dev Res 1990; 19:301–314.
57. Nickolson VJ, Tam SW, Myers MJ, Cook L. DuP 996 [3,3-bis(4-pyridinylmethyl)-1-phenylindolin-2-one] enhances the stimulus-induced release of acetylcholine from rat brain in vitro and in vivo. Drug Dev Res 1990; 19:285–300.
58. Wesseling H, Agoston S, Van Dam GBP, Pasma J, DeWit DJ, Havinga H. Effects of 4-aminopyridine in elderly patients with Alzheimer's disease. N Engl J Med 1984; 310:988–989.
59. Whitehouse PJ, Martino AM, Wagster MV, Price DL, Mayeux R, Atack JR, Keller KJ. Reductions in [^{3}H]nicotinic acetylcholine binding in Alzheimer's disease and Parkinson's disease: an autoradiographic study. Neurology 1988; 38:720–723.
60. Gage FH, Chen KS, Buzsaki G, Armstrong D. Experimental approaches to age-related cognitive impairments. Neurobiol Aging 1988; 9:645–655.
61. Snider WD, Johnson EM. Neurotrophic molecules. Ann Neurol 1989; 26: 489–506.
62. Zornetzer SF. Catecholamine system involvement in age-related memory dysfunction. Ann NY Acad Sci 1985; 444:242–254.
63. Arnsten AFT, Goldman-Rakic PS. α_2-Adrenergic mechanisms in prefrontal cortex associated with cognitive decline in aged nonhuman primates. Science 1985; 230:1273–1276.
64. Arnsten A, Cal J, Goldman-Rakic PS. The alpha-2 adrenergic agonist guanfacine improves memory in aged monkeys without sedative or hypotensive side effects: evidence for alpha-2 receptor subtypes. J Neurosci 1988; 11:4287–4298.
65. Davis RE, Callahan MJ, Downs DA. Clonidine disrupts aged-monkey delayed response performance. Drug Dev Res 1988; 12:279–286.
66. Frith CD, Dowdy J, Ferrier IN, Crow TJ. Selective impairment of paired

associate learning after administration of a centrally acting adrenergic agonist (clonidine). Psychopharmacology 1985; 87:490–493.
67. Dehlin O, Hedenrud B, Jansson P, Norgard J. A double-blind comparison of alaproclate and placebo in the treatment of patients with senile dementia. Acta Psychiatr Scand 1985; 71:190–196.
68. Bergman I, Brane G, Gottfries CG, Jostell KC, Karlsson I, Svennerholm L. Alaproclate: a pharmacokinetic and biochemical study in patients with dementia of Alzheimer type. Psychopharmacology 1983; 80:279–283.
69. Cutler NR, Haxby J, Kay AD, Narang PK, Lesko LJ, Costa JL, Ninos M, Linnoila M, Potter WZ, Renfrew JW, Moore AM. Evaluation of zimeldine in Alzheimer's disease: cognitive and biochemical measures. Arch Neurol 1985; 42:744–748.
70. Tariot PN, Sunderland T, Weingartner H, Murphy DL, Welkowitz JA, Thompson K, Cohen RM. Cognitive effects of L-deprenyl in Alzheimer's disease. Psychopharmacology 1987; 91:489–495.
71. The Parkinson Study Group. Effect of deprenyl on the progression of disability in early Parkinson's disease. N Engl J Med 1989; 321:1364–1371.
72. Tetrud JW, Langston JW. The effect of deprenyl (selegiline) on the natural history of Parkinson's disease. Science 1989; 245:519–522.
73. Cutler NR, Haxby JV, Narang PK, May C, Burg CO, Reines SA. Evaluation of an analog of somatostatin (L-363,586) in Alzheimer's disease. N Engl J Med. 1985; 312:725.
74. Wolters EC, Riekkinen P, Lowenthal A, Van der Plaats JJ, Zwart JMT, Sennef C. DGAVP (Org 5667) in early Alzheimer's disease patients: an international double-blind, placebo-controlled, multicenter trial. Neurology 1990; 40:1099–1011.
75. Tariot PN, Sunderland T, Murphy DL, Cohen MR, Welkowitz JA, Weingartner H, Newhouse PA, Cohen RM. Design and interpretation of opiate antagonist trials in dementia. Prog Neuropsychopharmacol Biol Psychiatry 1986; 10:611–626.
76. Serby M, Resnick R, Jordan B, Adler J, Corwin J, Rotrosen JP. Naltrexone and Alzheimer's disease. Prog Neuropsychopharmacol Biol Psychiatry 1986; 10:587–590.
77. Johnson G. Recent advances in excitatory amino acid research. Annu Rep Med Chem 1989; 24:41–50.
78. Greenamyre JT. The role of glutamate in neurotransmission and in neurologic disease. Arch Neurol 1986; 43:1058–1063.
79. Perry TL, Yong VW, Bergeron C, Hansen S, Jones K. Amino acids, glutathione, and glutathione transferase activity in the brains of patients with Alzheimer's disease. Ann Neurol 1987; 21:331–336.
80. De Boni U, McLachlan DR. Controlled induction of paired helical filaments of the Alzheimer type in cultured human neurons, by glutamate and aspartate. J Neurol Sci 1985; 68:105–118.
81. Morris RGM, Anderson E, Lynch GS, Baudry M. Selective impairment of learning and blockade of long-term potentiation by an *N*-methyl-D-aspartate receptor antagonist, AP5. Nature 1986; 319:774–776.

82. Reimherr FW, Wood DR, Wender PH. The use of MK-801, a novel sympathomimetic, in adults with attention deficit disorder, residual type. Psychopharmacol Bull 1986; 22:237–242.
83. Mattson RJ, Moon SL. Agents for the treatment of cognitive disorders. Annu Rep Med Chem 1988; 23:29–38.

13

Trophic Factors and Invasive Procedures

Franz F. Hefti and Lon S. Schneider *Andrus Gerontology Center, University of Southern California, Los Angeles, California*

I. INTRODUCTION

Currently used drugs and most pharmacologic compounds being developed to treat cognitive disorders influence mechanisms related to neuronal impulse flow and transmission at the synapse. They do not affect the structural features of the central nervous system, and there are no known clinically effective compounds that are reliably able to promote regeneration, plasticity, and maintenance of structural integrity of selected neuronal systems. Neurobiological research carried out in recent years has revealed that proteins, called neurotrophic factors, have a major influence on development, maintenance of function, and regeneration of neurons. The discovery of these neurotrophic factors may lead to such a new, structurally oriented neuropharmacology.

Nerve growth factor (NGF) is the first and best characterized among this group of molecules. Because of its pronounced and rather selective trophic action on cholinergic neurons of the basal forebrain, NGF presently is being considered as a potential experimental treatment in Alzheimer's disease (AD). The rationale and potential problems of its clinical use are discussed in detail in the first part of this chapter because NGF may become paradigmatic for therapeutic applications of other neurotrophic factors. The second part of the chapter summarizes knowledge about neurotrophic factors other than NGF. Since neurotrophic factors do not cross the blood–brain barrier, the route of administration represents a major issue, which is addressed in the third part of the chapter.

II. NERVE GROWTH FACTOR AND ALZHEIMER'S DISEASE

A. The Cholinergic Deficit

Alzheimer's disease is associated with a pronounced loss of cholinergic neurons of the basal forebrain located in the nucleus basalis and diagonal band of Broca. A large body of evidence supports the view that these cholinergic neurons are involved in functions related to cognition and memory (1,2). The massive decline of the cholinergic basalocortical projection in AD is well established. Early findings of reductions in the activity of cerebral cortical choline acetyltransferase (ChAcT), the key enzyme in acetylcholine synthesis (3–5), were followed by the demonstration of a massive loss of cholinergic cell bodies in the nucleus basalis (6–8). Further studies then revealed correlations between cortical ChAcT reduction or nucleus basalis cell reduction and plaque densities in cortical areas (9–11). Besides cholinergic neurons, many other neuronal systems are affected (12,13), and the cholinergic deficit may represent a degenerative process of secondary importance when compared with the appearance of classic neuropathological structures, neuritic plaques, and neurofibrillary tangles (14,15). Nevertheless, the cholinergic deficit represents the most pronounced transmitter deficit and, probably, one of the early events in the disease process (16).

If the cholinergic deficit is responsible for cognitive or behavioral changes typical of AD, one would expect cholinomimetic drugs to be effective in its treatment. Thus far, there have been three main cholinergic approaches to the treatment of AD: the use of precursor loading, cholinesterase inhibition, and direct cholinergic agonists. Numerous trials with precursors have been unimpressive, failing to reliably improve cognitive function in AD patients. Modest, but reliable, improvement in memory have been produced by the acetylcholinesterase inhibitor physostigmine (17–20). Dramatic improvements had been claimed for another choinesterase inhibitor, tacrine (21), but subsequent pilot studies have shown more modest effects (22). Studies with direct cholinergic agonists so far have failed to produce conclusive results (23–25).

B. Trophic Actions of Nerve Growth Factor on Basal Forebrain Cholinergic Neurons

Nerve growth factor is necessary for normal development of peripheral sympathetic and sensory neurons and the cholinergic neurons of the basal forebrain (26–28). During adult life, forebrain cholinergic neurons remain responsive to NGF. In the forebrain of adult rats, primates, and humans, expression of NGF receptors seems to be limited to the population of cholinergic neurons (29–37). Concentrations of NGF as well as mRNA coding for NGF are highest in the hippocampus and cortex, and hippocampal target cells of the cholinergic neurons have been shown to express NGF and mRNA (38–40). In olfactory bulb and the brain stem of adult rats, NGF receptors are also located on several populations of noncholinergic cells. The NGF seems to play a less selective role during early development.

The finding that adult cholinergic neurons express NGF receptors and that this population of cells degenerates in human AD prompted several research groups to study the effects of NGF in animals with experimental lesions of forebrain cholinergic neurons. Intraventricular infusions of NGF prevented degenerative changes and loss of cholinergic cell bodies in the septum of rats with transections of the septohippocampal pathway (29,41, 42). Such infusions also stimulated expression of ChAcT and low-affinity NGF receptors by remaining cholinergic cell bodies (43,44) and synthesis and release of acetylcholine in their hippocampal terminals (45). These changes in biochemical parameters were associated with the acceleration in recovery from behavioral deficits (46). Intraventricular administration of NGF was also found to counteract reductions of cortical ChAcT activities following ibotenic acid-induced lesions of the nucleus basalis (48), but failed to attenuate reductions in ChAcT activity induced by administration of the ethyl choline mustard aziridinium ion (49). Intraventricular administration of NGF improved spatial performance of rats following nucleus basalis lesioning (47). Treatment with NGF failed to prevent the loss of septohippocampal GABAergic neurons or dopaminergic nigrostriatal neurons (50). The NGF treatment prevented the lesion-induced loss of septal cholinergic neurons in old rats as effectively as in young animals (51). These findings suggest that NGF prevents the lesion-induced loss of septal cholinergic neurons by directly acting on NGF receptors expressed by cholinergic cells, and that NGF does not simply protect any neuron with an axonal lesion.

Levels of NGF and its mRNA were found diminished in the brain of aged rats (52), and there is an age-related decrease in the intensity of low-affinity NGF receptor immunoreactivity in the basal forebrain of aged rats and humans, suggesting a down-regulation of receptor synthesis (37,53). Gage and collaborators selected behaviorally impaired aged rats that performed poorly in a swimming maze paradigm. The size of cholinergic cell bodies in the forebrain of the impaired animals was smaller than in nonimpaired aged rats, again supporting the view that cholinergic neurons play an important role in cognitive functions. Intraventricular NGF infusions counteracted both the morphological atrophy of cholinergic neurons and the behavioral deficits (54,55). According to these findings it seems likely that intraventricular infusions of NGF are able to counteract age-related atrophic changes of cholinergic neurons in the mammalian brain and improve those behavioral functions that are dependent upon an intact cholinergic system.

C. Nerve Growth Factor Mechanisms in Alzheimer's Disease

The originally published hypothesis (relating NGF to AD) focused on the possibility that NGF administration may counteract diminished function of one of the NGF-related mechanisms (56). So far, only a very few studies have assessed NGF-related functions in AD, and there is no direct evidence supporting a primary involvement of NGF in the pathogenesis of AD. Normal levels of mRNA coding for NGF were obtained in cortical samples from AD (57). The NGF receptor mRNA levels in the basal forebrain were normal when studied with northern blotting techniques (58) and decreased when studied with in situ hybridization techniques (59).

The foregoing animal studies suggest that NGF administration will counteract cholinergic atrophy, irrespective of the actual cause. Accordingly, it is important to consider administration of NGF to patients with AD not as replacement therapy, but rather, as a pharmacologic attempt to induce hypertrophy of cholinergic neurons surviving in the AD brain. In experimental studies, NGF-induced hypertrophy is manifest by increases in the expression of structural and transmitter-specific proteins. Administration of NGF reverses age-related degenerative changes of cholinergic neurons, and NGF-induced hypertrophy increases their resistance to experimental insults. Behavioral studies suggest that hypertrophy increases the ability of cholinergic neurons to influence their postsynaptic neurons. Given these considerations, it can be anticipated that NGF administration would attentuate the rate of degeneration of cholinergic neurons surviving in AD brains and improve their functional performance. Accordingly, NGF treatment may attenuate the deterioration of, or eventually improve, those aberrant behaviors that are a consequence of the cholinergic deficit.

D. Considerations in the Organization of Clinical Trials with Nerve Growth Factor

To be able to reach neuronal populations in the brain, NGF will have to be given intracerebrally, since the protein does not cross the blood–brain barrier. Problems associated with this intraventricular application and possible alternatives are the subject of this section. Although it is possible to administer purified mouse NGF to the human brain, it seems more prudent to use recombinant human NGF to diminish the possibility of immunological responses.

The organizational design of NGF clinical trials must be carefully considered in accord with ethical, scientific, and Food and Drug Administration (FDA) guidelines. The work group convened by the National Institute on Aging recommended an initial, open toxicity study, followed by a 3- to 4-month therapeutic trial, and then by a controlled long-term study to assess differential deterioration (60).

Issues in sample selection involve age, duration, severity, and the clinical heterogeneity of the illness itself. A differential response among subtypes might occur. It may be desirable to choose, or screen, potential subjects for NGF, based on their clinical response to acetylcholinesterase inhibitors. More severely demented patients have more cholinergic impairment and have been considered less likely to respond to cholinesterase inhibitors. Similarly, NGF, acting on surviving cholinergic neurons, may be more effective at early stages of the disease. Early controlled Phase II studies of NGF will provide estimates of NGF's effect on short-term clinical improvement. For placebo-controlled studies attempting to demonstrate that NGF retards AD progression, a larger sample size is likely to be needed (61). Sample size determination will depend, in part, on interindividual variation, the sensitivity and reliability of the instrument used to measure change, the study duration, and the magnitude of NGF's effect. Objective proof of NGF's efficacy will likely need to be in the form of improvement in cognitive function, rather than in behavior, functional activities, or survival.

Detrimental effects of NGF are concerns when considering its clinical use in humans. Long-term administration in humans may induce aberrant cholinergic sprouting, as observed in lesioned rodents (41). The NGF treatment may be associated with behavioral toxicity not previously recognized in animals, such as depression or psychosis. Since intraventricular NGF administration to neonatal animals elevates brain levels of amyloid precursor protein mRNA (62), it must be determined whether application of NGF to the adult brain elevates amyloid precursor protein levels and whether such elevations produce pathological changes typical for AD. Furthermore, since some nonneuronal cells are responsive to NGF (28), the possibility of undesired proliferation has to be considered. Infusions of NGF may act on intracerebral sympathetic neurons and produce changes in local blood flow (63).

III. NEUROTROPHIC FACTORS OTHER THAN NERVE GROWTH FACTOR

Several neurotrophic factors, with a spectrum of responsive neurons different from those of NGF, have been characterized. The following section provides a brief synopsis of the present knowledge of neurotrophic factors.

It attempts to provide information about receptive neuronal populations, since the spectrum of actions on responsive cells will determine the therapeutic usefulness of any given neurotrophic factor. Trophic factors acting on motoneurons should be useful in the treatment of amyotrophic lateral sclerosis, whereas factors supporting dopaminergic mesencephalic neurons might be useful for Parkinson's disease. Less selective neurotrophic factors may be useful in the treatment of general neurodegenerative disorders, including AD.

So far, there is no formal definition of the term *neurotrophic factor.* Proposed definitions are generalizations of the knowledge of NGF and infer that neurotrophic factors are "endogenous, soluble proteins promoting survival and function of neurons." This definition does not include molecules, like laminin, that are bound to cellular surfaces and mediate cell adhesion, nor nonproteineous molecules, like steroid and thyroid hormones, that also affect neuronal survival and differentiation. Neurotrophic factors occur in minimal quantities, making their isolation difficult. During the past decade, many laboratories attempted to purify factors from various sources using neuronal tissue cultures as assay systems. This approach resulted in the purification of brain-derived neurotrophic factor (BDNF) and ciliary neurotrophic factor (CNTF). These proteins have been characterized and corresponding cDNAs have been cloned. The sequence of BDNF is closely related to that of NGF, suggesting the existence of other related neurotrophic molecules. A third member of this group, neurotrophin-3 (NT-3) was recently discovered. Many other factors have been partially purified. Some putative neurotrophic factors turned out to be identical with previously characterized growth factors, in particular to basic fibroblast growth factor (bFGF). Furthermore, other previously characterized growth factors, including insulin-like growth factors (IGFs) and transforming growth factors (TGFs) were found to exert trophic actions on neurons. The factors are listed in Table 1 and, for further information, the reader is referred to the references given in the table.

A. Brain-Derived Neurotrophic Factor and Neurotrophin-3

The BDNF was purified from pig brain using survival of cultured chick sensory neurons as a bioassay (64). It is chemically similar to NGF, and its sequence shows a high degree of homology to that of NGF (65). BDNF promotes survival and fiber growth of neurons from most chick sensory ganglia, but fails to affect chick or rat sympathetic neurons (64). Binding studies resulted in the characterization of high- and low-affinity receptors on chick dorsal root ganglion cells (70). Injections of BDNF to quail embryos prevents the normally occurring neuronal death in sensory ganglia

TABLE 1 Molecules Exhibiting Neurotrophic Activities

Growth factor	Refs.
Proteins initially characterized as neurotrophic factors	
Nerve growth factor (NGF)	26–28
Brain-derived neurotrophic factor (BDNF)	64,65
Neurotrophin-3 (NT-3)	67–69
Ciliary neurotrophic factor (CNTF)	75,76
Growth factors with neurotrophic activity	
Fibroblast growth factor (FGF)	80,88,92
Insulin-like growth factors (IGFs), insulin	97,98
Epidermal growth factor (EGF)	86
Transforming growth factor-α (TGFα)	7,102
Interleukin-1 (IL-1)	111
Interleukin-3 (IL-3)	108
Interleukin-6 (IL-6)	109
Protease nexin I and II	110–113
Cholinergic neuronal differentiation factor	103

References given refer to recent reviews or recent key publications.

(71). BDNF was found to support survival and axonal elongation of rat retinal ganglion cells in culture (70). A function of BDNF in the adult brain was suggested by the facts that BDNF has been purified from the brain of adult pigs and that its mRNA seems to be predominantly expressed in the brain (65). Recent findings indicate that BDNF promotes the developmental growth of forebrain cholinergic neurons in a way similar to NGF (66). These findings make it likely that BDNF will be among the most interesting molecules when considering pharmacologic applications to the brain.

The extensive homology between BDNF and NGF led several research groups to use the polymerase chain reaction (PCR) methodology to search for additional members of a postulated group of NGF-related molecules. So far, this approach led to the discovery of NT-3 which shares approximately 50% of its amino acids with both NGF and BDNF. Similar to BDNF, NT-3 acts on subpopulations of sensory neurons, and its mRNA is heterogeneously distributed in the brain, suggesting a neurotrophic function for populations of central neurons (67–69).

B. Ciliary Neurotrophic Factor

The CNTF was purified from chick eye and rat sciatic nerve tissue using chick embryonic ganglion cells as a bioassay (73,74), and it has recently been cloned (75,76). Besides acting on ciliary parasympathetic neurons, it supports survival of various chick and rodent sensory and sympathetic ganglia (73) and promotes differentiation of chick sympathetic neurons (77). It affects cholinergic neurons in cultures of chick retinal cells (78), but fails to affect rat brain cholinergic neurons (79). Highest concentrations of CNTF mRNA were found in the adult sciatic nerve, supporting the speculation that it plays a role in peripheral nerve regeneration processes (76).

C. Fibroblast Growth Factor

Basic fibroblast growth factor (bFGF) and acidic fibroblast growth factor (aFGF) were originally purified together and were later found to have a high degree of homology (80,81). There is evidence for the existence of tissue-specific forms of the FGFs (82). Two different FGF receptors have been tentatively characterized, which both recognize aFGF and bFGF, one with a preference for aFGF the other with a preference for bFGF (83). In many cell types, these receptors mediate very potent mitogenic effects of FGF (80,84). The bFGF and its receptor occur in the brain (85). Both forms of FGF influence neuronal survival and differentiation during development. Both aFGF and bFGF support initial survival and subsequent fiber outgrowth of dissociated rodent fetal neurons in culture (86,87). Although neurons from many brain regions are affected, the proportion of neurons surviving varies among brain regions, suggesting that subpopulations of neurons are responsive to FGF (88). Similar to NGF, FGF induces cell division and neurite outgrowth from cultured neonatal adrenal chromaffin cells; however, in contrast with NGF, it does not support the survival of sympathetic neurons derived from chromaffin cells (89,90). Basic FGF promotes survival and differentiation of cholinergic neurons of the rat basal forebrain and of mesencephalic dopaminergic neurons (91,92). The presence of FGF in the adult brain suggests that this factor, similar to NGF, remains important for maintenance of function of responsive neuronal populations. Pharmacologic administration of bFGF to transected neuronal pathways attenuates the loss of neuronal cell bodies. Local administration of bFGF to the proximal nerve stump of a transected sciatic nerve partially prevents the loss of dorsal root ganglion neurons in adult rats (93). In adult rats with fimbrial transections, chronic intraventricular infusions of bFGF attenuate the loss of septal cholinergic neurons, similar to the effects produced by NGF (94,95). Given the broad spectrum of bFGF responsive neurons, this protein may beneficially influence the recovery from lesions of many neuronal systems.

D. Insulin and Insulin-like Growth Factors

Insulin and the structurally related insulin-like growth factors I and II (IGF-I and IGF-II) are involved in the regulation of metabolism and cellular growth of many tissues. The three proteins exhibit overlapping specificities for receptors (96). There is abundant evidence for the existence for insulin and IGF receptors in the brain, and the IGFs have been shown to be synthesized in the brain (97). The function of insulin and IGFs in the brain is not clear, despite the many findings showing that they affect various brain cell populations in vitro. Insulin, IGF-I, and IGF-II promote survival and stimulate neurite outgrowth from cultured central and peripheral neurons (98,99). Besides stimulating survival and initial growth of cultured neurons, insulin and the IGFs promote their differentiation and maturation. Insulin, IGF-I, and IGF-II promote the differentiation of septal and pontine cholinergic neurons and dopaminergic neurons of the mesencephalon (92). The neuronal actions of IGFs seem to be relatively nonselective and to involve a majority of neuronal populations.

E. Epidermal Growth Factor and Transforming Growth Factor-α

Epidermal growth factor (EGF), which is a potent mitogen for several cell types, enhanced survival and neurite growth of cultured subneocortical and cerebellar neurons of the neonatal rat brain (86). Immunoreactivity of EGF and the EGF receptor was demonstrated in the rat brain (100). Transforming growth factor-α (TGF-α) shows structural homology to EGF; it is present in several brain areas and synthesized in cell bodies of selected rat forebrain regions (101,102). Both EGF and TGF-α promote the differentiation of mesencephalic dopaminergic neurons in culture, probably by acting on the same receptors (Knusel et al., unpublished observations).

F. Cholinergic Neuronal Differentiation Factor, Interleukins

Cholinergic neuronal differentiation factor is known to regulate the neurotransmitter phenotype of sympathetic neurons in culture. This factor was purified, partially sequenced and found to be identical with the leukemia inhibitory factor, which regulates growth and differentiation of stem and myeloid cells (103). Its actions have been compared with those of interleukins (IL). Interleukin-1 is a potent mitogen for astroglial cells, and its synthesis is induced after experimental injury in the brain (104). This protein is able to elevate the expression of NGF in sciatic nerve explants and seems to be responsible for the large increases in NGF synthesis observed after transection of peripheral nerves (105). Injections of IL-1 into the brain elevate NGF mRNA levels in the hippocampus (106). Interleukin-2 promotes division and maturation of oligodendrocytes, and similar to IL-1, was detected in the vicinity of experimental brain lesions (107). Interleukin-3 and IL-6 were reported to promote survival of cultured postnatal forebrain cholinergic neurons (108,109).

G. Protease Nexins

Several findings point to an important role of proteases and protease inhibitors in neuronal growth. Natural and artificial protease inhibitors stimulate neurite outgrowth from cultured neurons, and it has been speculated that neurite outgrowth and stabilization of axonal terminals at their target cells requires a delicate balance between activities of proteases and protease inhibitors (110). A glia-derived neurotrophic factor was found to be identical to protease nexin I (110), and this molecule is induced in peripheral nerves after experimental lesions (111). The amyloid precursor protein has been reported to trophically affect cultured neurons (112), and the secreted part containing the Kunitz domain is identical to protease nexin II (113).

H. Trophic Factors for Motor Neurons and Mesencephalic Dopaminergic Neurons

Factors for these neuronal populations are of obvious interest given their selective degeneration in amyotrophic lateral sclerosis and Parkinson's disease, respectively. Attempts by several research groups to purify neurotrophic factors for motoneurons suggest the existence of various factors with distinct effects on neurite outgrowth and cholinergic differentiation (114,115). Appel and collaborators were able to separate a protein that stimulates neurite growth from other factors that stimulate cholinergic properties. One of these latter factors was purified to homogeneity, partially characterized, and named *choline acetyltransferase development factor* (116). Several studies provide indirect evidence for the existence of such a factor (117,118); however, no selective dopaminergic neurotrophic factor has been purified so far. It has been found that dopaminergic neurons developing in culture respond to IGFs, bFGF, EGF, and TGF-α (92,119).

It seems clear from this summary that the field of neurotrophic factors is still in its infancy, making it difficult to draw a generally valid conclusion. Most of the findings were obtained on experimental systems reflecting developmental processes. Very little is known about the function of neurotrophic factors in the adult and aging brain, i.e., when therapeutic applications are likely to be sought. The degree of selectivity of the factors needs to be determined. The data available at the present time are compatible with the concept that there are many of highly selective neurotrophic factors, or, alternatively, that the neurotrophic actions represent a functional part of more generally acting protein hormones.

IV. PHARMACOLOGY OF NEUROTROPHIC FACTORS

Neurotrophic factors should become useful in the treatment of diseases involving structural disintegration of nervous tissue, since they play a major

TABLE 2 Possibilities of Pharmacologic Manipulations Based on Neurotrophic Factor Actions

Intracerebral application of native or recombinant trophic factors
Delivery by
Intraventricular infusion pumps
Slow-releasing polymer implants
Genetically engineered cells
Intracerebral application of modified neurotrophic factors and active peptide fragments or analogues
Delivery by
Intraventricular infusion pumps
Slow-releasing polymer implants
Systemic application of nonpeptide neurotrophic factor mimetics
Modification of synthesis and metabolism of endogenous neurotrophic factors

role in brain development and function. Moreover, they have been shown to attenuate age-related and experimentally induced degeneration and behavioral deficits in animals. The following section discusses pharmacologic strategies that could be pursued to exploit neurotrophic factor mechanisms. Table 2 shows a summary of these strategies.

A. Intracerebral Infusion

Neurotrophic factors must be given intracerebrally, since these proteins are not able to cross the blood–brain barrier. In experimental animals, NGF has been injected intraventricularly through permanently implanted cannulas or has been continuously infused with the help of osmotic minipumps. In humans, NGF may be continuously infused into the brain with the help of similar mechanical pump devices. Subcutaneous pumps are available that deliver drugs through a small tube to the cerebral ventricles (120). Pumps and the intraventricular delivery systems are well tolerated in animals (121) and, apparently, are at least adequately tolerated in humans, but are not without risk of infection and perioperative complications such as hemorrhage and seizure (120). Studies addressing the bioavailability of infused neurotrophic factors should precede clinical trials. Degradation of the molecules within the CSF and the brain parenchyma as well as their penetration into the brain tissue will affect the amounts reaching responsive neurons.

Sufficient quantities of well-characterized neurotrophic factors are a prerequisite for pharmacologic and toxicologic studies. The scarcity of natural molecules will make it necessary to produce recombinant proteins. Large quantities of recombinant IGFs, bFGF, and TGF-α have become available during the past years. Several groups have reported the production of recombinant human NGF (rhNGF). The rhNGF is equally as effective as natural murine NGF in promoting survival and function of rat forebrain cholinergic neurons (Knusel et al., unpublished observations).

Stability of the neurotrophic factors during storage in these pump devices may require special preparations. In the case of bFGF, a more stable molecule was produced by single amino acid substitutions (122). Self-assembly may become a problem when proteins are packed at high concentrations in pumps or polymers. For insulin, this problem was solved by substitution of single amino acids (123).

B. Release from Implants and Genetically Engineered Cells

The demonstration that intraventricular infusion of a neurotrophic factor is clinically effective is likely to stimulate research into alternative methods of administration. It seems possible to develop slow-releasing intracerebral implants. Such implants contain the active protein embedded in a biodegradable polymer matrix. Existing polymers provide stable release rates over a period of several weeks (124). Combinations of modified neurotrophic factors with polymer matrix materials will offer vast possibilities of patent protection and may be an attractive avenue for commercial exploitation. Slow-releasing polymers could be implanted in a simple neurosurgical session and pose less risk than a intraventricular pump.

The grafting of brain tissue to replace degenerated cells is frequently proposed as a potential approach to treat brain dysfunction. Such techniques are not limited to natural cells, but can include genetically modified cells, which selectively secrete a desired neurotrophic factor. Rosenberg (125) and Ernfors (126) showed that the implantation of cells producing recombinant NGF evokes trophic actions on NGF responsive cholinergic neurons. It is possible to produce cells that do not proliferate after implantation, are well tolerated by the host, and in which the synthesis of the desired growth factor is under the control of a promoter regulated by drugs. However, such cells may release a multitude of other active molecules, making it difficult to control their actions.

C. Production of Peptide Fragments and Nonpeptide Mimetics

Rather than administering entire trophic factor molecules, it may be possible to use active fragments or molecules mimicking the active sites of neurotrophic factors. Currently, very little is known about the possibility of producing active fragments of NGF or other neurotrophic factors. A trypsin fragment of NGF, claimed to be effective several years ago, was later shown to be inactive (127). More recently, Longo (128) reported the production of peptide fragments that inhibit biological actions of NGF. Fragments of EGF, bFGF, IGF-I, and IGF-II appear to retain activity (82, 129–132). A synthetic peptide analogue of TGF-α was shown to specifically inhibit EGF and TGF-α growth stimulatory actions on responsive cell lines (133). Although effective concentrations of the active peptides were often much higher than those of the native proteins, these reports demonstrate the feasibility of the approach that attempts to reduce trophic factors to smaller and smaller molecules, exerting the same actions on the specific receptors.

Studies with peptide fragments and modified peptides will provide a basis for molecular-modeling studies attempting to replace peptides with nonpeptide effectors. Theoretical feasibility of this approach is illustrated by the example of endorphins and morphine, which act on the same receptors. Although this approach has the potential to lead to trophic factor agonists that can be administered systemically, it must be noted that the systemic administration of such active molecules may substantially elevate the possibility of undesired side effects. Actions on neurons of the peripheral nervous system may lead to undesired stimulatory actions on the autonomic nervous system. Furthermore, since NGF is involved in the function of the immune and reproductive system (134,135), it is likely that neurotrophic factors exert a variety of nonneuronal actions that may limit the possibilities of systemic administration.

D. Pharmacologic Manipulation of Neurotrophic Factor Synthesis

A feasible approach to influence neurotrophic actions may be to search for ways to specifically manipulate the synthesis of endogenous neurotrophic factors. Currently, very little is known about the regulation of synthesis of NGF or other neurotrophic factors, and the mechanisms controlling the selective expression of their genes are poorly understood. The gene promoter regions of NGF were recently isolated and cloned from rodent genomic libraries as a first step in the analysis of the transcriptional regulation of NGF expression (136).

Molecules probably involved in the regulation of neurotrophic factor expression are IL-1, retinoic acid, and thyroid hormones. Interleukin-1 elevates expression of NGF in sciatic nerve and hippocampus (106,107). Retinoic acid has recently been reported to increase the number of receptors for NGF in neuroblastoma cells (137) and to elevate the levels of NGF and its mRNA in L cells (138). Morphological and biochemical differentiation of human neuroblastoma cells is affected by retinoic acid (139,140).

Two human genes for the retinoic acid receptor, which show extensive similarity with the steroid and thyroid hormone receptor genes, have been identified (142).

Thyroid hormones are essential for the normal development of the brain, and these hormones have been reported to influence axonal regeneration in adult animals (143). Several findings suggest a relationship between thyroid hormones and NGF, at least in relation to cholinergic neurons of the basal forebrain. Thyroid deficiency is associated with a reduction of ChAcT activity in the brain of experimental animals (144,145). Triiodothyronine (T_3) has increased ChAcT activity in various cultures system with rat neurons (29,146,147). Recent structural data on thyroid hormone analogues indicate the existence of tissue-specific receptors (148), and novel analogues have been described that differentiate between receptors of various peripheral organs (149). These discoveries may make it possible to develop thyroid hormone analogues selectively regulating the expression of neurotrophic factors.

E. Side Effects of Neurotrophic Factors

Given the multitude of systems affected by neurotrophic factors, one has to consider the possibility that pharmacologic use of growth factors and trophic agents may be detrimental to neuronal function, contrary to the beneficial role implied by the term *trophic*. Such detrimental actions have to be considered and ruled out before clnically using trophic molecules. Neurotrophic agents may, by promoting the function of selective neuronal systems, alter the balance among various systems within neuronal networks. Trophic agents may induce the formation of aberrant synaptic connections that may disrupt normal signal flow. They may induce the expression of abnormal proteins by neuronal and nonneuronal cells and stimluate pathological proliferation of nonneuronal cells.

Detrimental actions of trophic factors are concerns when considering the clinical use of NGF in AD. The notion the NGF will be useful is based on substantial biochemical and anatomical evidence indicating trophic stimulation of forebrain cholinergic neurons and behavioral findings showing that the cholinergic hypertrophy is accompanied by behavioral improvement. Given these findings, it seems unlikely that NGF-mediated cholinergic stimulation is functionally detrimental. However, long-term administration may induce aberrant cholinergic sprouting, as observed in lesioned rodents (150). The NGF infusions may increase the sympathetic innervation of the cerebral vasculature and produce alterations in cerebral blood flow (63). Since intraventricular NGF administration to neonatal animals elevates brain levels of amyloid precursor protein mRNA (62), it has to be determined whether application of NGF to the adult brain elevates amyloid precursor protein levels and whether such elevations produce pathological changes typical for AD. Furthermore, since several nonneuronal cell populations are responsive to NGF (135,136), the possibility of undesired proliferation has to be considered.

Application of neurotrophic factors by using pumps or slow-releasing polymers raises the issue of termination of application, if indeed there are side effects. Mechanical pumps, but not osmotic pumps, can be turned off after implantation. Termination of the action of implanted polymers will require a second surgical intervention. These problems again emphasize the necessity for a careful and stepwise development of the clinical use of such compounds. Mechanical pump devices seem to be most suited for initial trials establishing safety and efficacy.

Although representing a novel therapeutic approach, clinical application of NGF and other neurotrophic factors will have to follow general rules applied to the development of drugs. To rule out unacceptable actions of NGF, clinical application will have to be preceded by toxicology studies. Effective and safe dosages will have to be established. Guidelines for the use of NGF in AD have been formulated by an ad hoc committee of the National Institute of Aging (60).

V. CONCLUSIONS

Neurotrophic factors play a major role in brain development and function. Since administration of these factors can attenuate age-related and experimentally induced degeneration and behavioral deficits in animals, such molecules may become useful in the treatment of diseases involving structural disintegration of nervous tissue. There are various pharmacologic strategies that will result in the production of clinically useful molecules.

REFERENCES

1. Russell RW. Cholinergic system in behavior: the search for mechanisms of action. Annu Rev Pharmacol Toxicol 1982; 22:435–463.
2. Smith G. Animal models of Alzheimer's disease: experimental cholinergic denervation. Brain Res Rev 1988; 13:103–118.
3. Bowen DM, Smith CB, White P, Davison AN. Neurotransmitter-related enzymes and indices of hypoxia in senile dementia and other abiotrophies. Brain 1976; 99:459–496.
4. Davies P, Maloney AJF. Selective loss of central cholinergic neurons in Alzheimer's disease. Lancet 1976; 2:1403.

5. Perry EK, Perry RH, Tomlinson, BE. Necropsy evidence of central cholinergic deficits in senile dementia. Lancet 1977; 1:189.
6. Whitehouse PJ, Price DL, Struble RG, Clarke AW, Coyle JT, DeLong MR. Alzheimer's disease and senile dementia: loss of neurons in the basal forebrain. Science 1982; 215:1237–1239.
7. Nagai T, McGeer PL, Peng JH, McGeer EG, Dolman CE. Choline aetyltransferase immunohistochemistry in brains of Alzheimer's disease patients and controls. Neurosci Lett 1983; 36:195–199.
8. Arendt T, Bigl V, Tennstedt A. Loss of neurons in the nucleus basalis of Meynert in Alzheimer's disease, paralysis agitans and Korsakoff's disease. Acta Neuropathol 1983; 61:101–108.
9. Arendt T, Bigl V, Tennstedt A, Arendt A. Correlation between cortical plaque count and neuronal loss in the nucleus basalis in Alzheimer's disease. Neurosci Lett 1984; 48:81–85.
10. Arendt T, Bigl V, Tennstedt A, Arendt A. Neuronal loss in different parts of the nucleus basalis is related to neuritic plaque formation in cortical target areas in Alzheimer's disease. Neuroscience 1985; 14:1–14.
11. Etienne P, Robitaille Y, Wood P, Gauthier S, Nair NPV, Quirion R. Nucleus basalis neuronal loss, neuritic plaques and choline acetyltransferase activity in advanced Alzheimer's disease. Neuroscience 1986; 19:1279–1291.
12. Katzman R. Alzheimer's disease. N Engl J Med 1986; 314:964–973.
13. Price DL. New perspectives on Alzheimer's disease. Annu Rev Neurosci 1986; 9:489–512.
14. Muller-Hill B, Beyreuther K. Molecular biology of Alzheimer's disease. Annu Rev Biochem 1989; 58:287–307.
15. Glenner GG, Murphy MA. Amyloidosis of the nervous system. J Neurol Sci 1989; 94:1–28.
16. Francis PT, Palmer AM, Sioms NR, Bowen DM, Davison AN, Esiri MM, Neary D. Neurochemical studies of early-onset Alzheimer's disease. Possible influence on treatment. Lancet 1985; 2:7–11.
17. Davis KL, Mohs RC. Enhancement of memory processes in Alzheimer's disease with multiple-dose intravenous physostigmine. Am J Psychiatry 1982; 139:1421–1424.
18. Thal LJ, Fuld PA. Memory enhancement with oral physostigmine in Alzheimer's disease. N Engl J Med 1983; 308:720.
19. Stern Y, Sano M, Mayeux R. Effects of oral physostigmine in Alzheimer's disease. Ann Neurol 1987; 22:306–310.
20. Thal LJ, Masur DM, Sharpless NS, Fuld PA, Davies P. Acute and chronic effects of oral physostigmine and lecithin in Alzheimer's disease. Prog Neuropsychopharmacol Biol Psychiatry 1986; 10:617–636.
21. Summers WK, Majovski LV, Marsh GM, Tachiki K, Kling A. Oral tetrahydroaminoacridine in long-term treatment of senile dementia, Alzheimer type. N Engl J Med 1986; 315:1241–1245.
22. Gauthier S, Bouchard R, Lamontagne A, Bailey P, Bergman H, Ratner J, Tesfaye Y, Saint-Martin M, Bacher Y, Carrier L, Charbonneau R, Clarfield

AM, Collier B, Dastoor D, Gauthier L, Germain M, Kissel C, Krieger M, Kushnir S, Masson H, Morin J, Nair V, Neirinck K., Suissa S. Tetrahydroaminoacridine–lecithin combination treatment in patients with intermediate-stage Alzheimer's disease. N Engl J Med 1990; 322:1272–1289.

23. Penn RD, Martin EM, Wilson RS, Fox JH, Savoy SM. Intraventricular bethanechol infusion for Alzheimer's disease: results of double-blind and escalating dose trials. Neurology 1988; 39:219–222.
24. Caine ED. Cholinomimetic treatment fails to improve memory disorders. N Engl J Med 1980; 303:585–586.
25. Davis KL, Hollander E, Davidson M, et al. Induction of depression with oxotremorine in patients with Alzheimer's disease. Am J Psychiatry 1987; 144:468–471.
26. Thoenen H, Bandtlow C, Heumann R. The physiological function of nerve growth factor in the central nervous system: comparison with the periphery. Rev Physiol Biochem Pharmacol 1987; 109:145–178.
27. Whittemore SR, Seiger A. The expression, localization and functional significance of beta-nerve growth factor in the central nervous system. Brain Res Rev 1987; 12:439–464.
28. Hefti F, Hartikka J, Knusel B. Function of neurotrophic factors in the adult and aging brain and their possible use in the treatment of neurodegenerative diseases. Neurobiol Aging 1989; 10:515–533.
29. Hefti F. Nerve growth factor (NGF) promotes survival of septal cholinergic neurons after fimbrial transections. J Neurosci 1986; 6:2155–2162.
30. Riopelle RJ, Richardson PM, Verge VMK. Distribution and characteristics of nerve growth factor binding on cholinergic neurons of rat and monkey forebrain. Neurochem Res 1987; 12:923–928.
31. Eckenstein F. Transient expression of NGF-receptor-like immunoreactivity in postnatal rat brain and spinal cord. Brain Res 1988; 446:149–154.
32. Kordower JH, Bartus RT, Bothwell M, Schatteman G, Gash DM. Nerve growth factor immunoreactivity in the non-human primate (*Cebus apella*): distribution, morphology, and colocalization with cholinergic enzymes. J Comp Neurol 1988; 277:465–486.
33. Kordower JH, Mufson EJ. NGF and Alzheimer's disease: unfulfilled promise and untapped potential. Neurobiol Aging 1990; 10:543–544.
34. Schatteman GC, Gibbs L, Lanahan AA, Claude P, Bothwell M. Expression of NGF receptor in the developing and adult primate central nervous system. J Neurosci 1988; 8:860–873.
35. Yan Q, Johnson EM. An immunohistochemical study of the nerve growth factor receptor in developing rats. J Neurosci 1988; 8:3481–3498.
36. Batchelor PE, Armstrong DM, Blaker SN, Gage FH. Nerve growth factor receptor and choline acetyltransferase co-localization in neurons within the rat forebrain: response to fimbria–fornix transection. J Comp Neurol 1989; 284:187–204.
37. Hefti F, Mash DC. Localization of nerve growth factor receptors in the normal human brain and in Alzheimer's disease. Neurobiol Aging 1989; 10:75–87.

38. Shelton DL, Reichardt LF. Studies on the expression of beta NGF gene in the central nervous system: level and regional distribution of NGF mRNA suggest that NGF functions as a trophic factor for several neuronal populations. Proc Natl Acad Sci USA 1986; 83:2714–2718.
39. Rennert PD, Heinrich G. Nerve growth factor mRNA in brain: localization by in situ hybridization. Biochem Biophys Res Commun 1986; 138:813–818.
40. Ayer-Lelievre C, Olson L, Ebendal T, Hallbook F, Persson H. Nerve growth factor mRNA and protein in testis and epididymis of mouse and rat. Proc Natl Acad Sci USA 1988; 85:2628–2632.
41. Williams LR, Varon S, Peterson GM, Wictorin K, Fischer W, Bjorklund A, Gage FH. Continuous infusion of nerve growth factor prevents basal forebrain neuronal death after fimbria fornix transection. Proc Natl Acad Sci USA 1986; 83:9231–9235.
42. Kromer LF. Nerve growth factor treatment after brain injury prevents neuronal death. Science 1987; 235:214–216.
43. Hefti F, Dravid A, Hartikka J. Chronic intraventricular injections of nerve growth factor elevate hippocampal choline acetyltransferase activity in adult rats with septo-hippocampal lesions. Brain Res 1984; 293:305–311.
44. Higgins GA, Mufson EJ. NGF receptor gene expression is decreased in the nucleus basalis in Alzheimer's disease. Exp Neurol 1989; 106:222–236.
45. Lapchak PA, Junard EO, Hefti F. Recombinant human nerve growth factor enhances presynaptic cholinergic function in cholinergic neurons surviving partial septo-hippocampal lesions: chronic NGF treatment. Neuroscience 42:639–649 (1991).
46. Will B, Hefti F. Behavioral and neurochemical effects of chronic intraventricular injections of nerve growth factor in adult rats with fimbria lesions. Behav Brain Res 1985; 17:17–24.
47. Mandel RJ, Gage FH, Thal LJ. Spatial learning in rats: correlation with cortical choline acetyltransferase and improvement with NGF following NBM damage. Exp Neurol 1989; 104:208–217.
48. Haroutunian V, Kanof PD, Davis KL. Partial reversal of lesion-induced deficits in cortical cholinergic markers by nerve growth factor. Brain Res 1986; 386:397–399.
49. Johnson GVW, Simonato M, Jope RS. Dose- and time-dependent hippocampal cholinergic lesions induced by ethylcholine mustard aziridinium ion: effects of nerve growth factor, GM1 ganglioside, and vitamin E. Neurochem Res 1988; 13:685–692.
50. Montero CN, Hefti F. Rescue of lesioned septal cholinergic neurons by nerve growth factor: specificity and requirement for chronic treatment. J Neurosci 1988; 8:2986–2999.
51. Montero CN, Hefti F. Intraventricular nerve growth factor administration prevents lesion-induced loss of septal cholinergic neurons in aging rats. Neurobiol Aging 1989; 10:739–743.
52. Lärkfors L, Ebendal T, Whittemore SR, Persson H, Hoffer B, Olson L. Decreased level of nerve growth factor (NGF) and its messenger RNA in the aged rat brain. Mol Brain Res 1987; 3:55–60.

53. Koh S, Loy R. Age-related loss of nerve growth factor sensitivity in rat basal forebrain neurons. Brain Res 1988; 440:396–401.
54. Fischer W, Wictorin K, Bjorklund A, Williams LR, Varon S, Gage FH. Amelioration of cholinergic neurons atrophy and spatial memory impairment in aged rats by nerve growth factor. Nature 1987; 329:65–68.
55. Fischer W, Gage FH, Bjorklund A. Degenerative changes in forebrain cholinergic nuclei correlate with cognitive impairments in aged rats. Eur J Neurosci 1989; 1:33–45.
56. Hefti F. Alzheimer's disease caused by a lack of nerve growth factor? Ann Neurol 1983; 13:109–110.
57. Goedert M, Fine A, Hunt SP, Ullrich A. Nerve growth factor mRNA in peripheral and central rat tissues and in the human central nervous system: lesion effects in the rat brain and levels in Alzheimer's disease. Mol Brain Res 1986; 1:85–92.
58. Goedert M, Fine A, Dawbarn D, Wilcock GK, Chao MV. Nerve growth factor receptor mRNA distribution in human brain: normal levels in basal forebrain in Alzheimer's disease. Mol Brain Res 1989; 5:1–7.
59. Higgins GA, Mufson EJ. NGF receptor gene expression is decreased in the nucleus basalis in Alzheimer's disease. Exp Neurol 1989; 106:222–236.
60. Phelps CH, Gage FH, Growdon JH, Hefti F, Harbaugh R, Johnston MV, Khachaturian ZS, Mobley WC, Price DL, Raskind M, Simpkins J, Thal LJ, Woodcock J. Potential use of nerve growth factor to treat Alzheimer's disease. Neurobiol Aging 1989; 10:205–207.
61. Overall JE. Estimating sample size for logitudinal studies of age-related cognitive decline. J Gerontol 1987; 2:137–141.
62. Mobley WC, Neve RL, Prusiner SB, McKinley MP. Nerve growth factor induces gene expression for prion and Alzheimer's beta-amyloid proteins. Proc Natl Acad Sci USA 1988; 85:9811–9815.
63. Isaacson LG, Saffran BN, Crutcher KA. Intracerebral NGF infusion induces hyperinnervation of cerebral blood vessels. Neurobiol Aging 1990; 11:51–55.
64. Barde Y-A, Davies AM, Johnson JE, Lindsay RM, Thoenen H. Brain-derived neurotrophic factor. Prog Brain Res 1989; 71:185–189.
65. Leibrock J, Lottspeich F, Hohn A, Hofer M, Hengerer B, Masiakowski P, Thoenen H, Barde YA. Molecular cloning and expression of brain-derived neurotrophic factor. Nature 1989; 341:149–152.
66. Knusel B, Winslow JW, Rosenthal A, Burton LE, Seid DP, Nikolics K, Hefti F. Promotion of central cholinergic neuron differentiation by brain-derived neurotrophic factor but not neurotrophin-3. Proc Natl Acad Sci USA 1991; 88:961–965.
67. Maisonpierre PC, Belluscio L, Squinto S, Ip NY, Rurth ME, Lindsay RM, Yancopoulos GD. Neurotrophin-3: a neurotrophic factor related to NGF and BDNF. Science 1990; 247:1446–1449.
68. Rosenthal A, Goeddel DV, Nguyen T, Lewis M, Shih A, Laramee GR, Nikolics K, Winslow JW. Primary structure of a novel human neurotrophic factor. Neuron 1990; 4:767–773.
69. Hohn A, Leibrock J, Beiley K, Barde YA. Identification and characterization

of a novel member of the nerve growth factor/brain-derived neurotrophic factor family. Nature 1990; 344:339–341.
70. Rodrigeuz-Tebar A, Barde YA. Binding characteristics of brain-derived neurotrophic factor to its receptors on neurons from the chick embryo. J Neurosci 1988; 8:3337–3342.
71. Hofer MM, Barde YA. Brain-derived neurotrophic factor prevents neuronal death in vivo. Nature 1988; 331:261–262.
72. Thanos S, Bahr M, Barde YA, Vanselow J. Survival and axonal elongation of adult rat retinal ganglion cells. In vitro effects of lesioned sciatic nerve and brain derived neurotrophic factor. Eur J Neurosci 1989; 1:19–26.
73. Barbin G, Selak I, Manthorpe M, Varon S. Use of central neuronal cultures for the detection of neuronotrophic agents. Neuroscience 1984; 12:33–43.
74. Manthorpe M, Skaper SD, Williams LR, Varon S. Purification of adult rat sciatic nerve ciliary neuronotrophic factor. Brain Res 1986; 367:282–286.
75. Lin L-FH, Mismer D, Lile JD, Armes LG, Butler ET III, Vannice JL, Collins F. Purification, cloning, and expression of ciliary neurotrophic factor (CNTF). Science 1989; 246:1023–1025.
76. Stockli KA, Lottspeich F, Sendtner M, Masiakowski P, Carroll P, Gotz R, Lindholm D, Thoenen H. Molecular cloning, expression and regional distribution of rat ciliary neurotrophic factor. Nature 1989; 342:920–923.
77. Ernsberger U, Sendtner M, Rohrer H. Proliferation and differentiation of embryonic chick sympathetic neurons: effects of ciliary neurotrophic factor. Neuron 1989; 2:1275–1284.
78. Hofmann HD. Development of cholinergic retinal neurons from embryonic chicken in monolayer cultures: stimulation by glial cell-derived factors. J Neurosci 1988; 8:1361–1369.
79. Knusel B, Hefti F. Development of cholinergic pedunculopontine neurons in vitro: comparison with cholinergic septal cells and response to nerve growth factor, ciliary neuronotrophic factor, and retinoic acid. J Neurosci Res 1988; 21:365–375.
80. Gospodarowicz D. Brain and pituitary fibroblast growth factors. In: Li CH, ed. Hormonal proteins and peptides, vol 12. New York: Academic Press, 1985:205–230.
81. Gospodarowicz D, Neufeld G, Schweigerer L. Molecular and biological characterization of fibroblast growth factor, an angiogenic factor which also controls the proliferation and differentiation of mesoderm and neuroectoderm derived cells. Cell Differ 1986; 19:1–17.
82. Klagsburn M, Smith S, Sullivan R, Shing Y, Davidson S, Smith JA, Sasse J. Multiple forms of basic fibroblast growth factor: aminio-terminal cleavages by tumor cell- and brain-derived acid proteinases. Proc Natl Acad Sci USA 1987; 84:1839–1843.
83. Neufeld G, Gospodarowicz D. Basic and acidic fibroblast growth factors interact with the same cell surface receptors. J Biol Chem 1986; 261:5631–5637.
84. Baird A, Esch F, Mormede P, Ueno N, Ling N, Bohlen P, Ying SY, Wehrenber WB, Guillemin R. Molecular characterization of fibroblast growth factor.

Distribution and biological activities in various tissues. Recent Prog Horm Res 1986; 42:143–205.

85. Logan A, Logan SD. Distribution of fibroblast growth factor in the central and peripheral nervous system of various mammals. Neurosci Lett 1986; 69:162–165.
86. Morrison RS, Keating RF, Moskal JR. Basic fibroblast growth factor and epidermal growth factor exert differential trophic effects on CNS neurons. J Neurosci Res 1988; 21:71–79.
87. Walicke PA, Baird A. Neurotrophic effects of basic and acidic fibroblast growth factors are not mediated through glial cells. Dev Brain Res 1986; 40:71–79.
88. Walicke PA. Basic and acidic fibroblast growth factors have trophic effects on neurons from multiple CNS regions. J Neurosci 1988; 8:2618–2627.
89. Claude P, Parada IM, Gordon KA, D'Amore PA, Wagner JA. Acidic fibroblast growth factor stimulates adrenal chromaffin cells to proliferate and to extend neurites, but is not a long-term survival factor. Neuron 1988; 1:783–790.
90. Stemple DL, Mahanthappa NK, Anderson DJ. Basic FGF induces neuronal differentiation, cell division, and NGF dependence in chromaffin cells: a sequence of events in sympathetic development. Neuron 1988; 1:517–525.
91. Grothe C, Otto D, Unsicker K. Basic fibroblast growth factor promotes in vitro survival and cholinergic development of rat septal neurons: comparison with the effects of nerve growth factor. Neuroscience 1989; 31:649–661.
92. Knusel B, Michel PP, Schwaber JS, Hefti F. Selective and nonselective stimulation of central cholinergic and dopaminergic development in vitro by nerve growth factor, basic fibroblast growth factor, epidermal growth factor, insulin and the insulin-like growth factors I and II. J Neurosci 1990; 10:558–570.
93. Otto D, Unsicker K, Grothe C. Pharmacological effects of nerve growth factor and fibroblast growth factor applied to the transectioned sciatic nerve on neuron death in adult rat dorsal root ganglia. Neurosci Lett 1987; 83:156–160.
94. Anderson KJ, Dam D, Lee S, Cotman CW. Basic fibroblast growth factor prevents death of lesioned cholinergic neurons in vivo. Nature 1988; 332: 360–362.
95. Schwaber JS, Due B, Junard EO, Sharma A, Hefti F. Analysis of NGF- and bFGF-mediated rescue of septal cholinergic neurons following partial fimbrial transection by computerized data acquisition using a digital brain atlas. J Comp Neurol 1991; 309:27–39.
96. Rechler MM, Nissley SP. The nature and regulation of the receptors for insulin-like growth factors. Annu Rev Physiol 1985; 47:425–442.
97. Rotwein P, Burgess SK, Milbrandt JD, Krause, JE. Differential expression of insulin-like growth factor genes in rat central nervous system. Proc Natl Acad Sci USA 1988; 85:265–269.
98. Aizenman Y, Weischsel ME Jr, De Vellis J. Changes in insulin and transferrin requirements of pure brain neuronal cultures during embryonic development. Proc Natl Acad Sci USA 1986; 83:2263–2266.
99. Recio-Pinto E, Ishii DN. Insulin and insulin-like growth factor receptors regu-

lating neurite formation in cultured human neuroblastoma cell. J Neurosci 1988; 6:1211–1219.

100. Fallon JH, Seroogy KB, Loughlin SE, Morrison RS, Bradshaw RA, Knauer DJ, Cunningham DD. Epidermal growth factor immunoreactive material in the central nervous system: location and development. Science 1984; 224: 1107–1109.
101. Code RA, Seroogy KB, Fallon JH. Some transforming growth factor-alpha connections and their colocalization with enkephalin in the rat central nervous system. Brain Res 1987; 421:401–405.
102. Derynck R. Transforming growth factor alpha. Cell 1988; 54:593–595.
103. Yamamori T, Fukada K, Aebersold R, Korsching S, Fann MJ, Patterson PH. The cholinergic neuronal differentiation factor from heart cells is identical to leukemia inhibitory factor. Science 1989; 246:1412–1416.
104. Nieto-Sampedro M, Chandy KG. Interleukin-2-like activity in injured rat brain. Neurochem Res 1987; 12:723–727.
105. Lindholm D, Heumann R, Meyer M, Thoenen H. Interleukin I regulates synthesis of nerve growth factor in non-neuronal cells of rat sciatic nerve. Nature 1987; 330:658–659.
106. Spranger M, Lindholm D, Bandtlow C, Heumann R, Gnahn H, Naher-Noe M, Thoenen H. Regulation of nerve growth factor (NGF) synthesis in the rat central nervous system: comparison between the effects of interleukin-1 and various growth factors in astrocyte cultures and in vivo. Eur J Neurosci 1990; 2:69–76.
107. Nieto-Sampedro M, Berman MA. Interleukin-1-like activity in rat brain: sources, target, and effect of injury. J Neurosci Res 1987; 17:214–219.
108. Kamegai M, Niijima K, Kunishita T, Nishizawa M, Ogawa M, Araki M, Ueki A, Konishi Y, Tabira T. Interleukin 3 as a trophic factor for central cholinergic neurons in vitro and in vivo. Neuron 1990; 2:429–436.
109. Hama T, Miyamoto M, Tsukui H, Nishio C, Hatanaka H. Interleukin-6 as a neurotrophic factor for promoting the survival of cultured basal forebrain cholinergic neurons from postnatal rats. Neurosci Lett 1989; 104:340–344.
110. Monard D. Role of protease inhibition in cellular migration and neuritic growth. Biochem Pharmacol 1987; 36:1389–1392.
111. Meier R, Spreyer P, Ortmann R, Harel A, Monard D. Induction of glia-derived nexin after lesion of a peripheral nerve. Nature 1989; 342:548–550.
112. Whitson JS, Selkoe DJ, Cotman CW. Amyloid beta protein enhances the survival of hippocampal neurons in vitro. Science 1989; 246:243–249.
113. Oltersdorf T, Fritz LC, Schenk DB, Lieberburg I, Johnson-Wood KJ, Beattie EC, Ward PJ, Blacher RW, Dovey HF, Sinha S. The secreted form of the Alzheimer's amyloid precursor protein with the Kunitz domain is protease nexin-II. Nature 1989; 341:144–147.
114. Dohrmann U, Edgar D, Sendtner M, Thoenen H. Muscle-derived factors that support survival and promote fiber outgrowth from embryonic chick spinal motor neurons in culture. Dev Biol 1986; 118:209–221.
115. Smith RG, Vaca K, McManaman J, Appel SH. Selective effects of skeletal

muscle extract fractions on motoneuron development in vitro. J Neurosci 1986; 6:439–447.
116. McManaman JL, Haverkamp LJ, Appel SH. Developmental discord among markers for cholinergic differentiation: in vitro time courses for early expression and responses to skeletal muscle extract. Dev Biol 1988; 125: 311–320.
117. Shalaby IA, Kotake C, Hoffmann PC, Heller A. A release of dopamine from coaggregate cultures of mesencephalic tegmentum and corpus striatum. J Neurosci 1983; 3:1565–1571.
118. Tomozawa Y, Appel SH. Soluble striatal extracts enhance development of mesencephalic dopaminergic neurons in vitro. Brain Res 1986; 399:111–124.
119. Ferrari G, Minozzi MC, Toffano G, Leon A, Skaper SD. Basic fibroblast growth factor promotes the survival and development of mesencephalic neurons in culture. Dev Biol 1989; 133:140–147.
120. Harbaugh RE, Reeder TM, Senter HJ, Knopman DS, Baskin DS, Pirozzolo F, Chui HC, Shetter AG, Bakay RAE, Leblanc R, Watson RT, DeKosky ST, Schmitt FA, Read SL, Johnston JT. Intracerebroventricular bethanechol chloride infusion in Alzheimer's disease: results of a collaborative double-blind study. J Neurosurg 1989; 71:481–486.
121. DeYebenes JG, Fahn S, Lovelle S, Jackson-Lewis V, Jorge P, Mena MA, Reiriz J, Bustos JC, Magarinos C, Martinez A. Continuous intracerebroventricular infusion of dopamine and dopamine agonists through a totally implanted drug delivery system in animal models of Parkinson's disease. Mov Disord 1987; 2:143–158.
122. Seno M, Sasada R, Iwane M, Sudo K, Kurokawa T, Ito K, Igarashi K. Stabilizing basic fibroblast growth factor using protein engineering. Biochem Biophys Res Commun 1988; 151:701–708.
123. Brange J, Ribel U, Hansen JF, et al. Monomeric insulins obtained by protein engineering and their medical implications. Nature 1988; 333:679–691.
124. Leong KW, Brott BC, Langer R. Bioerodible polyanhydrides as drug-carrier matrices. I. Characterization, degradation, and release characteristics. J Biomed Mater Res 1986; 20:51–64.
125. Rosenberg MB, Friedmann T, Robertson RC, Tuszynski M, Wolff JA, Breakefield XO, Gage FH. Grafting genetically modified cells to damaged brain: restorative effects of NGF expression. Science 1989; 242:1575–1578.
126. Ernfors P, Ebendal T, Olson L, Mouton P, Strnmberg I, Peersson H. A cell line producing recombinant nerve growth factor evokes growth responses in intrinsic and grafted central cholinergic neurons Proc Natl Acad Sci USA 1989; 86:4756–4760.
127. Romani S, Moroder L, Gohring W, Scharf R, Wunsch E, Barde YA, Thoenen H. Synthesis of the trypsin fragment 10-25/75-88 of mouse nerve growth factor. Int J Protein Res 1987; 29:107–117.
128. Longo FM, Vu TH, Mobley WC. In vitro biological effect of nerve growth factor inhibited by synthetic NGF peptides. Soc Neurosci Abstr 1989; 15:17.
129. Baird A, Schubert D, Ling N, Guillemin R. Receptor- and heparin-binding

domains of basic fibroblast growth factor. Proc Natl Acad Sci USA 1988; 85:2324–2328.

130. Ballard FJ, Francis GL, Ross M, Bagley CJ, May B, Wallace JC. Natural and synthetic forms of insulin-like growth factor-1 (IGF-1) and the potent derivative, destripeptide IGF-1: biological activities and receptor binding. Biochem Biophys Res Commun 1987; 149:398–404.

131. Komiriya A, Hortsch M, Meyers C, Smith M, Kanety H, Schlessinger J. Biologically active synthetic fragments of epidermal growth factor: localization of a major receptor-binding region. Proc Natl Acad Sci USA 1984; 81:1351–1355.

132. Konishi Y, Kotts CE, Bullock LD, Tou JS, Johnson DA. Fragments of bovine insulin-like growth factors I and II stimulate proliferation of rat L6 myoblast cells. Biochemistry 1989; 28:8872–8877.

133. Eppstein DA, Marsh YV, Schryver BB, Bertics PJ. Inhibition of epidermal growth factor/transforming growth factor-alpha-stimulated cell growth by a synthetic peptide. J Cell Physiol 1989; 141:420–430.

134. Matsuda H, Coughlin MD, Bienenstock J, Denburg JA. Nerve growth factor promotes human hemopoietic colony growth and differentation. Proc Natl Acad Sci USA 1988; 85:6508–6512.

135. Persson H, Ayer-Le Lievre C, Söder O, Villar MJ, Metsis M, Olson L, Ritzen M, Hökfelt T. Expression of beta nerve growth factor receptor mRNA in Sertoli cells downregulated by testosterone. Science 1990; 25:704–710.

136. Zheng M, Heinrich G. Structural and functional analysis of the promoter region of the nerve growth factor gene. Mol Brain Res 1988; 3:133–140.

137. Haskell BE, Stach RW, Werrbach-Perez K, Perez-Polo JR. Effect of retinoic acid on nerve growth factor receptors. Cell Tissue Res 1987; 247:67–73.

138. Wion D, Houlgatte R, Barbot N, Barrand P, Dicou E, Brachet P. Retinoic acid increases the expression of NGF gene in mouse L cells. Biochem Biophys Res Commun 1987; 149:510–514.

139. Thiele CJ, Reynolds CP, Israel MA. Decreased expression of N-*myc* precedes retinoic-acid induced morphological differentiation of human neuroblastoma. Nature 1985; 313:404–406.

140. Casper D, Davies P. Stimulation of choline acetyltransferase activity by retinoic acid and sodium butyrate in a cultured human neuroblastoma. Brain Res 1989; 478:1989 74–84.

141. Bedo G, Santisteban P, Aranda A. Retinoic acid regulates growth hormone gene expression. Nature 1989; 339:231–237.

142. Brand N, Petkovitch M, Krust A, Chambon P, de The H, Marchio A, Tiollais P, Dejean J. Identification of a second human retinoic acid receptor. Nature 1988; 332:850–853.

143. Grave GD. Thyroid hormones and brain development. New York: Raven Press, 1977.

144. Kalaria RN, Prince AK. The effects of neonatal thyroid deficiency on acetylcholine synthesis and glucose oxidation in rat corpus striatum. Dev Brain Res 1985; 20:271–279.

145. Kojima M, et al. Effect of thyroidectomy on choline acetyltransferase in rat hypothalamic nuclei. Brain Res 1981; 209:227–230.
146. Honegger P, Lenoir D. Triiodothyronine enhancement of neuronal differentiation in aggregating fetal rat brain cells cultured in a chemically defined medium. Brain Res 1980; 199:425–434.
147. Hayashi M, Patel AJ. An interaction between thyroid hormone and nerve growth factor in the regulation of choline acetyltransferase activity in neuronal cultures, derived from the septal-diagonal band region of the rat. Dev Brain Res 1987; 36:109–120.
148. Nakai A, Seino S, Sakurai A, Szilak I, Bell GJ, DeGroot LJ. Characterization of a thyroid hormone receptor expressed in human kidney and other tissues. Proc Natl Acad Sci USA 1988; 85:2781–2785.
149. Underwood AH, Emmett JC, Ellis D, Flynn SB, Leeson PD, Benson GM, Novelli R. A thyromimetic that decreases plasma cholesterol levels without increasing cardia activity. Nature 1986; 324:425–429.
150. Junard EO, Montero CN, Hefti FF. Long-term administration of mouse nerve growth factor to adult rats with partial lesions of the cholinergic septohippocampal pathway. Exp Neurol 1990; 110:25–38.

14

Clinical Trials Issues: The Example of Dementia

Paul D. Leber, M.D. *Potomac, Maryland*

I. INTRODUCTION

> Throw out opium, . . . throw out a few specifics which our art did not discover, and is hardly needed to apply; throw out wine, which is a food, and the vapors which produce the miracle of anesthesia, and I firmly believe that if the whole materia medica, as now used, could be sunk to the bottom of the sea, it would be all the better for mankind, . . . and all the worse for the fishes (1).

Much has changed in the century that has passed since Oliver Wendell Holmes, physician and father of the famous Supreme Court Justice of the same name, made these damning remarks about the pharmacopoeia. The worthless poultices, liniments, and alcohol-laden tonics that constituted the bulk of the armamentarium as recently as 50 years ago are now largely gone, replaced by drug products that the medical profession can be certain are not only effective, as their vendors claim they are, but reasonably safe for use under the conditions of use recommended in their labeling.

Two major factors account for the change. One, the more obvious, is the astounding advance of scientific knowledge, not only in medicine, but in

NOTICE: Dr. Leber is with the Food and Drug Administration, Rockville, Maryland. However, this chapter was written by Dr. Leber in his private capacity. No official support or endorsement by the Food and Drug Administration is intended or should be inferred.

virtually every field of endeavor, physics, chemistry, genetics, mathematics, that has made it possible to design and develop effective drugs for the management of an increasing number of conditions afflicting mankind. The second, often totally unappreciated, is society's decision to control the content of the armamentarium through a system of federal regulation that requires that the safety and efficacy of drug products be documented before marketing. Without this regulatory safeguard, much of the armamentarium would still deserve burial, although perhaps not at sea, given our new-found appreciation of the importance of protecting the environment from toxic waste.

This chapter considers what is the most critical, and perhaps most poorly understood, facet of the federal drug regulatory process: the premarket assessment of drug efficacy.* In particular, it deals with the design and conduct of clinical trials carried out to document the efficacy of drug products being advanced for the treatment of dementia.

The choice of clinical antidementia drug treatments as the major focus of this chapter might appear to restrict its scope unnecessarily. However, the matters to be considered have generic implications for treatments being developed for virtually any cognitive impairment associated with a chronic neurological or systemic illness. Moreover, any loss of generality that may result from focusing exclusively on dementia is offset by the opportunity to discuss specific issues of immediate practical importance. Dementia is not only a prototype of conditions causing cognitive impairment, but a major public health problem for which a number of new treatments are now under active development.

The chapter reviews aspects of clinical trial design and conduct that I believe are important (ca. 1990) to a successful demonstration of the efficacy of investigational treatments advanced for use in dementia. The advice offered applies to this area of drug development *at this point in time.* One recognizes, as should the reader, that many of the recommendations made are at risk of becoming obsolete as new information is gained about the etiology and pathogenesis of the dementia syndrome.

For example, what we currently view as a single, albeit heterogeneous, entity may actually be a large number of different conditions that present with a common clinical phenotype. If this is so, the development of biological markers and nonclinical tests for the subclassification of dementia will radically affect how new treatments are identified, developed, and tested.

*Importantly, proof of effectiveness is not the only requirement of marketing, but it is, on logical grounds, the most important. Obviously, if a drug does not work, there is little point in administering it to anyone, no matter how little it costs, how well it is made, or how safe it is. Moreover, from a practical perspective, no active pharmacologic substance is absolutely safe; consequently, the marketing of an ineffective drug can never be in society's collective interest.

On the other hand, no qualifying disclaimer is offered about the epistemological basis for the recommendations. The philosophical position espoused holds that the value of putative remedies for the treatment of human disease can be established only in valid, controlled, *clinical* experiments. It is acknowledged that other, often less rigorous, strategies for the assessment of the efficacy of new treatments have been proposed and have, at one time or another, gained a modicum of popularity, often, perhaps, because their weaknesses are not readily apparent to those untutored in the methods of scientific inquiry. However, popularity cannot be permitted to become a test of scientific validity. If we are to determine whether or not a drug is what its proponents claim it to be, if we are to ensure that the armamentarium remains free of ineffective and, worse, dangerous drugs, there is no alternative to the adequate and well-controlled trial. The suggestions that follow are the result of applying this guiding tenet to the design, planning, and conduct of clinical trials of putative antidementia agents.

II. BASIC PRINCIPLES

By law, the efficacy of an investigational drug may be documented only with evidence adduced from bona fide, epistemologically valid, clinical experiments (i.e., with "substantial" evidence of efficacy).* Accordingly, the choice of an experimental design for a clinical investigation intended to support the efficacy of a drug is a fundamental and critical step for a sponsor seeking marketing approval for an investigational drug product.

The choice of trial design is almost never a matter of personal preference or taste alone. In fact, an experiment's purpose, the desired precision of its results, and the nature of the disease, and the patient population involved usually limit, and may even dictate, the choice of experimental strategy that can be deemed acceptable.

For example, the US Food and Drug Administration's (FDA's) regulations identify five different types of "adequate and well-controlled" clinical trial designs† that are deemed capable of generating 'substantial' evidence of efficacy; however, these designs are not deemed equivalent in the

***Substantial evidence* is a term of 'art.' It is defined in the *Federal Food, Drug and Cosmetic Act,* as "evidence consisting of adequate and well-controlled investigations, including clinical investigations, by experts qualified by scientific training and experience to evaluate the effectiveness of the drug involved, on the basis of which it could fairly and responsibly be concluded by such experts that the drug will have the effect it purports or is represented to have under the conditions of use prescribed, recommended, or suggested in the labeling or proposed labeling thereof" [Sect. 505(d)].

†21 CFR 314.126 enumerates the following types of controls: placebo, fixed dose, active, historical, and no-treatment control.

strength of evidence they produce nor are they viewed as equally appropriate for use in all circumstances.

The three designs that employ concurrent randomized controls (i.e., placebo, active, and fixed dose) and blind both subjects and assessors to the nature of the assigned treatments are equivalent, in theory, in their power to document efficacy when they find a statistically significant between-treatment difference favorable to the investigational agent (2). A similar statistically significant difference in a no-treatment, concurrent, randomized control is ordinarily considered less persuasive because systematic bias may inflate the estimate of the treatment effect (i.e., because neither subjects nor assessors are blind to the nature of the treatment assignment). Of course, the extent of bias may be so slight that it is irrelevant if the outcome assessment cannot be influenced substantially by knowledge of treatment assignment (e.g., cardiac output).

Of the five controlled designs, historical controls are least reliable because their interpretation depends entirely upon the accuracy of an assumption that ordinarily cannot be verified, that is, that a group of patients undergoing open treatment are identical in all respects, save treatment, to some group (i.e., the control) evaluated in the past. In some situations, this is a safe assumption; in most situations, it is not. Consequently, the historical control is appropriate only in a very limited number of clinical settings.

A. General Considerations About the Practical Conduct of Clinical Trials

1. Laying the Foundation for a Valid Clinical Experiment

Countless factors undoubtedly influence how the results of a particular experiment are received by the scientific community. Certainly, the structure of an experiment (i.e., its design) is of paramount importance, but, by itself, structure cannot possibly guarantee an experiment's validity. Clearly, a valid experiment is one that is not only structurally sound, but competently carried out. Thus, if the results of a study are to gain acceptance, those conducting it must be able to provide documentation that the study was, in fact, performed as it was designed to be.

The fundamental documentation for a study consists of two parts: 1. the protocol (i.e., a prospectively written plan describing the study), and 2. records documenting that the plan was faithfully carried out.

a. The Research Plan It is by now standard practice to set out in written form a detailed plan for the conduct and analysis of any clinical experiment. In fact, a prospectively drafted, detailed protocol is ordinarily a sine qua non of an "adequate and well-controlled investigation," the only type of clinical investigation, importantly, that may serve for regulatory purposes as a source of substantial evidence of an investigational new drug's efficacy [See 21 CFR 314.126(b)(1)]. Admittedly, a perfectly valid experiment might be carried out without a prospectively written protocol, but the absence of the protocol places the investigator in an exceedingly difficult, sometimes embarrassing, position if he or she is called upon to defend the study and its results in a public or regulatory forum. Indeed, in the absence of a prospectively written protocol, there is little to distinguish a bona fide clinical experiment from a report of a series of patients who have been managed with a new treatment under open conditions. (A pundit once defined such a case series as a sequence of patients that begins with the first observed success of the new treatment and ends immediately before its first subsequent failure.)

*b. Records of Trial Conduct** Records serve as a tangible trace of the persons, actions, and events that are the constitutive elements of any clinical investigation. To be useful, records must be contemporaneously made, complete, legible, logical in organization, cumulative in nature, and contain sufficient information and links to corroborating evidence (e.g., laboratory reports, x-ray films, clinic appointment books) to provide, if need be, robust substantiation that the maneuvers called for in the study protocol were actually performed as required. For example, the individual record kept on each subject who participates in an investigation should identify the patient fully and make clear what examinations and tests were performed, where and by whom they were done, and on what calendar dates and times of day. On face, without additional post hoc, retrospective explanation, the records should be sufficient to substantiate why the individual was a suitable subject for entry into the study and show how, and on the basis of what data, that judgment was made. The individual subject's record should show when and to what treatment he or she was randomized and provide a full accounting of the subsequent administration of that treatment by dose (or plasma concentration), day, and time.

Original records for a study are also expected to include documents that deal with the study as a whole. For example, in addition to the original protocol and amendments to it (all should be dated), there should be a document describing the randomization scheme for the study and records

*The recommendations enumerated are not intended to constitute an exhaustive list of any set of official regulatory requirements. The suggestions offered are intended to convey the scope and level of detail of comprehensive record keeping that may prove useful in clinical trial records. Readers seeking formal advice about official regulatory requirements governing records that must be maintained should rely upon the FDA's official regulations, guidelines, and policy statements. Explicit advice on specific matters is ordinarily best obtained through direct consultation with the appropriate FDA organizational unit responsible for the matter.

that show precisely how, when, and by whom each treatment assignment was made. There should also be a record of the staff involved in a study that indicates the period of their involvement, their duties, and their role vis-à-vis record keeping, patient assessment, and treatment allocation. Clearly, individuals with knowledge of treatment assignment should not be involved in the assessment of response to treatment in any study that is identified as one conducted under "blind" conditions.

Much of the documentation that the author recommends to be collected as a matter of routine ordinarily will not be of particular value in the analysis of most clinical studies. Nonetheless, detailed, easily retrievable records of the sort recommended can be invaluable should the need arise to investigate why a particular study failed to show expected results or to defend the study's interpretation in face of challenges to its validity.

III. SPECIFIC CONSIDERATIONS IN THE PLANNING AND DESIGN OF CLINICAL TRIALS OF ANTIDEMENTIA AGENTS

A. Definition of Dementia

Dementia, as used throughout this chapter, refers to an irreversible neurological condition of unknown etiology that is ordinarily characterized by a progressive decline of intellectual and cognitive abilities. In particular, this chapter considers clinical studies intended to evaluate the efficacy of drugs proposed for use in the management of patients with Alzheimer's dementia (AD), the type of dementia likely to be found with the highest prevalence in typical samples of elderly patients presenting clinically with signs of a dementing illness.

B. The Nature of Dementia's Manifestations That Are the Legitimate Targets of a Drug Exerting an Antidementia Action

The central issue, one yet to be fully resolved, is what defines an antidementia drug. In the absence of a recognized or approved treatment for dementia, advice based on precedent is unavailable. Logically, of course, a drug that reversed or slowed the dementing process or, even better, one that prevented its occurrence, would qualify. It is also logical that a drug that improved a subject's performance or behavior in those areas of function that are characteristically and progressively impaired by the dementing process should also be viewed as exerting an antidementia action.

The nexus of the question, therefore, is which manifestations of dementia a drug must affect, at a minimum, to be deemed an antidementia treatment. Experts who gathered to discuss the subject at an FDA symposium held in 1989 (3), agreed that any treatment worthy of an antidementia designation should exert a beneficial effect on the core manifestations of dementia. Although there are some minor disagreements about the identity of the core phenomena and their relative importance, these experts generally agreed that a treatment cannot be considered to exert an "antidementia" action unless it beneficially affects a demented patient's ability to learn new and retrieve old, previously learned, information.

This does not gainsay the value of developing drugs that affect other aspects of the dementing process (i.e., failed self-care, disturbed mood, loss of control over impulses, and such), but it does have import for the manner in which such effects might be described in the labeling of marketed drug products. This leads directly to the controversial subject of "pseudospecificity" of claimed indications.

C. The Nature of a Drug's Claimed Effect: The Problem of Pseudospecificity

Not surprisingly, experimental designs and protocols are ordinarily constructed with the nature of the claim the investigator hopes to make, if the investigation succeeds, in mind. This holds whether the experiment poses a purely academic or commercial question. There is, however, a potential trap that uniquely awaits those seeking to develop commercial drug products for use in the management of patients with AD. It arises because a drug may confer benefit without having any biological or logical link to dementia, as the drug would benefit any human being with the target condition, whether or not they had AD. The author coined the term *pseudospecificity* to refer to this problem (4).

A claim for a product is pseudospecific when the relationship between the pharmacological effect and the characteristic of the population to which it is linked arises solely because the product was selectively tested in patients with the pseudospecific characteristic. For example, a demonstration that penicillin cures pneumococcal pneumonia in patients who are selected for evaluation because they have both pneumonia and AD does not justify a claim linking penicillin and dementia.

Although the logical flaw in the example given to illustrate the problem is self-evident, pseudospecificity may occur in far less obvious circumstances. For example, impulsive behavioral acts are common in advanced dementia; if their incidence can be reduced by judicious use of a neuroleptic, is the neuroleptic exerting an antidementia action? The issue is vexing, especially if its recognition discourages development of new symptomatic treatments for the management of patients with advanced dementia.* Logically, however, the flaw remains.

In any event, an unmodified claim for efficacy in dementia can be readily justified only if 1. a drug beneficially affects a "core" sign or symptom of dementia {see foregoing}, or if 2. the effect of the drug is only expressed, or differentially expressed, in patients with dementia. For example, if a drug acted as an hypnotic only in the insomnia seen in dementia, it would be entitled to a dementia-related claim. However, if a benzodiazepine hypnotic were evaluated only in demented patients (by virtue of the sponsor's drug development decision) and was found to be effective in reducing sleep latency, the sponsor would *not* be entitled to a claim linking the drug to dementia. Importantly, however, if the product met requirements for marketing as a general use hypnotic, the studies in demented patients, provided they were adequate and well controlled, could be described in the marketed product's labeling as among those supporting the product's claims of effectiveness in insomnia.

D. The Study Participants

Obviously, the efficacy of an antidementia agent cannot be properly assessed in an experiment in which a substantial number of subjects do not have dementia.† Thus, the subject selection process should be designed to capture only those individuals in whom the diagnosis is unequivocal and fully documented.

As a first step, patients selected for study should meet widely accepted clinical diagnostic criteria for AD. For example, patient classification can

*The argument has been advanced that commercial sponsors are less willing to investigate a drug that might, because of some attribute, be especially useful in the elderly if pseudospecific claims are denied. The rejoinder, however, is that the "special advantage" to the elderly demented patient cannot be advanced or implied in labeling without probative clinical evidence. Thus, a sponsor seeking to promote the product as uniquely valuable for a demented patient would, in the end, have to conduct what would be essentially the very same clinical experiments required to examine the product's pseudospecific claim.

†However, studies in nondemented patients, in particular the elderly, could contribute useful information about the safety and biopharmacokinetic performance of a drug, at least insofar as one is willing to assume that the elderly population, as a whole, is a reasonably representative surrogate for demented patients. Of course, because the demented state might render individuals uniquely susceptible to some adverse action of a drug, the bulk of clinical evidence amassed to document a drug's safety would still have to be gained in demented patients.

Another exception is studies conducted to evaluate treatments intended to delay the onset or block the occurrence of dementia. Obviously, such experiments would have to enroll nondemented subjects.

be based on *DSM-III-R* criteria for primary degenerative dementia of the Alzheimer's type (5) or the NINCDS–ADRDA criteria for dementia (6). However, mere specification of diagnosis is not enough. The protocol must enumerate in detail the set of maneuvers and criteria that will be employed to screen, reject, and select patients for study.

Special efforts should be taken to ensure that the patients selected do *not* suffer from a condition that may be confused clinically with dementia. In particular, it is important to be certain that patients do not suffer from retarded depression (i.e., pseudodementia), delirium, or some primary neurological or systemic illness that can mimic dementia (e.g., normal pressure hydrocephalus, Parkinson's disease, brain tumor, myxedema, drug-induced deliriform illness, or other). Strategies for evaluating patients to exclude those with the more frequent of the conditions mistaken for AD are well known (e.g., 7).

The extent of functional cognitive impairment among patients enrolled should be characterized using measures and instruments that have documented reliability and validity. Unfortunately, a single standardized system for assessing the severity of dementia has yet to be adopted by the community of experts. Nonetheless, it seems reasonable to recommend that the extent of each study participant's clinical impairment be assessed using *both* a clinical-staging device like the Global Deterioration Scale (GDS) (8) and a standardized comprehensive test that employs objective measures of cognitive performance. Examples of the latter include the Mini-Mental Status Examination (MSSE) (9), the Alzheimer's Disease Assessment Scale (ADAS) (10), the Memory Information Test (MIT) (11), and the Dementia Rating Scale (DRS) of Mattis (12).

E. Enrichment Maneuvers

In several recent (ca. 1990) antidementia drug trials involving drugs thought to exhibit an inverted U-shaped dose–response relationship, patients were selected for entry into the randomized phase of the experiment if, and only if, they exhibited, during a prerandomization phase, an apparently positive response to treatment with the investigational drug. These patients were then randomized and assigned either to placebo or to the dose of drug to which they had shown the "best" apparent response.

The maneuver just described was undertaken to increase the efficiency of the experiment. In theory, such an enrichment maneuver makes considerable sense, especially if 1. dementia is a heterogeneous condition, and 2. only a subset of the demented population has the capacity to respond to the treatment being tested. In the example cited, a subject's response to the experimental drug was presumed to signal his or her capacity to respond to treatment. Of course, any trait or measurable attribute predicting treatment response can be used for the same purpose. Indeed, using a marker other than response to the investigational drug has advantages. First, it does not increase the likelihood, as does prior exposure to drug, that the subject will recognize his treatment assignment. Second, if the experimental drug being tested induces physical dependence, a trial design that rerandomizes apparent treatment responders may be demonstrating only a withdrawal phenomena when it finds a between-treatment difference favoring subjects assigned to the investigational drug.

In any event, an enrichment maneuver may be counterproductive if the presumed predictor is unreliable. In such a case, the maneuver may actually undermine the efficiency of the trials, because it will lead to the needless rejection of perfectly good study candidates.

F. The Choice of Clinical Trial Design

1. The Need for Concurrently Randomized Controlled Designs

As noted in the introduction, the advice and counsel offered in this chapter derives from the philosophical conviction, endorsed by law, that evidence of a drug's efficacy can be adduced only in adequate and well-controlled clinical studies. For drugs advanced for the treatment of dementia, proof of efficacy consists of showing that the experimental treatment is superior to some control treatment.

Although the issue was touched upon in an earlier section of this chapter, it may not be evident, so far at least, why evidence derived from all experimental designs identified in Federal Regulations (i.e., 21 CFR 314.126) as "adequate and well controlled" and capable of serving as sources of substantial evidence of drug efficacy is not automatically acceptable. In particular, why will a historical (i.e., external) control study not suffice to establish the efficacy of an antidementia drug? The answer lies in the nature of the dementing process.

The extent of variation among samples of patients drawn from the population of individuals with dementia is far too great to permit the use of nonconcurrent (i.e., external) controls. Over the interval of time corresponding to the duration of the typical clinical dementia drug study (e.g., several months), it is impossible to predict precisely how much deterioration, if any, will be seen in the clinical state of a particular sample of demented patients. In fact, over a period of weeks, some samples of demented patients may be expected to show improvement, perhaps as a result of being exposed to the novel, relatively enriched and, therefore, therapeutic, environment created by the conduct of the experiment. In the long run, typical samples of demented patients will deteriorate. The critical point for the designer of clinical trials is that the rate of deterioration is highly variable and irregularly irregular.

Consequently, each clinical study intended to document the efficacy of an antidementia drug must include an appropriate "internal" control as a means to determine whether the study's outcome, if nominally positive, can be unambiguously attributed to the effects of treatment with the experimental drug, rather than to the variation among samples of demented patients or spontaneous fluctuations in the severity of the manifestations of the dementing process in the particular sample of patients evaluated.

2. Placebo Is the Preferred Choice for an Internal Control

For studies evaluating antidementia treatments, placebo is the obvious choice for an internal control; however, a subtherapeutic dose of the investigational drug or some less-than-optimal therapeutic dose of some other pharmacologically active agent might, provided certain conditions are met, be used instead. (It must be certain that exposure to the control does not make the patients worse than they might have been had they received no treatment at all. If this is not so, a demonstration that an experimental drug is superior to the control is not clear proof of efficacy; the experimental drug may only be less toxic than the control.) Regardless of the type of control employed, evidence of efficacy derives from a showing that patients randomized to the investigational drug fare significantly better than those concurrently randomized to the control.

3. The Added Advantage of Fixed Treatment Level Designs

Beyond demonstrating that a product is "effective," it is important to understand the link between *dose* (or drug plasma concentration), *dosing regimen* (drug plasma level fluctuations) and clinical responses, both therapeutic and untoward. Obviously, a design employing but a single level of a treatment is not able to address the issue. A study allowing flexible titration, based on clinical response of patients, may provide some information, but such a design may produce a distorted picture of the overall dose–response relationship. First, patients showing inadequate responses tend to be titrated to the highest clinically tolerable dose. As a consequence, dose–response relationships based on open titration often reveal an artifactual inversion (negative slope) at the higher end of the recommended dose range. Titration is also likely to overestimate the dose required to produce a response if there is a substantial latency to the development of a maximum response following the administration of a given dose. Such delays in response can occur for pharmacokinetic (e.g., long half-life of the drug or its active metabolites) or pharmacodynamic (effector system undergoes time-dependent changes) reasons. In such circumstances, if the latency to maximum effect is not recognized, the dose may be advanced before the full response at the dose (or steady-state plasma level) is achieved.

Consequently, dose–response relationships are best evaluated with study designs that randomize patients to two or more fixed "levels" of experimental treatment. Critically, "fixed treatment level" designs do *not* require that patients be randomized to their final, full predetermined dose on the very first dose or day of treatment. Indeed, such a rigid dosing policy can, if a drug has many dose-related side effects, cause a fixed treatment level design to fail (patients assigned to the higher dose levels selectively dropout for adverse reactions). In such circumstances, if there is any chance that tolerance to dose-related side effects will develop, patients assigned to higher treatment levels should be gradually titrated to their predetermined dose or plasma concentration. This strategy is acceptable as long as 1. the levels of treatment (dose or concentration) assigned are specified before beginning the experiment; 2. the outcome assessment for each treatment level is made after steady-state is achieved and sufficient time has elapsed to allow the full therapeutic response to develop under these stabilized conditions; and 3. a similar dosing strategy is employed uniformly among all treatment groups (i.e., to maintain the blind).

4. *Parallel and Crossover Designs*

Ordinarily, parallel designs are considered superior to crossover designs for the study of antidementia treatments. In theory, however, a crossover design may be employed if its treatment periods are relatively short and carryover effects or withdrawal effects associated with the use of the drug are so insignificant that they are unlikely to confound the experiment's interpretation. Unfortunately, the existence of carryover and withdrawal effects are commonly discovered only after the completion of a study at the time its results are being analyzed. In any event, if a sponsor does conduct a study using a crossover design, it must be carried out in a manner that will permit its assumptions (i.e., no carryover, no withdrawal, no treatment by period interactions) to be reliably evaluated from evidence developed in the experiment (i.e., a sufficient number of subjects must be enrolled to provide adequate power to test for the presence of these confounding effects).

Additionally, those electing to use a crossover design in any study lasting more than a week or so, must be prepared to defend the suitability of the design for the evaluation of an antidementia drug, especially one that is intended for long-term administration. In particular, if the study is to be accepted as valid, there must be evidence to document that patients entering any period of the design, other than the first, have returned to the clinical state they exhibited before the start of that first period. If this cannot be demonstrated, the investigator conducting the study will be hard pressed to defend any favorable interpretation attached to the results observed. Given the issues discussed, the often cited theoretical advantage of the crossover design (i.e., a reduction in variance contributed by between-subject differences) may not be sufficient to warrant its use.

5. *The Choice of Experimental Conditions*

a. Settings. A controlled trial of a new drug can be carried out in virtually any setting given appropriate planning and resources. Often, however, especially early in Phase II, concerns about the potential risks of the drug preclude its testing in ambulatory patients living outside a medically supervised environment. The problem ordinarily is not that a drug is known affirmatively to be dangerous, but that the limited experience gained during Phase I clinical testing cannot provide sufficient reassurance about the drug's safety "for use," at least under minimally supervised or unsupervised conditions.

However, investigators are understandably reluctant to ask ambulatory demented patients to enter medically supervised environments for the sole purpose of participating in a study. The hardship imposed upon such patients may be somewhat reduced if testing is split between inpatient and ambulatory environments. For example, induction and dose titration can be accomplished within a medically supervised environment. After a time judged sufficient to establish steady-state plasma concentrations at the maximum dose to be given, patients may be discharged to their usual place of domicile, provided that monitoring of treatment continues at frequent intervals. Ideally, monitoring would include frequent sampling of blood levels of the drug to mitigate any risks that might be associated with accumulation of the drug.

An alternative strategy is to initiate controlled Phase II testing of a new antidementia drug in more severely impaired patients who are already institutionalized. Some may fault this approach, arguing that it is more difficult to document drug effects, at least on the core phenomena of dementia, in such advanced patients. On the other hand, even if such studies fail to provide definitive evidence of an antidementia effect, they may provide valuable insights about the nature of the drug's therapeutic action (i.e., positive trends) and insights into the nature of the drug's dose-related toxicities. This information may then serve as a basis for the initiation of trials that can be conducted in ambulatory settings with less impaired patients.

b. Choosing the Dose and Dosing Regimen to Study. Obviously, if a clinical experiment is to succeed, the experimental drug should be administered in a manner that allows plasma concentrations presumed necessary to produce a therapeutic effect to be attained without undue degrees of toxicity or dysphoric effects. Clearly, knowledge of a drug's metabolism, systemic bioavailability, rate of elimination, and the relationship between plasma drug concentrations and dysphoric or untoward pharmacologic effects would be invaluable in determining how often a drug can or must be given. The problem, however, is that such information is not always available.

In fact, what concentration of drug (or active metabolite) is required to achieve a desired therapeutic effect is never known at the initiation of a clinical drug development program. Thus, selecting the dose(s) of the experimental drug and the regimen for its administration in clinical trials is invariably a problematic undertaking. In general, two strategies are used. One, the empirical, proceeds upon the assumption that the best dose to employ is the one that has been found to be *maximally tolerated* in Phase I clinical testing. This strategy implicitly assumes that the dose and therapeutic response exhibit a monotonic and positive correlation. However, some dose–response relationships are biphasic; that is, they exhibit an inverted U-shaped profile. Moreover, volunteers and patients may differ in their sensitivity to drug, either by virtue of the disease process or as a function of the conditions of treatment under which they are evaluated. (For example, a parkinsonian patient may be less sensitive to side effects induced by a dopamine agonist than a normal individual. A chronic insomniac may be more tolerant to the sedative effects of a benzodiazepine than a naive subject. Thus, higher doses than those identified during Phase I single-dose studies as toxic can sometimes be administered without ill effect to patients.) To adjust for such uncertainty, empirical dose-finding strategies regularly begin therapeutic assessment trials at doses (or drug plasma concentrations) lower than those found to be maximally tolerated. However, to avoid missing important therapeutic effects, such studies also assess, with appropriate safeguards, the consequences of employing doses exceeding those 'found' in Phase I to be maximally tolerated, provided that 1. the apparent therapeutic response is less than that sought; and 2. the patients involved are tolerating the presumed 'maximally tolerated' dose without significant ill effect.

The second strategy, the rational, attempts to predict the required human dose or minimum effective plasma levels on the basis of data derived from preclinical models. The approach assumes that the concentration of drug that must be obtained in the "biophase" of the preclinical animal to achieve a surrogate therapeutic effect is approximately the level required in humans. Whether this strategy will have application in antidementia drug development is now uncertain.

c. Enhancing Compliance. Because poor compliance may lead to failed clinical trials, every effort should be made to ensure that subjects comply fully with their treatment regimen. Although good study protocols mandate routine checks on patient compliance (plasma or urine sampling), it may also be helpful to take steps to enhance compliance before a trial is actually begun.

For example, both product formulations and dosing regimens should be designed with patient compliance in mind. The palatability (i.e., taste, appearance, smell, consistency) of the dosage form should be considered, as well as its ease of administration and consumption. The elderly individual, even if not demented, may be physically impaired to the extent that it becomes difficult for him or her to open a container of drugs. Similarly, visual impairments may make it impossible for many older patients to identify the contents of a container or follow the dosing recommendations written upon them. The timing and complexity of a regimen may also create difficulties, especially for those with emotional and physical impairments. For these reasons, among others, experts urge that ambulatory dementia patients living outside special care environments not be enrolled in clinical trials unless they live with a competent adult who agrees to cooperate in the clinical trial process.

G. Efficacy Assessment

1. Prospective Identification of Major Outcome Assessment Variables: The Avoidance of Multiplicity

The protocol for a clinical study should prospectively identify which outcome variables among the many assessed will be employed to evaluate the clinical investigation's overall outcome vis-à-vis the efficacy of the drug. Prospective designation of outcome variables is necessary to prevent the overall experiment's type I error rate from being grossly inflated over the nominal "alpha" level at which each outcome variable assessed is tested. However, provided that the designation is made prospectively, this recommendation allows use of summed scores or factors derived from appropriate multivariate analyses to be used as the primary outcome measures of a study. The epistemological point is that outcome variable(s) must be specified before an experiment is analyzed, preferably at the time of its planning. The outcome measures should *never* be selected on the basis of an evaluation of the data developed in a study.

2. The Measurement of Antidementia Drug Effects in Clinical Trials

As noted earlier, experts more or less uniformly endorse the principle that a drug can be considered to have an 'antidementia' action only if it exerts a clinically meaningful effect on the core manifestations of dementia. This consensus, however, is restricted to principle; there is considerably less agreement among experts about which specific tests or batteries of tests should be used to measure "clinically meaningful antidementia" treatment effects.

Experts generally agree that a comprehensive cognitive performance assessment instrument with an established capacity (reliability, validity) to assess changes in the severity of the core manifestations of dementia is a sine qua non of any outcome assessment battery. If such a performance-based test is not employed, uncertainties will invariably exist about whether between-treatment differences detected during the course of a controlled clinical investigation are or are not reflections of an 'antidementia' action. However, experts question the wisdom of relying exclusively on performance-based assessments.

At the 1989 FDA-sponsored symposium on the assessment of antidementia treatment effects (3), experts expressed the concern that so-called comprehensive-based assessments might detect drug-induced changes in the performance of demented subjects on tests that, despite their nominal face validity, are largely irrelevant to a patient's clinical state or well-being. In other words, the concern is that performance-based test batteries may be too sensitive and, as a consequence, their use as the sole device to assess antidementia drug efficacy might lead to the approval of products without clinically meaningful effects.

To reduce the likelihood that products with clinically trivial effects would be inappropriately declared effective as antidementia agents, experts at the symposium recommended that clinical trials of investigational antidementia drugs regularly employ a "clinical global assessment" as well as a comprehensive performance-based assessment. A clinical global assessment is one made by a skilled clinician familiar with dementia and its manifestations. Presumably, if a disinterested clinician, blind to treatment assignment, can detect a beneficial effect of a treatment, the effect is clinically meaningful.

Thus, trials intended to provide "substantial" evidence of an investigational drug's antidementia efficacy should employ both a clinical global and a comprehensive performance-based cognitive test battery as outcome assessments. Statistically significant between-treatment differences on the former establish that the treatment effects have clinical meaning. Significant differences on the performance-based assessment document that the drug's effects are directed against the manifestations of dementia deemed key to a bona fide antidementia claim.

3. *The Choice of Domain-Specific Cognitive Performance-Based Assessment*

The identity of the specific performance-based assessment instrument (e.g., the ADAS, the Blessed, or other) is not important as long as it is accepted as valid and reliable by a substantial proportion of experts working in the fields of dementia and neuropsychological assessment.

It is important to match the difficulty of a test and the level of pathology it assesses to the severity of illness exhibited by the patients studied. In particular, an instrument that works well with patients early in the course of dementia may be much too difficult for patients with advanced disease.

4. The Choice of a Global Assessment Measure

There are two general types of global assessments that can be applied by professional staff conducting an experiment:* One type, the *clinical global improvement rating,* is designed to capture the extent of overall improvement or deterioration that the clinician perceives has occurred in the patient's status since an earlier evaluation (i.e., usually, a baseline evaluation). The second type, the *absolute global severity assessment,* is intended to capture the absolute severity of the medical condition affecting the patient. The degree of severity is judged in relation to the full range of pathology exhibited by patients suffering from the disease for which the experimental treatment is being evaluated.

Which of the two types of global assessments is best? There is no simple answer.

Global ratings intended to reflect the absolute severity of a patient's pathology are probably less sensitive to variation in the skills and experience of clinical raters than are global assessments based on perceived improvements in a patient's clinical state. In part, this is a reflection of our ability to tie specific global severity assessment scores to examples of patients representing each of the ordered categories that compose the typical global severity scale. Clearly, it is virtually impossible to create a system for anchoring the points along a global improvement scale in the same manner as is done with global severity assessments, especially when the disease being assessed is not known to show a substantive response to treatment.

*Although family or significant others can offer global opinions concerning their demented relative or loved one, their judgments are not readily translated into meaningfully valid ratings for use in assessing the outcome of clinical trials. To begin, the scope of experience of the significant other/family member is severely limited. Specifically, it is unlikely that the significant other/family member has a past body of experience with demented patients that can be used to anchor his or her assessment. Similarly, the family member will have little basis for weighing in quantitative terms with public meaning the extent of changes seen or believed to be seen in his relative or loved one. Finally, the blinding of family or significant others to the nature of the treatment assignment may be very difficult, if not impossible, to maintain, especially if the experimental drug causes very untoward and unique side effects. These factors make the use of family- or significant other-based globals problematic for use a primary assessment measures.

On the other hand, global severity categories tend to be relatively broad, and it is conceivable that improvements in the condition of patients of sufficient magnitude to be detected by an astute clinician might be too small to be registered on a global severity assessment. However, there is a price to pay for the greater "sensitivity" of the global improvement assessment. Because they encourage the clinician to offer ratings for clinical changes of relatively small magnitude, global improvement assessments are likely to exhibit greater variation within and among raters than do global severity assessments offered for the same patient. Thus, a conundrum arises. If a drug has a small treatment effect, the global improvement is more likely than the global severity assessment to detect it; however, because the treatment effect is small, the variation associated with the global improvement assessment scores (among and between raters) may preclude attainment of statistically significant differences on the assessment, especially in small studies.

Consequently, it is especially important to minimize or eliminate sources of variation that may add to the variation of global assessments. One source, all too often ignored, is that arising from the use of inconsistent raters (i.e., different raters on different assessment occasions). Because globals depend upon the personal judgment of individual raters, the advantages of having the same individual rate a patient on each occasion are obvious. In theory, because of the availability of clinical anchor points, the use of consistent assessors is not mandatory for global severity assessments, but it clearly is for assessments of improvement. In fact, it is logically difficult to understand how a rater could conclude a patient has improved if he or she has not seen the patient at an earlier point.

Before leaving the topic of global assessment measures, it is critical to note that neither type provides a valid measure of a patient's clinical state when used by raters aware of the treatment assignment of the patients being rated. Consequently, special precautions should be taken to enhance the likelihood that treatment assignments will not become known to those making global assessments. Beyond the usual precautions ordinarily taken, raters responsible for providing global assessments should be denied access to information about untoward clinical responses reported by, or abnormal laboratory test results obtained on, the subjects being assessed. In fact, it might be useful to have those providing global assessments base their ratings on video-taped interviews presented to them in some random, nonchronological, permuted sequence.

In sum, it is not now possible to endorse one of the two types of global assessment in preference to the other. Either or both can be used. However, if both are used, the protocol for the study should specify which of the two globals will be considered the primary one to be used in association with the comprehensive performance-based assessment instrument to judge the overall outcome of the investigation.

H. Safety Assessments

Ordinarily, beyond tests required to establish their suitability as subjects, patients entering a clinical trial should have a full physical and neurological examination and a comprehensive battery of medical laboratory and special tests performed. Testing of this scope is readily justified. First, it may protect the patient with unrecognized illness from possible harm should his undiscovered illness make him more susceptible to the untoward actions of the investigational drug. Second, it protects the drug from being misidentified as the cause of the undetected illness, protection that the sponsor of an investigational drug sorely needs. Finally, such testing contributes importantly to the assessment of a drug's safety. In particular, randomized controlled trials often provide the only source of information that can be used to determine the "attributable" risk for events seen in the diseased population being treated.

Accordingly, it seems prudent to recommend that every participant in a controlled trial be evaluated at or immediately before actual treatment exposure.* Baseline assessments, logically, are critical to determining whether abnormalities detected during drug exposure can reasonably be attributed to the assigned treatment. (Logically, a treatment-emergent adverse event consists either of an event arising de novo following the initiation of drug treatment, or an event that, although present before drug administration, increases in severity after drug treatment begins.) Subsequently, additional safety evaluations should made, periodically, at reasonable intervals, throughout both the period of treatment exposure and the period immediately following drug discontinuation (i.e., to determine if the use of the drug is associated with withdrawal-emergent adverse events).

I. Pharmacokinetic Screening

Although not primarily intended for the purpose, controlled trials provide an opportunity to collect information that may be useful in identifying

*The critical point is to obtain data on subjects as close to the time of, but not after, their initial exposure to the assigned treatment. The concern addressed is that some protocols allow patients to be given their treatment assignments well in advance of the time of their initial treatment exposure. This creates a situation in which a spontaneously untoward event or abnormality, unrelated to treatment assignment, may be incorrectly attributed to the assigned treatment. The possibility for such an error can be virtually eliminated by making the act of randomization virtually simultaneous with the initial exposure of the subject to treatment.

causal associations between pharmacokinetic and various clinical phenomena. Plasma samples obtained from patients exposed to a new drug over an extended period may also help identify factors contributing to the variability of a drug's pharmacokinetic performance within the population. Thus, the collection of two or more samples of blood from patients who are on stable dosing regimens at known times following administration of a particular dose of their drug is encouraged in every Phase III trial.

J. The Duration of Clinical Studies

One of the most vexing questions affecting the testing of all drug products is the interval over which their efficacy should be evaluated. For drugs that are used to treat acute, transient illness, there is never much of a controversy; the drug is evaluated for at least as long as it likely to be used to produce its desired effect. Thus, an injectable analgesic, intended to be used for 1 or 2 days in most cases, might be evaluated in efficacy studies lasting as long as several days to a week. Similarly, an antibiotic intended to treat streptococcal pharyngitis need only be evaluated over the interval needed to eradicate the streptococcal infection.

Drugs intended for palliation of chronic illness, however, pose an entirely different set of problems. Ideally, the efficacy of such drugs ought to be demonstrated over the full interval of their probable duration of use. However, practical considerations have made this goal regularly unattainable. For example, antidepressants, drugs that are routinely administered for periods of 6 months to 2 years in the management of an episode of depression, are evaluated for efficacy in studies lasting but 4–8 weeks.

Understandably, therefore, it is impossible to specify precisely how long a drug intended to treat dementia should be evaluated. In principle, the longer the study, the better, but in practice, this may not be realized. In particular, patient recruitment may suffer. Patients willing to accept the possibility of randomization to placebo for a matter of weeks may balk at participating in an experiment that may lead to them being denied access to an active, albeit only putatively effective, treatment for 6 months. Moreover, the longer the duration of any study, the smaller the proportion of subjects that are likely to complete the study as planned, an outcome that invariably complicates the study's eventual analysis.

On the other hand, if a treatment merely retards the rate of functional deterioration of the core manifestation of dementia, the size of the average treatment effect will be a direct function of the duration of the study. Under these circumstances, a statistically significant effect on a multi-item comprehensive cognitive performance instrument or a global might be found with a 6-months long, but not with a 3-months long, study.

At the time this manuscript is being written (ca. 1990), therefore, it is not possible to make a specific recommendation for the duration of trials. It seems unlikely, however, that experts will judge studies of fewer than 3 months adequate to support claims of efficacy.

K. Special Issues

1. Protecting a Drug's Reputation: Controlled Safety Assessment Studies

Evaluating new drugs in patient populations that are at high risk of suffering spontaneous untoward clinical events poses numerous risks to the commercial developer of a new drug. Specifically, any and all events occurring, even those seeming readily explained by alternative causes, must be considered as possibly drug related. There is no escape; without a control group, there is simply no way to evaluate the attributable risk for the drug.

One possible, but certainly expensive, strategy for dealing with the problem is the controlled safety study wherein the control group provides a basis for assessing the spontaneous incidence of adverse clinical events of all types occurring in the high-risk population. (Unfortunately, such an approach is only useful for assessing the cause of relatively common events. A control group provides few protections, for example, if only one or two catastrophic events are observed and each has occurred in a drug-exposed patient.) The choice of a control treatment poses a problem, however. Ideally, placebo should be used; however, as noted earlier, because patients are unlikely to be willing to accept long-term assignment to an inert substance, some active, potentially therapeutic agent must be used instead. Possible candidates are very much lower doses of the investigational agent, or some other drug product already legally marketed for use in virtually the same population of high-risk, elderly patients (e.g., ergoloid mesylates).

2. Extended Efficacy Studies: Rerandomization Designs

The practical factors limiting the duration of randomized, parallel, placebo-controlled efficacy trials was discussed earlier. One as yet unproved, but potentially useful, way to get at the same information is the so-called rerandomization design. In this approach, all patients are initially treated with the investigational agent. Those achieving an acceptable clinical response are maintained on the drug. At selected time points, a subset of the patients in the cohort is randomly selected, and its members are rerandomized to treatment with either the investigational drug or to placebo.

The nature of the events that occur following the rerandomization maneuver are the outcome of interest. If no clinical differences are observed between those rerandomized to placebo and to the investigational drug, questions must obviously be raised about the efficacy of the latter in extended use. On the other hand, if clinical deterioration is seen selectively among those rerandomized to placebo, it is evidence that the investigational drug is exerting some sustained pharmacological action. Importantly, however, the latter result is *not* unequivocal evidence that the investigational drug is actually exerting a beneficial therapeutic effect. It is always possible that the deterioration observed may only be a sign of physiological dependence, the clinical findings merely manifestations of a withdrawal reaction.

L. Analysis of Clinical Trial Outcomes

Solid design and competent execution will not protect a clinical study from being inappropriately or misleadingly analyzed.

It is not the immediate purpose of this chapter to review the numerous traps and pitfalls that await the unwary on the often difficult to negotiate road to valid statistical inference. However, there are some, egregious, all too common, analytical practices that deserve mention. Above all, data-conditioned subgroup analyses should never be advanced as a definitive finding of a prospectively controlled trial. Although investigators have the right to examine their data in any way they want, it is grossly misleading, indeed dishonest, to pretend that some data-conditioned subgroup analysis answers the research question that caused the study to be initiated. Presenting "unadjusted" p values for such analyses is grossly misleading because the probability presented has no valid significance.

In my opinion, any fair analysis of a study must account for everyone who participated in it. That is not to say that there is necessarily widespread agreement on how this is to be accomplished when subjects in the study fail to complete their treatment assignments in the manner specified in the protocol. However, simply doing an analysis of those completing the study can be extremely misleading, especially if treatment assignment had a differential effect on the type and timing of dropouts.

Another concern are experiments wherein the choice of analysis determines whether or not the results are significant. In such instances, the assumptions of each analysis must be examined with great care; the outcome of a clinical experiment should depend upon the data it generates, not the sanguine assumptions of those who analyze it.

IV. CONCLUDING REMARKS

Alzheimer's dementia is a terrible disease, a tragedy for its victims and their loved ones, and a major public health concern. Understandably, everyone of good will hopes to find a way to prevent it, or to find its cure, or at least, to delay its progression and modify the severity of its effects. However, there will be no gain to anyone if ineffective treatments for AD find their way into the armamentarium. The hope such false remedies can provide will be transient, and their cost considerable, especially if they prove dangerous as well as ineffective. Moreover, making an exception to principle for the purpose of satisfying a particularly intense immediate need is rarely worthwhile in the long run. For example, declaring a putative treatment for dementia effective on less than adequate evidence would set a precedent that could lead to circumstances in which Oliver Wendell Holmes' remarks again became true. Indeed, it is my belief that it is our collective endorsement of the randomized control trial as the only acceptable measure of a drug's true therapeutic value that keeps the pharmacopoeia from being diluted with worthless, potentially harmful, substances.

Why the clinical investigation employing randomized controls is so important for this purpose, along with suggestions for the design, conduct and analysis of clinical trials for assessing the efficacy of putative treatments for dementia, has been the subject of this chapter.

REFERENCES

1. Holmes, Medical Essays, 1842–1882. (Boston, 1891), 202–3 as cited in Young JH. Pure food: securing the Federal Food and Drugs Act of 1906. Princeton: Princeton University Press, 1989.
2. Leber PD. Hazards of inference: the active control investigation. Epilepsia 1989; 30(suppl 1):S57–S63.
3. Ad Hoc FDA Dementia Assessment Task Force. FDA Antidementia Drug Assessment Symposium, June 15 and 16, 1989.
4. Leber PD. Establishing the efficacy of drugs with psychogeriatric indications, In: Crook T, Ferris S, Bartus R, eds. Assessment in geriatric psychopharmacology. New Canaan: Mark Powley Associates, 1983:1–12.
5. Spitzer R, Williams J. Diagnostic and statistical manual of mental disorders, 3rd ed. revised. Washington, D.C.: American Psychiatric Association, 1987.
6. McKhann C, Drachman D, Folstein M, Katzman R, Price D, Stadlan EM. Clinical diagnosis of Alzheimer's disease: report of the NINCDS–ADRDA work group under the auspices of Department of Health and Human Services Task Force on Alzheimer's Disease. Neurology 1984;34:939–944.
7. Wells CE. Dementia. Philadelphia: FA Davis, 1977.
8. Reisberg B. Alzheimer's disease; the standard reference. New York: Free Press, Macmillan, 1983.
9. Folstein MF, Folstein SE, McHugh PR. Mini-Mental State: a practical method for grading the cognitive state of patients for the clinician. J Psychiatr Res 1975;12:189–198.

10. Rosen W, Mohs R, Davis K. A new rating scale for Alzheimer's disease. Am J Psychiatry 1984; 141:1356–1364.
11. Blessed G, Tomlinson BE, Roth M. The association between quantitative measures of dementia and of senile change in the cerebral gray matter of elderly subjects. Br J Psychiatry 1968; 114:797–811.
12. Coblentz JM, Mattis S, Zingesser H, Kasnof SS, Wisniewski HM, Katzman R. Presenile dementia. Arch Neurol 1973; 29:299–308.

Index

About the Editors

Leon J. Thal is Professor of Neurosciences, University of California, San Diego, La Jolla, and Chief of the Neurology Service and Co-Director, Geropsychiatry Program, San Diego Veterans Affairs Medical Center, San Diego, California. The author or coauthor of over 125 journal articles, book chapters, and abstracts, he is a member of the American Academy of Neurology, American Neurological Association, and International Society for Neurochemistry, among others. Dr. Thal received the B.S. degree (1965) in biology/chemistry from Tufts University, Medford, Massachusetts, and M.D. degree (1969) from Downstate Medical Center, the State University of New York, Brooklyn.

Walter H. Moos is Vice President, Research and Development, and Director of Chemical Therapeutics, Chiron Corporation, Emeryville, California. The author or coauthor of nearly 90 journal articles, book chapters, patents, and abstracts, and coeditor of one book, he is a Fellow of the American Institute of Chemists, a charter member of the American Peptide Society, and a member of the American Chemical Society, Society for Neuroscience, and Protein Society, among others. Dr. Moos received the A.B. degree (1976) from Harvard University, Cambridge, Massachusetts, and Ph.D. degree (1982) from the University of California, Berkeley, both in chemistry.

Elkan R. Gamzu is President and Chief Operating Officer, Cambridge NeuroScience, Inc., Cambridge, Massachusetts. The author or coauthor of over 100 journal articles, book chapters, and abstracts, and coeditor of one book, he is a member of the American Academy of Neurology, American Psychological Association, Society for Neuroscience, and American Society for Pharmacology and Experimental Therapeutics, among others. Dr. Gamzu received the B.A. degree (1967) from Hebrew University, Jerusalem, Israel, and M.A. (1968) and Ph.D. (1971) degrees in psychology from the University of Pennsylvania, Philadelphia.